Paediatrics

*For Sheila Pereira
and Oliver, 1991–1995*

For Churchill Livingstone:

Commissioning editor: Ellen Green
Project development manager: Barbara Simmons
Project manager: Frances Affleck
Design: Erik Bigland
Artist: Peter Lamb

Churchill's Mastery of Medicine

Paediatrics

Simon Attard-Montalto

MBChB DCH FRCP FRCPCH
Chairman, Department of Paediatrics, St Luke's Hospital
Gwardamangia, Malta

Vaskar Saha

MBBS DCH FRCPCH MD PhD
Senior Lecturer and Honorary Consultant in
Paediatric Haematology and Oncology,
The Royal London Hospitals, London, UK

CHURCHILL
LIVINGSTONE

EDINBURGH LONDON NEW YORK PHILADELPHIA ST LOUIS
SYDNEY TORONTO 1999

CHURCHILL LIVINGSTONE
An imprint of Harcourt Publishers Limited
Churchill Livingstone, 1–3 Baxter's Place, Leith Walk, Edinburgh
EH1 3AF

ISBN 0443 055165

British Library of Cataloguing in Publication Data
A catalogue record for this book is available from the British
Library.

Library of Congress Cataloging in Publication Data
A catalog record for this book is available from the Library of
Congress.

Medical knowledge is constantly changing. As information
becomes available, changes in treatment, procedures, equipment
and the use of drugs become necessary. The authors and publisher
have, as far as it is possible, taken care to ensure that the
information given in the text is accurate and up-to-date. However,
readers are strongly advised to confirm that the information,
especially with regard to drug usage, complies with current
legislation and standards of practice.

Printed in China

Contributors

Denis Azzopardi MD MRCP
Senior Lecturer in Paediatrics and Neonatal Medicine,
Imperial College School of Medicine, Hammersmith
Hospital, London, UK

Mehul Dattani MBBS MRCP DCH MD
Senior Lecturer and Honorary Consultant in Paediatric
Endocrinology, Institute of Child Health and Great
Ormond Street Hospital for Children NHS Trust,
London, UK

Andrew Winrow BSc MBBS MRCP
Consultant Paediatrician, Kingston Hospital NHS
Trust, Kingston-upon-Thames, UK

Contents

Using this book

Philosophy of this book

Undergraduate medical teaching is changing from a lecture-based, didactic theoretical curriculum relying heavily on memorising facts to an applied, problem-orientated approach. Although this means less spoon-feeding of students, it translates into a far more interesting curriculum that mirrors what actually happens in 'real life' clinical practice. Ultimately this approach is designed to produce new graduates who have a true understanding of clinical medicine and who are not left floundering with the awesome realisation of the potential chasm that spans medical theory and reality.

Whatever approach is adopted, a sound background knowledge of the subject is necessary. Inevitably, this will entail some basic reading and fact finding. This core knowledge should then form the basis upon which applied clinical medicine can be developed. This book has been designed to provide the essential core knowledge of paediatrics and to present this in a problem-orientated fashion. It is by no means a comprehensive or all-inclusive tome of paediatrics, which is only necessary for further reading, research or sheer curiosity. At undergraduate level, the student is expected to grasp basic principles, have clear ideas of common conditions and have a sensible approach to their management. One needs to appreciate what constitutes a normal child and what symptoms and signs may be indicative of serious illness requiring urgent intervention. Hence, in this book, paediatric emergencies and common problems are covered in detail while less common diseases are mentioned only briefly and esoteric rarities are omitted altogether. The information is presented in a format conducive to revision and approximately a quarter of each chapter is devoted to self-assessment. The questions in this section are designed to reflect standards in current undergraduate examinations and cover the most important topics within each chapter. In some instances, additional topics that are not discussed in the text feature in the self-assessment, and this section should not be considered an 'optional extra'. Likewise, self-assessment should not be approached with trepidation but should be used to confirm and consolidate one's understanding of the subject while uncovering the inevitable weak points and gaps in knowledge, which can then be addressed by further reading.

Book design and layout

The book is divided into chapters each covering the major systems in paediatrics. Individual chapters are organised with an introductory 'key' that briefly highlights the goals of each chapter and the essential information which the student is expected to gain after reading the chapter. In general, the common symptoms and signs pertaining to the individual system are dis-

cussed and their clinical relevance outlined. This is then followed by a discussion of various disease states and conditions that affect the system in question. Where relevant, important facts regarding anatomy, physiology and basic science are included. Individual topics are presented in a standardised format, with attention given to maintain the sequence aetiology, history, examination, differential diagnosis, investigation, management and outcome. Discussion of treatment is limited to the most important measures: excessive detail (e.g. drug dosages) and anecdotal or pure research-based therapeutic approaches are excluded, or alluded to very briefly.

Tables are used liberally. They are designed not only to consolidate essential lists but also to insert information. Figures are used to clarify topics that may be easier to comprehend when presented in graphic or pictorial form. Boxes are used to list causes of specific conditions.

The sections on self-assessment include multiple choice questions, short notes, case histories, viva voce examinations and construct questions. Each of these examination formats tests knowledge from a different angle. They are representative of similar questions posed in undergraduate examinations. Factual answers as well as detailed explanations are provided for each question. For those topics previously covered in the text, the questions generally address the problem from a different angle and the answers serve as revision. However, many questions are not covered in the text and, for those, the detailed answers provide an important extension to the basic information supplied in the book.

Approaching the examinations

Sadly, one is repeatedly asked by undergraduates whether a topic or item of information is 'necessary for the exam?' Presumably if the answer is no, then the implication is that the topic will simply be omitted altogether during revision. In many ways, this attitude is not surprising given the way undergraduates are constantly inundated with examinations. However, it is important that students are not reduced to automatons who simply live to get past the next examination hurdle (and having done so, rapidly forget all!). Medical education should be an enjoyable process with the aim of, ultimately, producing safe clinicians. Indeed, the latter entails more than simply passing exams.

Despite all their faults, examinations remain an integral part of assessing students. There are several options open to examiners, all of which test knowledge and understanding of the subject in different ways and all require different skills in order to optimise performance. Some general measures are useful prior to any medical examination:

- discover the format of the exam: length, question form, i.e. multiple choice, essays, etc.
- plan revision to dovetail with the exam format
- read instructions *carefully* before attempting questions
- be absolutely clear about the instructions, e.g. choice offered, timing, etc.
- allocate *equal* time to each question (or according to weighting of marking if known).

Multiple choice questions

Multiple choice questions (MCQs) test factual recall. They cover a broad spectrum of topics, allowing a wide-ranging assessment of the student's knowledge. Given the right approach, even those with a fairly threadbare knowledge can obtain a pass in MCQ examinations since these generally include a sufficient number of straightforward questions. The 'trick' is to maximise one's score on the easier questions while avoiding unnecessary risks on those that are more difficult. MCQs are made up of a stem statement followed by a series of secondary statements. In the usual format, the second statement is true or false in the context of the stem and *negative* marks are awarded for incorrect answers. Despite the common stem, each subsidiary statement must be assessed in isolation. Guidelines to the MCQ examination would include the following 'dos and dont's':

DO
- read and understand the stem extremely carefully, two or three times
- leave out questions where reasonable uncertainty exists
- beware of sweeping statements such as 'never', 'always', etc.
- beware of results given in abnormal units
- plan your timing: calculate the average time to allocate to each stem at the outset and stick to this
- practise mock MCQs several times over – you can never do enough MCQs.

DO NOT
- guess or take risks at any time: this is usually fatal
- answer too many or too few questions
- forget the negative marking format.

Essay questions

Essay questions require a comprehensive grasp of the topic. The answer needs to be laid out in a logical, flowing pattern with an introduction, sequential discussion and conclusion. Time spent on outlining one's train of thought beforehand in a simple list or flow diagram is well spent. It is advisable to annotate these notes alongside your script as insurance in case you run out of time. Essay questions generally cover common broad topics and can be revised by listing the more likely topics within each system and producing a schematic essay outline

for each. The use of headings and subtitles will help to divide the essay into ordered, manageable sections and focus the examiner's thoughts. Guidelines to the essay examination would include the following 'dos and dont's':

DO
- read and understand the question carefully
- be absolutely sure about any choice of questions offered
- time yourself carefully
- construct the essay logically
- outline the essay plan before starting to write.

DO NOT
- allocate time disproportionately
- indulge in verbose prose or repetition
- digress and answer out of context.

Short notes

Short notes provide an ideal method for covering several topics in reasonable depth. Marks are awarded for relevant facts; none are given for extra or superfluous detail. One should aim to produce a structured, ordered list in logical sequence. However, since there is no negative marking in 'short notes', it is not unreasonable to include details even if there is some doubt to their relevance to the question in hand. Guidelines to the short notes would include the following 'dos and dont's':

DO
- read and understand the question extremely carefully
- be absolutely sure about any choice
- answer succinctly, while avoiding irrelevant facts
- ensure a logical sequence of related facts.

DO NOT
- include irrelevant detail
- digress from the issue at hand
- allocate time disproportionately.

Data interpretation

Questions of data interpretation generally test the understanding of basic principles, normal values and pattern recognition. The erstwhile student does well to look at all the clues provided. Unless a single diagnosis comes to mind, then draw up a list of possible options and, depending on the clues available, decide on the best-fit scenario. This type of question usually does not include negative marking so it is important to provide an answer even if terribly unsure of its validity. Guidelines to the data questions would include the following 'dos and dont's':

DO
- read and understand the question extremely carefully
- look at all the clues provided
- choose the best-fit diagnosis.

DO NOT
- rush an answer before all the clues fit
- leave out any question
- allocate time disproportionately.

Viva voce

Many candidates expect an oral to be the most harrowing experience of the examination. The idea that the examiners 'are out to get you' is, frankly, a misconception. It is important to listen carefully to the questions asked, take time to construct your thoughts and speak clearly. Examiners are trying to ascertain your depth of knowledge and not trap you. They are human and you will gain sympathy by being courteous and maintaining eye contact. They will be irritated by a sub voce mumble aimed at the general direction of the floor. Avoid illogical statements, anecdotes and naming rare syndromes about which you know precious little. The last is invariably going to whet the examiners' interest, who will promptly ask about the syndrome! Above all, never bluff. The certainty of being caught out making things up is 100%. You will be much better off admitting that you do not know the answer to a certain question and moving on to some other, safer ground. Guidelines to the viva voce would include the following 'dos and dont's':

DO
- concentrate on the question
- structure your thoughts
- admit to not knowing.

DO NOT
- mumble, talk incoherently
- mention issues about which you have little knowledge
- bluff, or invent answers that you think the examiners want to hear.

Slide or picture examination

Slide and picture questions rely on recall and pattern recognition. A systematic approach is required and the whole picture, X-ray, etc. should be scrutinised very carefully for all the clues. This applies to any accompanying text, notes, captions, etc. Consider common problems first and query the possibility of a rare diagnosis only when you are in a distinction situation.

Guidelines to slides or pictures would include the following 'dos and dont's':

DO
- look at and understand all the clues extremely carefully
- focus on any obvious abnormality
- consider common conditions first
- base your answer on what you see and not what you think you should see.

DO NOT
- rush an answer before you have looked at all the clues
- guess or make up signs.

Problem-oriented questions

Problem-orientated questions present a mock, real-life situation via a brief history. The pattern of questioning may vary. In one method a series of questions is provided and a story unfolds. They epitomise the problem-orientated approach to examinations and test the candidate's ability to comprehend the salient clues provided and deal with the clinical situation. In another approach, you will be asked to manage a common medical problem. This may range from prescribing therapy or obtaining consent to advising a patient about their condition. This question asks for a constructed answer. In some cases, the various categories will be obvious from the question and should be dealt with accordingly. In others, you will be left to plan out a logical sequence of events. The guidelines for these types of question are:

DO
- make a stepwise plan before you start answering
- focus on the main problem in question
- identify investigations and procedures relevant to the case
- formulate a plan of management
- evaluate the short- and long-term implications of the case
- consider the main issues for communication and discussion with parents.

DO NOT
- get bogged down by detail
- repeat your observations disguised under different headings.

In this book we have attempted to provide different examples of these questions in different chapters. Remember the answers for these questions are only examples of how they can be answered. You are free to make your own strategy and as long as it is logical and practical you will be rewarded.

Self-appraisal and examination technique

Passing examinations does not depend solely on having sufficient core knowledge of the subject and being able to use this knowledge in applied clinical situations. It also relies on an understanding of the examination format and presentation, both on paper and verbally. This improves with confidence, which comes after sufficient reading around the subject and repeated practice of mock examinations. It is important to plan the revision for any examination and adjust the emphasis of the revision after gauging one's own depth of knowledge. An honest self-scoring exercise alone or with like-minded friends who are not hell bent on one-upmanship can be very useful. It is far better to have a working knowledge of most issues rather than an in-depth understanding of a few esoteric facts. Hence, revision should be planned with a broad list in mind and time allocated equally to all the major topics. A readable, medium-sized text is preferable to a comprehensive paediatric 'bible' or a rather artificial text comprising endless lists with little reference to clinical settings. Often personalised notes taken from lectures and texts leave lasting impressions and provide an efficient method for revision. At all times we would encourage participation during teaching sessions. Tutors welcome and respond to active dialogue, the two-way process generally enhancing the quality of the teaching as well as the impression left on the students.

Conclusion

The vast majority of undergraduates pass all the examinations set throughout the curriculum and eventually graduate successfully. Indeed, the system is designed to pass rather then to fail at this level. Those who do not succeed generally do so because they have not made a sufficient effort with background reading or have planned their revision badly. We hope that this book will help to address both these issues, while still allowing the student to appreciate the fascination of clinical paediatrics outside the examination setting.

Nutrition, normal growth and development

Key points

You should be familiar with:

- The basic nutritional requirements of neonates, infants and children
- The normal patterns of growth
- The milestones in normal development
- The common nutritional deficiency states.

1.1 Introduction

Childhood is a time of active growth in terms of physical size, mental, emotional and sexual maturation and psychological development. Normal growth is dependent on adequate nutrition and encompasses major transformations from birth to adulthood, progressing in an ordered, stepwise fashion. Although specific stages in physical and psychosocial maturation are attained at relatively fixed times in development, wide variations are observed from one individual to another. Despite this variation, there are, however, acceptable limits for the acquisition of developmental milestones, outside of which progress is considered to be delayed. The recognition of such delay is based on the identification of several absent or abnormal milestones following a comprehensive assessment of the whole child, taking into account several modalities of function and performance.

Major congenital anomalies, chromosomal defects and damage to the growing central nervous system (CNS) are likely to result in significant neurodevelopmental delay. The last is also associated with major disruption in the normal processes of growth and development, especially those affecting the central nervous system. Hence, severe hypoxic and hypotensive episodes, infections and metabolic derangement, especially if associated with intercurrent curtailment in adequate nutrition, can result in neuropsychomotor delay.

1.2 Nutritional requirements

Normal requirements

After birth, the fastest rate of growth (length increase per year) is observed in the newborn period. As shown in Figure 1, this rate falls steadily throughout childhood, until a second growth surge at puberty, before linear growth ceases. Consequently, newborns require more energy (measured in calories on joules) per kilogram weight than other stages in childhood (Table 1).

Preterm babies who have 'lost out' on the benefits of nine months of in utero feeding have increased calorific needs. As a result of their increased metabolic rate, surface area and heat loss, preterm babies have increased energy requirements and obtain the additional calories via an increased milk volume intake relative to their size (Table 2).

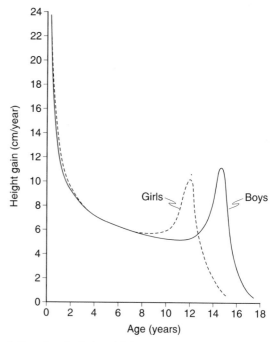

Fig. 1 Growth velocity from birth to adulthood.

Table 1 Changes in energy and protein requirements with age

Age (years)	Energy requirement		Protein requirement (g/kg)
	(kcal/kg)	(kJ/kg)	
0–1	120–90	500–380	3.5
1–7	90–75	380–300	2.5
7–12	75–60	300–250	2.0
12–18	60–30	250–125	1.5

Table 2 Daily volume intake of milk with weight and age

Weight (kg)	Daily intake of milk on days 1–14 after birth (ml/kg)*			
	1	3	10	14
<1.5	90	120	180	200
1.5–2.5	60	110	130	150
2.5–4.0	60	90	110	120
4.0–10.0	100 daily			
10.0–20.0	1000 ml + 50 ml/kg per kg over 10 kg			
>20.0	1500 ml + 25 ml/kg per kg over 10 kg			

* Breast milk contains up to 74 kcal/100 ml (300 kJ/100 ml) while average formula milk contains 67 kcal/100 ml (280 kJ/100 ml).

Milk feeds

The dictum *breast is best* remains true for almost all cases. Mature breast milk provides about 70–74 cal/100 ml presented in the ideal proportion of carbohydrate, fat and protein to ensure normal growth. Vitamins and minerals are provided in sufficient quantities and in

Table 3 Composition of various milk feeds

Content	Human milk		Formula milk		Cow's milk
	Term	Preterm	Term	Preterm	
Energy cal/100 ml	70	74	66	80	67
Carbohydrate (g/100 ml)	7.4	6.4	7.2	7.0	4.6
Fat (g/100 ml)	4.2	3.1	3.6	4.5	3.9
Protein (g/100 ml)	1.1	2.7	1.5	2.0	3.4
Casein:lactalbumin	2:3	2:3	2:2	2:3	4:1
Minerals					
Sodium (mmol/l)	6.4	17	7.6	20	23
Potassium (mmol/l)	15	17	15	20	40
Calcium (mg%)	35	29	40	70	124
Phosphate (mg%)	15	13	30	40	98
Ferrous iron (mg%)	0.08	0.15	0.65	0.65	0.05
Vitamins					
A (μg/100 ml)	60	–	80	96	28
D (μg/100 ml)	0.01	–	1.0	1.3	0.02
E (μg/100 ml)	350	–	700	1.5	90
Folic acid (μg/100 ml)	5.2	–	5.3	10	3.7

Table 4 Contraindications to enteral feeding

Contraindication	Examples
Prematurity	In severe prematurity delay for 24–48 hours*
Birth weight	Less than 1 kg, delay for 24–48 hours*
Gastrointestinal problems	The 3-hourly gastric aspirate is greater than the volume of milk given Ileus Mechanical obstruction Necrotising enterocolitis
Neurological problems	Feeding-associated apnoeas Uncontrolled convulsions
General illness	Acute phase of any major illness Septicaemia During major procedures (e.g. exchange transfusion)

*The delay varies from one unit to the next; many will commence enteral feeds within a few hours of birth (as there are no data to suggest which is better).

absorbable forms to ensure deficiencies do not arise. Bonding is easier in breast fed babies. 'Modern' *formula milks* emulate breast milk to a high degree (Table 3). Preterm infants require more calories, protein, vitamins and minerals (including sodium, calcium, phosphorus, magnesium, trace elements) in proportion to their weight, and this is indeed reflected in the composition of expressed breast milk. Preterm formulae are designed to take these needs into account.

Breast feeding is only contraindicated in mothers who are HIV positive, have active hepatitis B or C, or are taking lithium, immunosuppressants, cytotoxics or radio-pharmaceuticals.

Timing and route of feeds

Feeding should be commenced within the first 2 hours and continued 2-hourly in preterm and small-for-dates babies (especially if less than 1.5 kg). Term infants can be fed within 4 hours. *Enteral* feeding, preferably via the oral route, is ideal. Nasogastric tube feeding by gravity over 20 minutes is useful, especially in sick infants and those born at less than 30 weeks of gestation, when the sucking reflex is poorly developed. *Parenteral feeding* is reserved for infants who, as a result of illness or prematurity, are unable to tolerate enteral feeding (Table 4). In newborn infants, intravenous dextrose/saline solutions should only be used for about 48 hours before, if enteral feeding is still not possible, total parenteral nutrition (TPN) is commenced.

Weaning

Semi-solid food, usually a cereal with added iron and vitamin D, is introduced at around 4–6 months. By 6 months, infants can chew and drink from a beaker, and solid food, fruit juices, etc. can be given. At 1 year, chopped or liquidised adult food, including doorstep milk, provide an adequate diet.

Special feeds

Soy-based feeds are useful in proven cases of cow's milk allergy. Their protein provides less energy than breast milk and a corresponding 10% increase in volume is needed to make up the equivalent calorie content.

Elemental feeds contain partly predigested, absorbable nutrients and are, therefore, useful in children with short bowel syndrome and problems of absorption.

Specialised feeds are custom-made for patients with food intolerance (e.g. lactose-free milks for lactose intolerance), specific malabsorption (e.g. milk containing medium-chain triglycerides in certain postoperative situations) or metabolic disorders (e.g. low phenylalanine milk for phenylketonuria).

Intravenous feeding

Intravenous feeding is given to children who are unable to tolerate enteral feeds: 10% dextrose can be given to preterms for 1–3 days and term infants for 4–6 days, after which body energy stores are exhausted. Older children can be given combinations of 5–10% dextrose and 0.45–0.9% saline, with appropriate electrolyte supplementation (e.g. daily potassium, 2 mmol/kg). If intravenous feeding is prolonged, a comprehensive feed, including a nitrogen and fat source, should be used.

Total parenteral nutrition

Total parenteral nutrition is tailor-made according to the age, weight and needs of the individual patient. It provides calories in the form of carbohydrate, protein and fats, together with mineral requirements, vitamins and trace element supplements. It should be administered through an indwelling central venous (or umbilical) catheter, preferably used solely for TPN. Regular assessment of the serum glucose, pH, electrolyte and trace elements, urinary glucose and liver and renal function is necessary while on TPN. Complications of TPN include:

- catheter-related sepsis
- thromboses
- extravasation and scarring
- cholestatic jaundice
- hyperlipidaemia
- hyperglycaemia
- acidosis
- metabolic derangement.

Relative contraindications to the use of TPN include:

- uraemia
- jaundice
- acidaemia
- sepsis

- hypoxia
- thrombocytopenia.

1.3 Normal physical growth

Weight gain

Neonates lose up to 5–10% of their birth weight, though this is regained by 10 days (up to 3 weeks in preterms). Weight gain generally progresses at about 15 g/kg per day. In the fullterm infant, the birth weight is doubled around 5 months of age and tripled by 12 months. Steady weight gain is a reliable guide to the well being of the child and should always be documented on an appropriate centile chart (Fig. 2a). Excess weight-for-age is the most common nutritional disorder in developed countries. *Failure to thrive*, as manifest by insufficient weight gain resulting in a 'falling off' downwards across centile lines, should prompt a search for the conditions listed in Box 1.

Obesity

The prevalence of childhood obesity is approximately 8% in the UK and 13% in the USA. Up to 30% of these children become obese adults. The risk is greater with a family history of obesity, affluence, higher socioeconomic group, urban existence and increase in time spent on sedentary activities (e.g. watching television). This disorder is generally caused by excessive food intake coupled with insufficient energy expenditure during exercise. Pathological causes contribute less than 1% of cases. Obese children are often teased and may have psychological problems. Advice on dietary curtailment,

Fig. 2 Increase in (a) weight and (b) height from birth to adulthood.

BOX 1
Causes of failure to thrive

Neonatal period
Inadequate calorie intake: insufficient volume, incorrect formula, poor feeding technique
Infection (e.g. urinary tract)
Acidaemia
Anaemia

Childhood
Poor feeding: brain damage, endocrinopathy
Excess vomiting
Malabsorption: milk intolerance, coeliac disease, inflammatory bowel disease, cystic fibrosis
Systemic illness: heart failure, respiratory failure, renal disease, liver failure
Chronic infection
Social deprivation

---

exercise and modification of lifestyle should be given. The help of a dedicated, experienced dietician is essential, but treatment is rarely successful unless there is a firm commitment of both the child and the family to adhere to the recommended diet.

Linear growth

Linear growth progresses in a steady fashion throughout childhood, with a surge at puberty followed by a total cessation in the late teenage years. This is depicted graphically on centile charts, compiled from a large cohort of normal children and showing the growth 'lines' for the mean of the population (50th centile) as well as for normal short and tall individuals (Fig. 2b). A normal growth curve is one that runs approximately parallel to a centile line. Patients whose height plots outside these lines or is rapidly crossing the percentile lines warrants investigation for the causes of tall or short stature.

Sexual maturation

Gonadotrophins and growth hormone release from the anterior pituitary initiates puberty, which is accompanied by an acceleration in linear growth in both sexes. The latter starts earlier in girls and begins in the peripheries, giving adolescents a gawky appearance. Gonadotrophins stimulate the release of oestrogens and androgens from the respective gonads, which, in turn, orchestrate pubertal development.

Girls

The appearance of breast buds heralds puberty and usually occurs at the age of 8–9 years (Fig. 3). This constitutes Tanner stage I breast development and is followed by an increase in breast tissue (stage II), increase in areolar size (stage III), increase in breast size and areolar pig-

mentation (stage IV) and the adoption of the adult breast (V). Pubic hair follows the appearance of breast buds. Hair is usually fair and downy (stage I), then darkens (II), becoming curly (III), and more abundant (IV) until the adult triangular pubic pattern is assumed (V). Labial, clitoral, uterine and ovarian development are under the influence of oestrogen and follicle stimulating hormone. Menstruation is usually a late feature, when linear growth is decelerating, and early periods are often anovulatory and irregular.

Boys

An increase in testicular size is the first sign of male puberty, usually occurring by the age of 10 years (Fig. 3). These organs increase in volume from 1–3 ml in infants to 12–20 ml in adults. Penile enlargement follows: initially an increase in length (stage I), then penile thickness (II), pigmentation (III) and rugosity of skin (IV), before the adult form is attained (V). Pubic hair develops in tandem, as it does in females. The seminiferous tubules, epididymis, seminal vesicles and prostate gland develop under the influence of luteinising hormone and testosterone. Changes in body build, hirsutism, acne, vocal cords and dentition complete the process.

1.4 Normal development

Human development progresses through a sequence of events, during which specific functional skills are acquired. Despite individual variation, these landmarks ('milestones') should occur at approximately the same age for normal children and are, therefore, essential in the assessment of neurodevelopmental progress. Developmental milestones can be assessed in five major categories:

- gross motor
- fine motor
- special senses (vision, hearing, language)
- psychosocial
- educational.

It is easier to grasp development by using these major categories while focusing on specific key age groups, rather than trying to remember a progressive continuum of developmental parameters throughout childhood.

Development: from birth to 4 years

Motor skills are primarily acquired during the first few months of life, whereas psychosocial and educational milestones assume greater importance after the first 2 years. Table 5 shows important milestones that, on average, are attained at birth, 6 weeks, 6, 10, 13, 18 months, and 2, 3 and 4 years.

Fig. 3 Sexual maturation in boys and girls. I–IVA show the changes in sexual maturation in boys. An increase in testicular volume is followed by increase in penile length and girth. Pubic hair increases from a few pale straight hairs to assume the adult appearance with dark, curly hair in both boys and girls (A and B). I–V C show the progression in breast bud and areolae to the adult shape and size.

Development: 4 to 6 years

Children generally commence school at 4 years at which time they should be independent with regard to feeding, dressing, washing and toilet care. They are now more gregarious, mischievous and sociable, appreciating the need to share and play together. They consolidate their understanding of colours, numbers and drawing skills. Their depiction of 'a man' and 'a house'

improves steadily (Fig. 4). The vocabulary escalates and speech becomes more complex so that 'baby talk' disappears by 7 years. They become forever more inquisitive and questioning and, as their understanding and imagination increases, so does the complexity of play.

Abnormal development

Developmental delay in infancy is manifest by a failure

Table 5 Developmental milestones from birth to 4 years

Age	Category	Acquired skill	
Birth	Gross motor	Complete head lag, lies prone, hips flexed	
	Fine motor	Sucking reflex, fisting	
	Vision	Blinks to light	
	Hearing	Startles to noise	
6 weeks	Gross motor	Improving head control, prone, hips extended	
	Fine motor	Hands often open	
	Vision	Focuses object in 90° arc	
	Hearing	Settles to mother's voice	
	Psychosocial	Smiles	
6 months	Gross motor	Good head control, press-up if prone, sits using hands	
	Fine motor	Transfers between hands, palmar grasp	
	Vision	Focuses object in 180° arc	
	Hearing	Whisper at short distance	
	Language	Chuckles, babbles	
	Psychosocial	Indicates likes, dislikes	
10 months	Gross motor	Creeps, cruises around furniture, sits and pivots	
	Fine motor	Index finger approach	
	Vision	Small objects other side of room	
	Hearing	Whisper at a distance	
	Language	Vocalising, da-da, ma-ma	
	Psychosocial	Waves, plays pat-a-cake	
13 months	Gross motor	Walks unaided, casting of objects	
	Fine motor	Offers objects in play, places cube	
	Vision	Small objects end of room	
	Hearing	Distraction test	
	Language	1–2 words; jargon commences	
	Psychosocial	Stops mouthing, slobbering	
18 months	Gross motor	Walks upstairs, jumps	
	Fine motor	Uses spoon, tower three cubes, scribbles with pencil	
	Language	Two to three word sentences	
	Psychosocial	Dry by day, partly dresses self	
	Education	Identifies one picture, points to some objects/parts of body	

Table 5 *(cont'd)*

Age	Category	Acquired skill	
2 years	Gross motor	Runs, kicks ball	
	Fine motor	Screws top, tower six cubes, copies vertical line	
	Language	Four to six word sentences	
	Psychosocial	Dry by day and night, dresses self well	
	Education	Points four parts of body, identifies five pictures; names three	
3 years	Fine motor	Tower nine cubes, copies cross, circle	
	Language	Vocabulary accelerates	
	Psychosocial	Dresses self fully except laces	
	Education	Points ten parts of body, identifies twelve pictures and names eight, names three colours	
4 years	Fine motor	Cubes: imitates gate, copies square, places shapes into slots	
	Psychosocial	Dresses self fully	
	Education	Identifies, names several pictures, names several colours	

to acquire motor milestones such as adequate head control, the ability to sit and bear weight as well as social non-responsiveness, lack of interest in surroundings and an inability to respond to audiovisual stimuli. Persistence of premature reflexes such as the Moro reflex beyond 2–3 months is also abnormal. These and a delay in milestones require review and follow-up by a specialist neurodevelopmental team. This team normally comprises paediatrician, orthoptists, audiologist, physiotherapists, speech, occupational and educational therapists, and social workers, who perform a comprehensive assessment of motor, functional, audiovisual and cognitive ability.

1.5 Nutritional disorders

Protein energy malnutrition

Protein energy malnutrition (PEM) follows a prolonged period of nutritional deprivation. Total body protein and muscle mass decrease as a result of catabolism outstripping anabolic processes. Total body fat is decreased, though its deposition in the liver may be increased. Minerals, especially potassium, are reduced.

Total body water is increased, especially in the extracellular space. PEM often arises after weaning and presents with marasmus or kwashiorkor, or both. Patients with marasmus are alert and hungry but severely wasted and stunted with lack of subcutaneous fat. Children with kwashiorkor are lethargic, miserable, apathetic and have severe hair and skin changes. There is a lack of muscle bulk, generalised oedema, ascites and hepatomegaly. Both are associated with secondary anaemia, endocrinopathies, immunosuppression and vitamin deficiencies. Electrolyte disturbances, hypoglycaemia, hypothermia, dehydration, anaemia, infection and vitamin deficiencies (especially A, D, E) must be corrected together with nutritional supplementation. Intravenous fluids should be replaced by oral replacement as soon as possible. A high-calorie diet (150–200 kcal/kg per day) with a minimum of 2–3 g/kg milk or animal protein and vitamin and mineral supplements are required. Recovery is characterised by the 'nutritional recovery syndrome' with a progressive gain in weight (10 g/kg daily), and an increased interest in the surroundings.

Iron deficiency

Iron deficiency is the most common deficiency in devel-

4 years   5 years   6 years

Fig. 4 Depiction of a man by a child of 4, 5 and 6 years.

oped countries. It is usually a consequence of an inadequate dietary intake of foodstuff rich in iron, including meat and green vegetables. Iron stores are primarily built up toward the end of uterine life so that preterms often lack this important element. Iron-deficiency anaemia is common after prolonged feeding with breast or cow's milk since neither contains sufficient iron. Chronic blood loss, especially in those with oesophageal reflux and gastrointestinal ulceration, ultimately leads to depletion of iron stores and symptoms of anaemia, including pallor, lethargy and, occasionally, cardiac failure and pica. Investigation shows a microcytic, hypochromic anaemia associated with low ferritin levels. Thalassaemia should be excluded in patients from the Mediterranean basin and Indian subcontinent. Treatment involves a daily replacement of 6 mg elemental iron, given orally as a ferrous salt.

Vitamin D deficiency (rickets)

Vitamin D is essential for the normal mineralisation of bone. Its deficiency results from a diet inadequate in dairy products, a lack of sunlight, malabsorptive states and liver and renal disease. The skin contains 7-dehydrocholesterol, which is converted to vitamin D_3 by ultraviolet light. Dietary vitamin can be obtained from plant sources (ergocalciferol or D_2) or animal sources (cholecalciferol or D_3). The pro-vitamin is first metabolised in the liver to the monohydroxy derivative and in the kidney to the active metabolite 1,25-dihydroxy cholecalciferol ($1,25(OH)_2D_3$) or the inactive metabolite $24,25(OH)_2D_3$ (Fig. 5).

Deficiency results in the decreased absorption of calcium and phosphate, with decreased mineralisation of the bones especially at the growth plate. Affected patients develop softened bones (e.g. craniotabes in infants, bowing of tibiae), distension of the growing ends of the bones (wrists, knees, ribs producing a rickety rosary), short stature and generalised hypotonia. Investigation shows a decrease in phosphorus, low or normal calcium and increased alkaline phosphatase. As a result the metaphyses of the long bones are demineralised and the epiphyseal plates widened and become cupped. (Fig. 6). An intake of 10 µg vitamin D daily prevents rickets; treatment requires 250 µg daily.

Other vitamin deficiencies

Vitamin A deficiency

Vitamin A is a fat-soluble vitamin. It is plentiful in liver, milk, coloured vegetables and wheat. Vitamin A deficiency is common in rice-consuming populations who rarely consume animal fat. Retinol is the active derivative of vitamin A. It is the prosthetic group of the photosensitive pigment in the rods (light) and cones (colour) of the retina. The major difference between the two lies in the nature of the protein bound to the retinol. *All-trans* retinal isomerises in the dark to the 11-*cis* form. This combines with opsin (in the cones) to form rhodopsin. Energy in the form of light reconverts the 11-*cis* form back to the *all-trans* form. This energy exchange, transmitted to the brain via the optic nerve, results in the visual sensation.

Vitamin A deficiency results in night blindness, later conjunctival xerosis and corneal scarring. Dry silver plaques may appear on the bulbar conjunctiva (Bitot spots). In parts of the world where vitamin A deficiency is a major problem, 30 mg should be given orally at least twice a year. In children with corneal involvement (keratomalacia), initially 3 mg/kg is given intramuscularly then 1.5 mg a day by mouth until healing is complete. Vitamin A also plays a role in keratinisation, spermatogenesis and the epithelialisation of the respiratory and gastrointestinal systems. Subclinical deficiencies in malnourished children with diarrhoea and respiratory tract infections have been associated with increased morbidity in developing countries.

Vitamin B_1 deficiency

Thiamine is absent in boiled rice. Thiamine deficiency results in beri-beri in infants, presenting with cardiac failure, laryngeal oedema and distal nerve degenera-

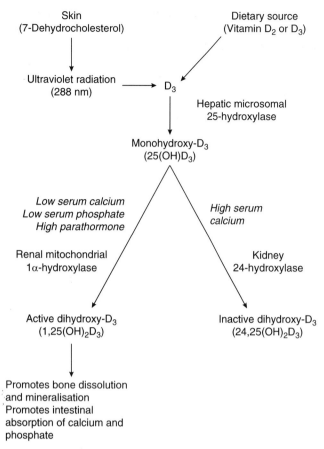

Fig. 5 Metabolism of vitamin D.

Fig. 6 Radiological changes in rickets.

tion. With Vitamin B_1 deficiency, up to 100 mg thiamine is first given, followed by 5–10 mg daily.

Vitamin B_2 deficiency

Riboflavin deficiency is usually associated with other coenzyme deficiencies. It causes an angular stomatitis, cheilosis and keratitis. Treatment of deficiency is with 3–10 mg daily.

Niacin deficiency

Niacin is present in small quantities in cereals. Hence, maize-eating communities may lack this coenzyme and develop pellagra, consisting of a symmetrical dermatitis on exposed surfaces, glossitis, fissuring of mucocutaneous junctions and neurological sequelae. Treatment of deficiency requires 50 mg daily.

Vitamin B_6 deficiency

Adequate functioning of the nervous system depends on pyridoxine, and its deficiency results in seizures and peripheral neuropathies and, occasionally, cheilosis and seborrhoea. Vitamin B_6 deficiency may occur in newborn infants and later, following malabsorption and destruction of pyridoxine by overheating milk and cereals. Treatment is with 100 mg intramuscularly for neonatal seizures, whereas a daily intake of 10–100 mg

by mouth generally suffices for pyridoxine-dependent children.

Vitamin B_{12} deficiency

Vitamin B_{12} deficiency is seen in patients taking a strictly vegan diet and in those with terminal ileal disease (e.g. Crohn's disease). It results in a macrocytic anaemia.

Vitamin C deficiency (scurvy)

Breast and formula milk, but not cow's milk, provide the daily requirement of 10 mg vitamin C deficiency results in symptoms initially observed at 6–12 months, with fretfulness, easy bruising, pseudoparalysis owing to subperiosteal haematomas, and bleeding gums. Investigation shows a hypochromic anaemia, bony atrophy, decalcification and subperiosteal calcification. Scurvy is effectively treated with 200 mg vitamin C daily.

Vitamin E deficiency

Vitamin E deficiency follows malabsorption and presents with haemolytic anaemia in preterm infants, and weakness, sometimes ataxia and neuropathy in children. Preterms are given 20 IU vitamin E supplements per day.

Vitamin K deficiency

Vitamin K is deficient in newborns, and in liver disease and malabsorption. Its deficiency results in haemorrhagic disease of the newborn (HDN), and hypoprothrombinaemia in children. An intramuscular injection of 1 mg vitamin K is given to all newborns to prevent HDN; 1–2 mg/day oral vitamin K also corrects any deficiency.

Self-assessment: questions

Multiple choice questions

1. The following statements describe developmental milestones:
   a. Infants do not smile socially before the age of 3 months
   b. Infants do not sit unaided till the age of 12 months
   c. Children walk without help at around 12–14 months of age
   d. Slobbering generally stops at 2 years of age
   e. An index finger approach is typical in a 10-month-old child

2. The following statements describe child development:
   a. Children voice words into simple sentences at around 18 months of age
   b. Children cannot build a tower of six bricks till they are about 6 years old
   c. Children can copy a circle at 18 months
   d. Picture cards provide a poor assessment of the power of comprehension
   e. Toilet training should begin at 12 months of age

3. With regard to normal growth in childhood:
   a. Growth velocity decreases in the first decade of life
   b. The pubertal growth spurt starts earlier in boys compared with girls
   c. Birth weight is doubled at 12 months
   d. Weight loss is the most common nutritional disorder in developed countries
   e. Puberty is commenced by the appearance of menstrual periods in girls

4. With regard to milk feeding in infancy:
   a. Preterm formulae contain additional calories compared with breast milk
   b. Breast milk is extremely rich in iron
   c. Expressed breast milk is usually sufficient to cater for the infant's needs
   d. Preterms require feeding at longer intervals to allow for slower gastric emptying
   e. Cow's milk is adequate for term but not for preterm babies

5. With regard to nutritional requirements and deficiencies in childhood:
   a. Iron deficiency may be associated with pica
   b. Rickets of prematurity presents with osteopenic bones, sometimes fractures
   c. Vitamin A deficiency is the commonest form of blindness, worldwide
   d. Infants require 4 mmol/kg body weight of potassium daily
   e. Protein and fat provide 4 kcal/g compared with 9 kcal/g from carbohydrate

Short notes

List the benefits and problems associated with breast feeding.

Viva voce question

Describe how you would perform a distraction test in an 18-month-old boy.

Case history

You are the senior house officer in paediatrics and have seen a 4-year-old girl in the outpatient department, referred by her general practitioner for poor weight gain. She is brought to clinic by her mother who is 8 months pregnant, her 2-year-old brother and her mother's friend. From the dietary history, you note that she has always been a 'difficult feeder'. She dislikes (and will throw up) almost all vegetables and most meat-containing foodstuffs, but likes potatoes, eggs, milk and fruit juice. She was breast fed for 1 week and then started on a standard formula milk and weaned onto semi-solids at 2 months. She is fully immunised. Mother kept an accurate record of her weight measurements and you note that she plotted on the 40th centile for weight at birth, and on the 10th at 3 months when she was changed to a soy-based preparation. Nevertheless, she plotted on the 3rd centile at 6 and 12 months. Her weight is now below the 3rd centile and her height on the 25th centile. A system review was unhelpful and examination confirms an unkempt, pale, boisterous, scrawny but otherwise normal girl.

1. What is the initial diagnosis?
2. What further details would you request about the child?
3. What further details would you request from the family and social history?

Mother is seriously concerned that her daughter has worms and would like X-rays, including a contrast study, of her bowels.

4. How would you counsel mother at this point?
5. What investigations are indicated?

You arrange to review the child in 1 month's time, when you discover that the haemoglobin is 8.5 g/dl, white cell count 16×10^9/l, MCV (mean cell volume) 72 fl and MCHC (mean corpuscular haemoglobin concentration) 25 g/dl. Urinalysis by dipstick showed 1+ protein and there were 10^4 cells per high power field with a mixed growth on culture.

---

6. What is the most likely diagnosis at this stage?
7. What therapeutic and follow-up arrangements measures are appropriate?

The child is not returned for follow-up on two occasions but returns unexpectedly to outpatients with both parents after another 7 weeks. Mother has been delivered of a baby boy in the interim and father claims he had misplaced the appointment card.

---

8. What important indices would you measure on this occasion?
9. What additional measures should you take for this child?
10. What additional measures should you take for this family?

Self-assessment: answers

Multiple choice answers

1. a. **False**. Smiles usually occur at 6 weeks.
   b. **False**. Infants can usually sit unaided at 6 months.
   c. **True**. The average age for unassisted walking is 13 months.
   d. **True**. Slobbering starts at 3–4 months and stops by 2 years.
   e. **True**. The primitive grasp reflex at birth disappears at 12 weeks; desire to go for objects is fulfilled by an inaccurate palmar grasp at 4 months. Deliberate, accurate grasp develops at 5 months. This improves steadily to enable picking up of ever smaller objects from 5–10 months when the index finger approach is established.

2. a. **True**. 'Da da' and 'ma ma' are voiced at around 8 months followed by single words from 10 months, culminating in simple, two-word sentences at 18 months.
   b. **False**. This occurs at around 2 years.
   c. **False**. A child can copy a circle at about 3 years.
   d. **False**. Picture cards test vision, recognition, association and speech and provide an excellent means of assessing comprehension.
   e. **False**. Toilet-training should not start before 18 months.

3. a. **True**. There is a second spurt at puberty.
   b. **False**. on average, the pubertal growth spurt starts 1–2 years earlier in girls.
   c. **False**. Birth weight is doubled at 5 months.
   d. **False**. Overweight and obesity are far more common in developed countries.
   e. **False**. Breast bud development is the first sign of puberty; periods appear toward the end of puberty.

4. a. **True**. Preterm formulae have 80 cal/100 ml compared with 70 cal/100 ml in breast milk.
   b. **False**. Breast milk is low in iron supply but its iron is readily absorbed.
   c. **True**. Although milk fortifiers may be added for preterm infants.
   d. **False**. Short intervals are used to prevent hypoglycaemia caused by increased requirements and low glucose stores in preterms.
   e. **False**. Cow's milk is not introduced before 12 months.

5. a. **True**. Inappropriate ingestion of inert material or faeces (pica) may be a presenting feature in children with iron deficiency.
   b. **True**. Generalised osteopenia, sometimes rendering bones virtually invisible on X-ray, and widespread fractures, especially of the ribs, are classical features of neonatal rickets.
   c. **False**. This is the most common cause of blindness in rice-dependent populations.
   d. **False**. They have a daily requirement of 2 mmol/kg potassium, 4 mmol/kg sodium and 1 mmol/kg calcium.
   e. **False**. Protein and carbohydrate provide 4 kcal/g; fat provides 9 kcal/g.

Short notes answer

The advantages of breast feeding include:

- correct amounts of protein, fat and carbohydrate for requirements
- appropriate ratio of casein:lactalbumin
- correct amounts of electrolytes
- iron presented in absorbable form
- contains vitamins, folic acid
- contains lipase, which helps digestion
- improved maternal bonding
- immune properties (e.g. IgA, lactoferrin, white cells, lysozyme)
- low pH encourages *Lactobacillus acidophilus* rather than *Escherichia coli* in stool
- economical, cheap.

Problems associated with breast feeding include:

- inability to assess exact amounts of feed taken
- increased unconjugated jaundice in the neonatal period: though never to kernicteric levels
- transfer of maternal medications and infections to infant.

Viva voce answer

The child should be seated on his parent's lap in a quiet room, preferably without too many visible distractions. The distractor positions himself (seated comfortably) a metre or so in front of the child, while the controller of the test stands behind the parent, out of sight of the child. The distractor is then told to gain the child's attention using a bright coloured object. Once the child's concentration is focused on this toy, the controller indicates by means of a sign to the distractor to hide the toy. At the moment when the child has lost the focus of his attention and is not yet distracted by some other object, the controller mouths a high-pitched (e.g. SSSHHH) or low-pitched (e.g. GGGOOO) noise at the level of the child's ear (while still out of sight). A positive distraction test is indicated by a clear appreciation of the sound by the child who then turns his head to seek out its origin. The test can be repeated for both ears using different sounds. The test is not applicable to children whose head and truncal control is underdeveloped such that they are unable to sit up (i.e. before 6 months), and it usually fails beyond 18 months or so when the child cannot be 'fooled' so easily.

Case history

1. Failure to thrive owing to an inadequate diet and probably a deficiency syndrome (especially iron). She was weaned too early and is now on an inadequate diet, mostly sustained with milk and fruit juice.
2. In addition to her medical history, it is important to enquire about her general behaviour, the presence of pica, global development, especially speech, language and learning, and social skills such as toilet training.
3. It is important to know the family setup, i.e. number of children and their ages, father's employment and family income, housing situation and social benefits, if any. The medical history of other family members and their heights and weights should be recorded.
4. Advise mother that the child's problem is likely to be related to her poorly balanced diet and that she is probably low in iron stores. Explain that this is not serious and is easily reversed with appropriate therapy and a good diet. Gently point out that X-ray imaging is unlikely to be helpful and would expose the child to unnecessary irradiation. Go on to explain what investigations are necessary, what they entail and why.
5. The following investigations are appropriate:

   - full blood count, differential and indices
   - electrolytes, calcium, phosphate, alkaline phosphatase, magnesium
   - iron, ferritin, folate
   - albumin, total protein
   - renal and liver function
   - urinalysis
   - bone age (X-ray left wrist and hand).

6. Iron-deficiency anaemia.
7. Commence iron supplements, repeat urinalysis and culture from a clean catch specimen (initial sample was contaminated). Arrange follow-up to monitor weight and response to treatment.
8. Check weight, (height), full blood count, iron, ferritin and urinalysis.
9. Refer the child to a professional dietician and, if appropriate, to a child guidance clinic.
10. Refer the family to social services to maximise state support and to supervise progress of the patient and siblings. The problem appears to be one of a chaotic family held together by a caring but overworked mother with too many young children. Her concern, fastidious recording of weight measurements and maintenance of an up-to-date vaccination schedule mitigate against child abuse by neglect.

Diseases of the newborn

Key points

You should have an understanding of:

- The care of healthy newborn infants and be able to perform an adequate examination of the newborn
- The causes, problems and complications of prematurity
- Inherited and congenital diseases that present in the neonatal period
- The diagnosis and management of acquired diseases of the newborn, especially infection
- The complications associated with multiple births.

2.1 Introduction

Of the 600 000 babies born each year in the UK, 4000 die during the first week of life. The causes of death are listed in Box 2. Though prematurity is the leading cause of morbidity, the outcome of premature birth has improved dramatically: 90% of those born after 28 weeks of gestation can be expected to survive without serious complications.

Definitions

Definitions related to growth

Term infant: infant born between 38 and 42 weeks of gestation (i.e. after 37 completed weeks)
Preterm infant: infant born before 37 completed weeks of gestation
Post-term infant: infant born after 42 weeks of gestation
Low birth weight (LBW): infant weighing 2500 g or less at birth
Very low birth weight (VLBW): infant weighing 1500 g or less at birth
Small for gestational age (SGA): infant weighing less than the 10th percentile
Large for gestational age (LGA): infant weighing more than the 90th percentile
Appropriate for gestational age (AGA): infant weighing >10th and <90th percentile for weight.

Causes of reduced intrauterine growth include maternal disease, placental dysfunction, fetal abnormalities and congenital infections. The most important cause of excessive growth is poorly controlled maternal diabetes.

Definitions related to outcome

Stillbirth: infant born dead after 24 weeks of gestation
Abortion: fetal death before 24 weeks of gestation
Perinatal mortality: the number of stillbirths and deaths during the first 1–6 complete days per 1000 total births
Neonatal mortality: deaths in the first 28 days of life per 1000 live births
Infant mortality: deaths occurring from birth to 12 months per 1000 live births.

The perinatal period refers to the first 7 days after birth; the neonatal period is the first 28 days after birth and the post-neonatal period spans 28 days to 12 months of life. The perinatal mortality rate for the UK has reduced greatly during the 1980s and 1990s and was approximately 8/1000 in 1993. The post-neonatal mortality rate has also fallen because of a great reduction in the number of cot deaths, probably as a result of the introduction of the supine sleeping posture.

The perinatal mortality rate is a measure of the quality of the antenatal care, management of labour and immediate resuscitation and care of the newborn. It also reflects the socioeconomic conditions affecting the general health of the mothers and the surroundings into which the babies are born. The infant mortality rate provides a more comprehensive overview and is low in the developed countries (less than 10 per 1000 live births) and high in some developing countries (30–200/1000 live births).

Prenatal diagnosis

Ultrasound is used routinely to assess fetal maturity and growth and to identify abnormalities such as cranial (e.g. hydrocephalus, anencephaly), thoracic (e.g. pulmonary and cardiac anomalies), gastrointestinal (e.g. obstruction, exomphalos), renal (e.g. agenesis, cysts or dilatation) and skeletal abnormalities (e.g. neural tube defects, achondroplasia). Other methods of prenatal diagnosis are used to obtain fetal cells for DNA or

---

BOX 2
Causes of death and morbidity in neonates

Fetal	Preterm infants	Term infants
Congenital anomalies	Congenital anomalies	Congenital anomalies
Placental insufficiency	Severe prematurity	Perinatal asphyxia
Abruptio placenta	Respiratory distress syndrome	Perinatal trauma
Umbilical cord accident	Bronchopulmonary dysplasia	Meconium aspiration
Hydrops fetalis	Intraventricular haemorrhage	Persistent fetal circulation
Intrauterine infection	Infection	Infection
	Necrotising enterocolitis	Metabolic diseases

Table 6 Methods and timing of prenatal diagnosis

Method	Timing
Ultrasound	6 weeks*
Chorionic villus sampling	12 weeks
Amniocentesis	16 weeks
Fetal blood sampling	after 20 weeks

*At 5 weeks using transvaginal probe.

biochemical analysis, allowing a large (and constantly increasing) number of metabolic, chromosomal and genetic disorders to be identified before birth (Table 6).

2.2 Assessment of the newborn

All newborn infants should be carefully examined after birth to exclude abnormalities and to reassure the parents. The first examination after birth is also a good opportunity to encourage the mother to breast feed the infant. The assessment should begin with a careful review of the maternal history and of the infant's behaviour. The examination is best done from 'top to toe' with the aim of excluding congenital abnormalities and searching for signs of ill health.

The history and examination

Maternal history

The following areas should be covered:

- Social, e.g. smoking, alcohol, drug abuse
- Genetic or familial disease, e.g. Down syndrome, cystic fibrosis
- Obstetric history, e.g. previous pregnancy loss
- Current pregnancy, e.g. blood loss, hypertension
- Results of investigations, e.g. ultrasound, serology, alpha fetoprotein.

Neonatal examination

The examination should be carried out with the infant undressed in the presence of the mother. Observe the infant's posture, movements and colour and exclude any characteristic disorder, e.g. Down syndrome. The infant's weight and head circumference should be plotted on appropriate centile charts.

Head and neck

Swellings may be caused by caput, a boggy swelling present from birth, subperiosteal cephalhaematoma, which is limited by sutures, or a subaponeurotic haematoma, an extensive boggy swelling that may cause hypovolaemia.

Abnormal shape may be caused by premature fusion of cranial sutures (craniosynostosis).

The head circumference may be abnormally small (microcephaly) or large (macrocephaly), e.g. as caused by hydrocephalus.

Clefts of lip and/or palate should be assessed with the mouth fully open.

Preauricular sinuses may be associated with branchial arch malformations.

Swellings, cysts or sinuses in the neck may be related to the thyroid gland if midline or to branchial cleft malformations if situated in the anterior triangle.

The eyes should be carefully examined to exclude cataracts or other abnormalities.

Chest

A respiratory rate greater than 60 breaths/minute, or central cyanosis, nasal flaring and costal recession should be investigated urgently.

Cardiovascular examination includes palpation of the peripheral pulses, including the femoral pulses (which may be absent in coarctation of the aorta) and auscultation for heart murmurs. However, a heart murmur may not be present even in major congenital heart abnormalities (see Chapter 4).

Abdomen

An exomphalos caused by failure of the midgut to return into the abdomen during fetal life or a **gastroschisis** resulting from herniation of abdominal contents through an anterior abdominal wall defect will be evident at birth. A simple umbilical hernia does not require treatment.

Abdominal distension may result from an enlarged organ or be caused by intestinal obstruction, e.g. from intestinal atresia or secondary to Hirschsprung's disease.

The genitalia should be examined, the testicular position noted in males and the anus checked for patency.

Hips

These should be examined for *congenital dislocation of the hips* (Section 2.3).

Back

A *myelomeningocele* (*spina bifida*) is usually diagnosed before birth, but less severe spinal abnormalities may be suspected because of a hairy patch or a lipoma on the lower back. A sacral dimple is not significant. A large swelling over the sacrum may be caused by a *sacrococcygeal teratoma*, which will require surgical excision shortly after birth.

Skin and mucous membranes

In dark-skinned babies and occasionally in Caucasians as well, blue-black pigmented areas or Mongolian spots are seen on the base of the back and buttocks. These usually fade after the first year. Urticaria, heat rash and white pimples (milia) are common transient phenomena. Often babies have small cysts in their mouths: Epstein pearls on the palate and epulis on the gums. Occasionally natal teeth may be present.

Table 7 Simplified neurological assessment

Examination	Observation
Spontaneous movements	Frequent
Posture	Flexed arms, extended legs
Upper limb tone	Resists lifting of arms
Lower limb tone	Resists hip abduction, popliteal extension
Truncal tone	Attempts to straighten back when lifted prone
Tendon reflexes	Brisk; some clonus common
Moro response	Abduction and extension then adduction and flexion
Response to objects	Fixes and follows bright objects
Response to sounds	Quietens or startles

Neurological assessment

A simplified neurological assessment is shown in Table 7. Spontaneous movements, posture, tone, the response to light, bright objects and to sounds should be noted and recorded. Tendon reflexes should be elicited. Clonus is often present in newborn infants. The Moro reflex, an 'embrace' elicited by removing support from under the infant's head, should be symmetrical and complete. Neurological disturbance may cause apathy or irritability and may result from cerebral malformations or be secondary to systemic illness such as infection or metabolic disease. Reduced tone and movements may be caused by neuromuscular diseases.

Assessment of maturity

Maturity may be assessed by physical and neurological

examination during the first 7 days of life. The method described by Dubowitz and colleagues in 1970 is commonly used and a simplified score is shown in Figure 7 and Table 8.

2.3 Congenital abnormalities

Congenital anomalies result from genetic, environmental or multifactorial causes. Structural defects of prenatal onset can be separated into those arising from a single primary defect in development and those representing multiple malformations, often associated together into characteristic *syndromes*.

Introduction

The most common *single primary defects* include congenital dislocation of the hip (p. 226) talipes equinovarus, (p. 226), cleft lip with or without cleft palate (p. 231) cardiac septal defects (p. 68) and neural tube defects (p. 105). Most single defects are acquired through multifactorial inheritance (p. 163). While the aetiology is often unknown, many can be categorised according to the error in morphogenesis. A specific, localised error results in a *malformation* (e.g. cardiac septal defect), whereas an alteration in shape or structure in a part that has already differentiated normally results in a *deformation*. The latter generally occur in the neuromuscular system and are probably

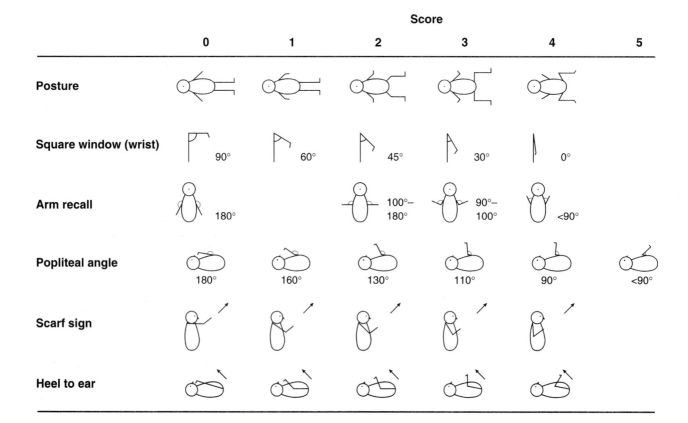

Fig. 7 Assessment of neuromuscular maturity. Score is used in the scale outlined in Table 8 to indicate maturity.

Table 8 Assessment of physical maturity

Assessments to produce maturity score

	Score					
	0	1	2	3	4	5
Skin	Gelatinous, red, transparent	Smooth, pink, visible veins	Superficial peeling and/or rash, few veins	Cracking, pale area, rare veins	Parchment, deep cracking no vessels	Leathery, cracked, wrinkled
Lanugo	None	Abundant	Thinning	Bald areas	Mostly bald	
Plantar creases	No crease	Faint red marks	Anterior transverse crease only	Creases anterior two thirds	Creases cover entire sole	
Breast	Barely perceptible	Flat areola, no bud	Stippled areola, 1–2 mm bud	Raised areola, 3–4 mm bud	Full areola, 5–10 mm bud	
Ear	Pinna flat, stays folded	Slightly curved pinna, soft, slow recoil	Well-curved pinna, soft but ready recoil	Formed and firm with instant recoil	Thick cartilage, ear stiff	
Genitals Male	Scrotum empty, no rugae		Testes descending, few rugae	Testes down, good rugae	Testes pendulous, deep rugae	
Female	Prominent clitoris and labia minora		Majora and minora equally prominent	Majora large, minora small	Clitoris and minora completely covered	

Use of score to indicate maturity rating

	Score									
	5	10	15	20	25	30	35	40	45	50
Maturity rating (weeks)	26	28	30	32	34	36	38	40	42	44

caused by intrauterine moulding. For example, reduced amniotic fluid results in a restriction in fetal movements and, in the first instance, may precipitate an abnormal presentation (e.g. breech). However, deformations such as talipes, hip dislocation, abnormal moulding of the head (e.g. dolicocephaly, plagiocephaly), underdevelopment or distortion of the chin (micrognathia, mandibular asymmetry) and torticollis may also arise.

Sometimes a single primary defect can result in a cascade, or *sequence*, of secondary and tertiary errors in morphogenesis. For example, in the Pierre–Robin sequence, there is an error in the development of the mandible with micrognathia. As a result, the tongue is relatively large for the distorted oral cavity and falls backwards (glossoptosis), blocking the closure of the posterior palatal shelves and giving rise to a large, U-shaped cleft palate. In Potter syndrome, renal agenesis/hypoplasia leads to oligohydramnios, which results in breech and other abnormal presentations, together with pulmonary hypoplasia.

Destruction of a normally formed part results in a *disruption*. This arises through amputation of a normal structure (e.g. a digit by an amniotic band) or infarction caused by interruption of the blood supply in utero (e.g. ileal atresia).

Malformations involving two or more systems usually have a common aetiological agent and are caused by related chromosomal and genetic defects or are the result of a common teratogen. Specific chromosomal disorders are discussed in Section 9.4.

Disorders associated with maternal abnormalities

Maternal disease (e.g. diabetes, thyroid disease, phenylketonuria and systemic lupus erythematosus), teratogens (e.g. alcohol, warfarin, phenytoin) and infection (e.g. cytomegalovirus, toxoplasmosis, rubella) may all result in a congenital abnormality in the fetus.

Infants of insulin-dependent diabetic mothers have an increased risk of hypoglycaemia in the neonatal period, are generally large for dates and may have associated malformations such as cardiovascular (cardiomyopathy), genitourinary and neural tube defects. Sacral agenesis results in a patulous anus and urinary incontinence.

Fetal alcohol syndrome results from maternal chronic alcoholism and is indicated by characteristic facies (long philtrum and thin smooth upper lip), growth retardation and microcephaly.

Congenital infections may cause hydrocephalus or microcephaly, cataracts, chorioretinitis, deafness, generalised neurodevelopmental delay, pneumonitis, congenital heart disease, hepatosplenomegaly, osteitis and myelosuppression, depending on the type of infection (see Section 2.6).

2.4 Birth asphyxia

Birth asphyxia is defined as a reduction of oxygen delivery and accumulation of carbon dioxide owing to cessation of blood supply to the fetus around the time of birth. The incidence is about 1:600 births, but the most serious consequence, brain injury, occurs in about 1:1000 births. Birth asphyxia may occur in a previously well infant, or follow neuromuscular, metabolic or infectious disease.

Diagnosis of birth asphyxia

The diagnosis of birth asphyxia is based on the presence of:

1. Evidence of fetal distress, such as an abnormal cardiotocograph.
2. Fetal metabolic acidosis, i.e. a pH <7.0 and a base deficit >15.
3. Abnormal neurological state, e.g. seizures, abnormal tone at and after birth.
4. Multiorgan involvement, e.g. transient renal failure.

Birth asphyxia is often first suspected when the infant unexpectedly fails to establish respirations after birth. In *primary apnoea*, the circulation is maintained and the heart rate is >100 beats per minute. Cessation of asphyxia at this stage is followed by spontaneous recovery of respiration. However, if asphyxia continues, *secondary apnoea* and circulatory failure develop. The heart rate is <100 beats per minute and immediate resuscitation is needed.

Apgar score

The Apgar score is commonly used to describe the condition at birth (Table 9) but a detailed clinical description is preferable. Details of any resuscitation required, particularly the time taken to establish respirations should be recorded. The cord arterial and venous blood gases should be measured to determine the occurrence of metabolic acidaemia. The Apgar score is usually recorded at 1, 5 and 10 minutes. A low Apgar score at 1–2 minutes indicates the need to initiate resuscitation, whereas a low score at 10 minutes is an indicator of a poor neurological outcome.

Management at birth

Most newborn infants will breathe vigorously by

1–2 minutes after birth and will not require resuscitation. The infant should be wiped dry, quickly inspected to exclude a major malformation and placed in the mother's arms. A breast feed may be offered after a few minutes. Approximately 1% of infants do not establish regular breathing and are still cyanosed after 1–2 minutes. These infants will require resuscitation, which should be initiated by those at the delivery, who, in turn, should also request assistance.

Ventilation

Ventilation is assisted with a well-fitting soft face mask attached to an oxygen source and blow off valve, but if this is not available, an infant ventilating bag may be used instead (Fig. 8). The first few assisted breaths should be of a long duration (>1 second) to achieve an adequate functional residual capacity. Ventilation should continue at about 40 breaths per minute until regular respirations are established.

Circulation

If the heart rate is <100 beats per minute, cardiac massage should be started. This is best performed by encircling the infant's thorax with both hands and using the thumbs to apply pressure on the lower sternum at a rate of about 100 thrusts per minute (Fig. 8).

Secondary apnoea

In secondary apnoea, the infant will have profound bradycardia or no audible heart sounds and will be limp, pale and apnoeic. The following action should be taken:

1. *Intubate* immediately and give intermittent positive pressure ventilation with oxygen, sufficient to achieve visible chest expansion. If unable to intubate, adequate ventilation can be achieved using a well-fitting face mask and infant ventilating bag.
2. *Cardiac massage* should be commenced.
3. *Adrenaline* (3 ml of 1:10 000 solution) should be given via the endotracheal tube.

With no improvement set up an intravenous cannula or an umbilical venous catheter.

4. Give 10 ml 4.2% *sodium bicarbonate* intravenously.
5. If peripheral pulses remain weak, give 30 ml (or 10 ml/kg) *albumin* or plasma expander.
6. If the infant is obviously pale, give 30 ml (or 10 ml/kg) *blood*.

The decision to discontinue resuscitation should be made by a senior paediatrician.

Management after resuscitation

The infant should be observed closely with particular attention to the following areas:

Table 9 The Apgar score

Score	0	1	2
Heart rate	0	<100	>100
Respiration	Absent	Irregular	Regular
Muscle tone	Limp	Reduced	Normal
Response to pharyngeal catheter	None	Grimace	Cough
Colour of trunk	White	Blue	Pink

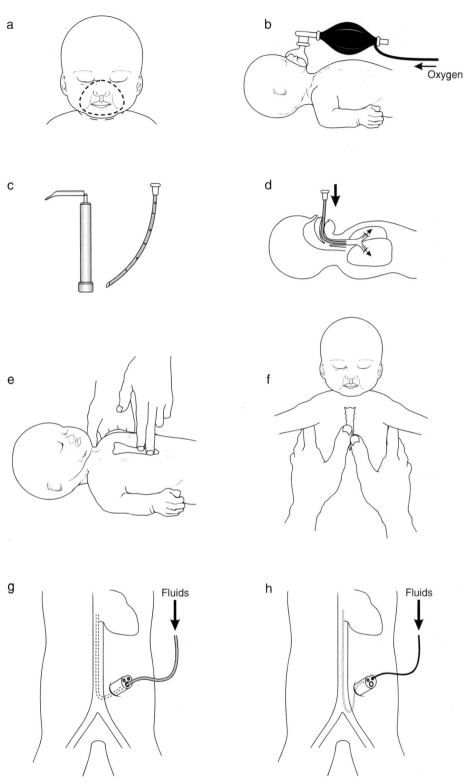

Fig. 8 Neonatal resuscitation. (a) The correct position of the face mask. (b) Face mask and bag ventilation. The laryngoscope shown in (c) is used to insert the endotracheal tube in the trachea for positive pressure ventilation (d). Cardiac massage can be applied using two fingers while supporting the back (e), or using bilateral chest compression (f). The umbilical vein allows the rapid insertion of a large catheter (g). The arteries are smaller and an umbilical arterial catheter dips into the pelvis before ascending the IVC (h).

Breathing is assessed by checking blood gases and mechanical ventilation is started if the infant has apnoea or the PCO_2 is >6 kPa.

Circulation is assessed by monitoring blood pressure, capillary return and central–peripheral temperature gap. Inotropes and colloid infusions may be required.

Fluid and electrolyte balance is monitored through urine output and plasma electrolyte concentration.

Moderate fluid restriction is often necessary because of transient renal impairment or excessive antidiuretic hormone secretion.

Seizures are common following moderately severe asphyxia. Anticonvulsant therapy is given if seizures are frequent and interfering with ventilation.

Complications of birth asphyxia

Birth asphyxia can lead to complications affecting different organ systems.

Central nervous system. Asphyxia may cause hypoxic–ischaemic encephalopathy (HIE), and impaired brainstem function.

Cardiovascular system. Ischaemic injury results in cardiac dysfunction and failure.

Pulmonary system. Pulmonary congestion and haemorrhage can occur.

Renal system. Transient renal failure is common.

Outcome following birth asphyxia

Clinical assessment and further investigations are needed to determine the neurological outcome following asphyxia.

Hypoxic–ischaemic encephalopathy

HIE describes the neurological syndrome that may develop following asphyxia. The severity of the neurological abnormality is variable and is related to the subsequent neurological outcome. Three grades are identified:

I.   Mild: infant is alert, irritable but has normal tone and no seizures.
II. Moderate: infant is lethargic, hypotonic, often has seizures.
III. Severe: infant is stuporose, flaccid, often apnoeic with persistent seizures.

Infants who only develop mild HIE recover completely, while about 20% of infants with moderate HIE have neurological complications. Most infants with severe HIE succumb or develop severe brain injury.

Brain activity

A normal electroencephalogram (EEG) during the first few days after asphyxia indicates a normal outcome, while a suppressed EEG or frequent seizure activity indicates a poor prognosis.

Brain damage: imaging assessment

Cranial ultrasound examination may demonstrate haemorrhage, infarction or suggest cerebral oedema. Cerebral artery blood flow velocity may be abnormally reduced following asphyxia. More detailed information can be obtained by nuclear magnetic resonance imaging (MRI) and spectroscopy.

2.5 Respiratory disease

Apnoea (cessation of breathing for >20 seconds, usually accompanied by bradycardia) and tachypnoea (respiratory rate >60 breaths per minute) indicate respiratory difficulty and require investigation. Central cyanosis may be difficult to recognise unless it is severe, and oxygen saturation should always be measured by pulse oximetry in those infants with respiratory difficulties. A 'grunting' sound is commonly heard in an infant with respiratory distress. The sound is caused by the infant breathing against a partially closed glottis, probably in an attempt to produce positive end expiratory pressure and prevent atelectasis (pulmonary collapse).

Causes of respiratory problems in the neonate

Respiratory distress is manifest by central cyanosis, tachypnoea, grunting, nasal flaring and intercostal and subcostal recession. Auscultation is often unhelpful in the premature and term infant. Respiratory distress is a sign of pulmonary disease but may also be a prominent feature of non-pulmonary pathology (Box 3).

BOX 3
Causes of respiratory distress

Pulmonary	Non-pulmonary
Surfactant deficiency	Infection
Pneumonia	Asphyxia
Aspiration: meconium, milk	Neuromuscular disease
Pneumothorax	Metabolic diseases with acidosis
Congenital abnormalities	Cardiac disease
Lung cysts	Left to right shunts
Tracheo-oesophageal fistula	Obstructed circulation
Diaphragmatic hernia	Arrhythmia (e.g. SVT)

Pneumonia

Pneumonia may present within hours of birth as a consequence of antepartum infection, or it may be acquired several days after birth as a complication of other illness. The most important cause of early onset pneumonia is infection with group B haemolytic streptococci. The infected infant develops increasing respiratory distress with tachypnoea and grunting. Generalised pulmonary opacification is present on the chest X-ray film similar to the appearance observed in surfactant deficiency. Septicaemic shock may develop rapidly, and prompt systemic antibiotic treatment and support of the circulation is essential. Intrapartum antibiotic therapy given to the mother may prevent neonatal infection.

Meconium aspiration

Meconium aspiration commonly occurs following intra-

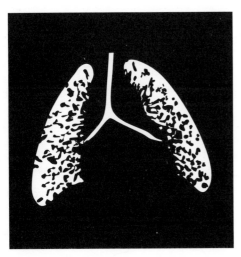

Fig. 9 Chest X-ray film showing changes occurring in surfactant deficiency disease.

Fig. 10 Chest X-ray film showing right tension pneumothorax.

partum asphyxia. Plugging of the airways by meconium causes distal atelectasis and/or hyperinflation through a ball valve effect. Inflammation and secondary infection of the affected lung tissue may occur. In severe cases, marked respiratory distress develops as a consequence of the ensuing hypoxia and pulmonary hypertension. Prompt suction of the airways at birth to remove as much meconium as possible may prevent respiratory complications.

Surfactant deficiency

Surfactant deficiency (hyaline membrane disease (HMD), or respiratory distress syndrome (RDS) is the most common cause of respiratory distress in premature infants. It is less likely to occur in small-for-gestational age infants because lung maturation is enhanced in this condition. The condition is caused by a deficiency of pulmonary surfactant, a phospholipid produced by type 2 alveolar cells. Surfactant lowers surface tension and its deficiency results in reduced lung compliance, increased work of breathing, atelectasis, hypoxia and respiratory acidosis. As a result, the infant develops tachypnoea, nasal flaring, grunting respirations and intercostal recession. The chest X-ray shows a characteristic diffuse granular appearance with a prominent air bronchogram (Fig. 9). Steroids given to the mother 24 hours before premature delivery promote lung maturity, encourage surfactant production and reduce the severity of the neonatal respiratory illness. Surfactant preparations given intratracheally have revolutionised the treatment of surfactant deficiency. Exogenous surfactant is effective in the prevention of this disease; it also reduces its severity, and has decreased the mortality of preterm infants with surfactant deficiency disease by about 40%.

Pneumothorax

A pneumothorax can occur spontaneously immediately after birth in otherwise healthy infants. The infant may be asymptomatic but may develop tachypnoea and

cyanosis. The diagnosis is confirmed by chest X-ray (Fig. 10). The condition often resolves spontaneously and a pleural drain is necessary only in those infants who develop severe respiratory difficulty.

Tension pneumothorax is an important, serious complication in infants requiring mechanical ventilation, especially preterm infants with surfactant deficiency and infants with meconium aspiration. Tension pneumothorax will cause lung compression, mediastinal shift and impairs venous return to the heart. Unless the situation is relieved by the immediate insertion of a pleural drain, profound hypoxia leading to cardiorespiratory arrest will ensue.

2.6 Infections

Newborn infants commonly develop minor infections such as conjunctivitis and skin pustules and are also more susceptible to serious infections, including septicaemia and meningitis. The early clinical features of serious infections are often non-specific and an increased awareness is essential if early diagnosis and prompt treatment are to be initiated and complications reduced.

Common minor infections

Conjunctivitis

A sticky eye is common after birth and usually results from irritation of the eye during delivery or is caused by a partially blocked tear duct. No treatment is required. Conversely, a purulent discharge may indicate bacterial or chlamydial conjunctivitis. The discharging eye should be swabbed and treated with appropriate antibiotic eye drops. Chlamydial conjunctivitis infection is an important cause of serious eye disease in developing countries and may be complicated by chlamydial pneumonitis. It causes a persistent discharge, and a swab obtained by scraping the conjunctiva is required to confirm the diagnosis. Erythromycin given systemically via the oral route is effective treatment for this condition.

Skin pustules

Skin pustules and paronychia are usually caused by staphylococci. If several lesions are present oral flucloxacillin is indicated to prevent dissemination and septicaemia.

Candidiasis

Candida albicans infection causes white patches on the inside of the cheeks and tongue while candidal dermatitis usually affects the nappy area. Treatment is with oral and topical nystatin.

Serious infections

Neonates are relatively immunosuppressed as a result of poor host barriers to infection and an immature immune system. Consequently, infection is a major cause of neonatal morbidity and may arise in utero or in the peri- and postnatal periods (Box 4).

Congenital infections

Congenital infections occur as a result of maternal infections during pregnancy. Although these infections may go unrecognised in the mother, who is often asymptomatic, they severely affect multiple organs in the fetus and tend to have a similar presentation. The clinical signs include low birth weight owing to prematurity or poor growth, microcephaly, hepatosplenomegaly, prolonged jaundice, petechiae caused by thrombocytopenia, choroidoretinitis and cataracts. Imaging may show cerebral atrophy, intracranial calcification, a pneumonitis and osteitis (Fig. 11) The diagnosis is usually confirmed by serological tests.

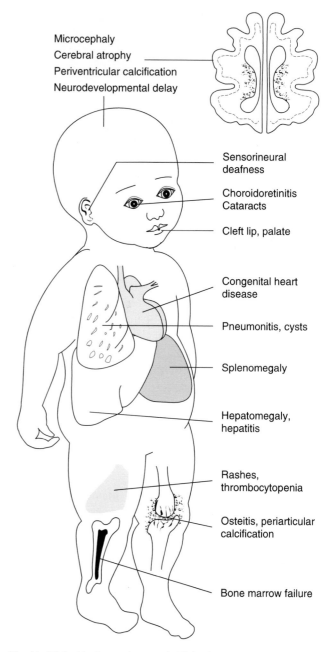

Microcephaly
Cerebral atrophy
Periventricular calcification
Neurodevelopmental delay

Sensorineural deafness

Choroidoretinitis
Cataracts

Cleft lip, palate

Congenital heart disease

Pneumonitis, cysts

Splenomegaly

Hepatomegaly, hepatitis

Rashes, thrombocytopenia

Osteitis, periarticular calcification

Bone marrow failure

Fig. 11 Clinical features of congenital infection.

BOX 4
Causes of infection in the newborn

Congenital	Perinatal	Postnatal
Toxoplasma (T)	Bacterial	Bacterial
Other (O)	septicaemia	septicaemia
Rubella (R)	Herpes simplex	Bacterial
Cytomegalovirus (C)	HIV	meningitis
Herpes, HIV (H)		
Syphilis (S)		

The congenital infections are often referred to as TORCHS, reflecting the causes

---

Cytomegalovirus infection

Cytomegalovirus (CMV) is the commonest congenital viral infection. Most infants are asymptomatic but CMV

infection may cause severe pneumonitis and survivors may develop intracranial calcification, microcephaly and severe neurological deficit. The diagnosis is confirmed by the presence of 'owl-eye' inclusion bodies in the urinary sediment, culture of urine for CMV and raised CMV-specific IgM in the serum.

Toxoplasmosis

Congenital toxoplasmosis is caused by primary maternal infection with the protozoan *Toxoplasma gondii*, following ingestion of meat contaminated by oocysts from cat faeces. The condition is rare in the UK but is more prevalent in continental Europe. Chorioretinitis may be the only manifestation, but the infection may cause growth retardation, and hydrocephalus and intracranial infection; the last have a poor prognosis despite antibiotic therapy. Repeated serological testing at a reference laboratory may be necessary to establish the diagnosis.

Rubella

Maternal infection with rubella during pregnancy has become exceptionally rare because of routine vaccination in childhood and routine screening in early pregnancy. Maternal infection in the first trimester poses the greatest risk to the infant. The complications include cataracts, cardiac defects (especially persistent ductus arteriosus), deafness, microcephaly and neurodevelopmental delay.

Congenital syphilis

Congenital syphilis is a rare illness since all pregnant women are screened for syphilis at presentation and treatment of affected mothers is effective in preventing vertical transmission of the spirochaete. However, maternal infection acquired later in pregnancy results in the occasional case of congenital syphilis. The affected newborn develops a rash, periostitis, nasal discharge, hepatomegaly and jaundice (caused by hepatitis). Treatment with penicillin is completely effective.

Perinatal HIV infection

The majority of HIV infections in children are acquired perinatally from mothers who may be asymptomatic. Infection is usually acquired during the last trimester or during the birth, but there is also a potential risk of transmission by breast feeding. Without preventive chemotherapy, about 25% of infants born to HIV-positive mothers become infected. Infected infants may become symptomatic weeks or months following birth. The presenting features are respiratory distress caused by *Pneumocystis carinii* infection or lymphoid interstitial pneumonitis, failure to thrive, enlarged lymph nodes or recurrent bacterial and fungal infections. Treatment of the mother with zidovudine (AZT) during pregnancy and delivery reduces the risk of perinatal infection.

Acquired infections

Infections acquired during birth are common when maternal infection occurs or there is prolonged rupture of the membranes. They usually present during the first 7 days, often within 48 hours of birth. Later onset infection occurs particularly in premature infants and hospitalised infants.

Acquired infections may progress rapidly if treatment is delayed, resulting in life-threatening septicaemia. Since the initial clinical features indicative of septicaemia are usually non-specific, infection should always be suspected in any infant who becomes unwell or develops symptoms and signs, as listed in Table 10.

Investigations are required to confirm the diagnosis. Thrombocytopenia may be present and there is increased toxic granulation, with a shift to the left seen on the blood film. Blood and urine should be cultured.

Table 10 Presenting features suggestive of infection

Symptoms	Signs
Change in behaviour (irritability, lethargy)	Poor perfusion
Poor feeding	Acidosis
Vomiting	Leucocytosis/penia
Apnoea or respiratory distress	Thrombocytopenia
Rash	Hypoglycaemia
Unstable temperature	

A lumbar puncture and culture of the CSF should be considered if there are neurological symptoms or apnoea. Treatment with dual broad-spectrum antibiotics to provide adequate Gram-positive and Gram-negative cover (usually cephalosporins) should be commenced while awaiting results of cultures.

Group B streptococcal infection

The most common acute neonatal bacterial infection involves group B streptococci. It is usually acquired during delivery from asymptomatic mothers. The infection presents within a few hours of birth with increasing respiratory distress, which may run a fulminating course unless prompt treatment is commenced. Late-onset disease after 7 days may be acquired in hospital and often presents with meningitis.

Herpes simplex infection

Herpes simplex infection may be acquired during birth if the mother has primary genital herpes infection; in this case, delivery by caesarean section is indicated. Early treatment with intravenous acyclovir may prevent the most serious consequences, meningoencephalitis and disseminated disease, which carry a high risk of mortality.

Hepatitis B infection

Vertical transmission of hepatitis B from mother to infant is likely where the mother is Hepatitis B e antigen (HBeAg) positive without having anti-HBe antibodies. Infants born to such mothers should be given both passive and active immunisation, a ploy that offers effective protection in more than 90% of susceptible infants. Hepatitis B immunoglobulin (HBIG) is given intramuscularly into one thigh soon after birth and hepatitis B vaccine (HBVac) in the contralateral thigh. The latter is repeated, 1 and 6 months later.

Other bacterial infections

Infection with *Listeria monocytogenes* accounts for about 5% of serious neonatal infections. It characteristically causes a severe pneumonia and, occasionally, meningitis. Treatment is with amoxycillin. Gram-negative infections (e.g. with *Escherichia coli*) can cause meningitis and septicaemic shock. Prompt treatment with antibiotics and circulatory support are essential. Repeated coagulase-negative staphylococcal infection is particularly common in preterm infants with an indwelling central venous catheter.

2.7 Jaundice in the newborn

Jaundice is very common, occurring in at least 50% of fullterm infants and in over 80% of preterm infants during the first week of life. The majority of jaundiced infants have physiological hyperbilirubinaemia and are otherwise healthy. Others are jaundiced as a result of neonatal illness such as hepatitis, biliary atresia, infection and haemolytic and metabolic disease. Unconjugated (indirect) bilirubin is fat soluble, may cross the blood–brain barrier and, unlike conjugated (direct) hyperbilirubinaemia, can cause brain injury, especially in the preterm infant with haemolytic disease. Unconjugated bilirubin deposits in parts of the brain including the basal ganglia, resulting in kernicterus. Initial hypotonia is usually followed by opisthotonus (marked extension of neck and back) and convulsions. Kernicterus has a high mortality rate; survivors may develop sensorineural hearing loss and athetoid cerebral palsy. Conjugated bilirubin is water soluble and excreted in the urine, where it imparts a dark colour (when compared with the usual, almost colourless appearance of normal urine in neonates). Hyperbilirubinuria, in conjugation with pale stools, is indicative of a biliary obstruction, with or without an associated hepatitic element.

Causes of jaundice

Physiological jaundice

Neonatal jaundice can be physiological or pathological. Physiological jaundice is caused by multiple factors, including immaturity of liver enzymes, an increased bilirubin load from excessive red cell degradation and increased absorption of bilirubin from the gut. Physiological jaundice develops after the first day and, though it persists for longer in preterm infants, it generally resolves after 10 days. The bilirubin level rarely exceeds 250 μmol/l. Prolonged physiological jaundice persisting for 3–4 weeks is common in breast fed infants, where the bilirubin level may exceed 250 μmol/l.

Pathological jaundice

Pathological jaundice may be unconjugated or conjugated in type (Box 5). Conjugated hyperbilirubinaemia (direct bilirubin >50 μmol/l) is abnormal and should prompt investigations to exclude biliary atresia.

Clinical assessment

Slightly jaundiced infants who are otherwise well do not require investigations; however, investigation is indicated in the following situations:

- Jaundice in the first 24 hours after birth (to exclude haemolytic disease)
- Moderately severe jaundice (bilirubin >200 μmol/l)

> **BOX 5**
> **Causes of neonatal jaundice**
>
> **Unconjugated hyperbilirubinaemia**
> Physiological jaundice
> Haemolysis
>   Blood group incompatibility (e.g. Rhesus, ABO, Kell)
>   Red cell enzyme defects (glucose 6-phosphate dehydrogenase (G6PD) or pyruvate kinase deficiency)
>   Red cell membrane defects (e.g. spherocytosis)
> Excess bilirubin
>   Large bruises/haematomas
>   Polycythaemia
> Inherited disorders of conjugation
>
> **Conjugated hyperbilirubinaemia**
> Obstructed biliary tract (e.g. biliary atresia, choledochal cyst)
> Hepatitis
> Hypothyroidism (initially unconjugated)
>
> **Combined hyperbilirubinaemia**
> Genetic disorders (e.g. cystic fibrosis, α_1-antitrypsin deficiency)
> Metabolic disorders (e.g. galactosaemia)
> Infection (e.g. septicaemia, urinary tract infection)

- Prolonged jaundice (persisting for more than one week).

Important points in the clinical history and examination are listed in Table 11.

Investigations

The total, direct and indirect bilirubin levels should be measured. Further investigations will depend on the type of hyperbilirubinaemia

Conjugated hyperbilirubinaemia

A conjugated (direct) bilirubin level >50 μmol/l is an

Table 11 Important symptoms and signs in the neonate with jaundice

	Symptoms and signs
History	
Positive family history of jaundice	Breast milk jaundice, Congenital spherocytosis G6PD deficiency (Asian, African and Mediterranean races)
Pregnancy and delivery	Maternal diabetes Evidence of congenital infection Operative or traumatic delivery
Examination	Apathy or irritability Excessive bruising or cephalhaematoma Hepatosplenomegaly Signs of congenital infection (e.g. cataracts, retinitis, rashes, etc.) Colour of urine and stools

indication to investigate for hepatic or biliary tract abnormalities, i.e. ultrasound scan of the liver, tests for biliary excretion and serological tests for congenital infection. If hepatic or biliary tract disease is suspected, the infant must be referred urgently to a specialist unit for treatment. Metabolic disease should also be considered and a positive urine test for reducing substances suggests galactosaemia.

Unconjugated hyperbilirubinaemia

In those with unconjugated (indirect) jaundice, haemolytic disease must be excluded by examining the blood count and film, the maternal and neonate's blood group and the Coombs test. Glucose 6-phosphate dehydrogenase (G6PD) deficiency should be excluded in infants of Asian, African or Mediterranean origin by measuring G6PD levels in serum.

Treatment

Phototherapy

Blue light (wavelength 450 nm) effectively converts unconjugated bilirubin to a non-toxic photoisomer that is excreted in bile. Exposure to blue light is indicated in:

- haemolytic disease, when it should be started as soon as possible
- preterm infants with rapidly rising bilirubin levels
- severe jaundice (bilirubin >250 µmol/l) in well fullterm infants.

Infants receiving phototherapy are often irritable, develop skin rashes and have loose stools. The eyes should be protected with covers and extra volume given to compensate for the increase in fluid losses while receiving phototherapy. Whenever possible the infant should be nursed at the mother's side.

Exchange transfusion

Exchange transfusion may be required to prevent kernicterus in the at-risk infant with rapidly rising unconjugated bilirubin levels. The procedure consists of withdrawing repeated portions of blood from the infant and replacing these with appropriately cross-matched blood. The volume of blood exchanged is usually twice the infant's blood volume (i.e. twice 85 ml/kg). Exchange transfusion may be indicated in the following situations:

- preterm infants especially if acidotic or hypoxic
- severe haemolytic disease, e.g. Rhesus incompatibility, G6PD deficiency.

2.8 Neonatal convulsions

Many normal newborn babies respond to minor stimuli with startle responses. It is often difficult to distinguish between these normal jitters from intermittent focal convulsions and generalised tonic spasms. Often neonatal convulsions are subtle, amounting to little more than a transient change in activity associated with minor eye movements, blinking, nystagmus, chewing, salivation, bicycling/pedalling movements, blanking episodes and brief alteration in breathing pattern. Convulsions must be considered in the differential diagnosis of recurrent apnoeas, cyanotic spells and bradycardias. The most common cause for neonatal seizures is hypoxic–ischaemic encephalopathy (HIE). Other causes are given in Box 6. The types of seizures occurring are described in Table 12.

BOX 6
Causes of neonatal seizures

Hypoxic–ischaemic encephalopathy (HIE): most common cause
Hypocalcaemia
Hypoglycaemia
Pyridoxine dependency
Infections (including congenital infections and meningitis)
Peri/intraventricular haemorrhage
Kernicterus
Drug withdrawal
Cytoarchitectural abnormalities
Inborn errors of metabolism

The precise diagnosis of neonatal convulsions requires a detailed neurological examination, metabolic screen including blood gas, electrolytes, glucose, calcium and magnesium, bilirubin, septic screen including blood count, blood, urine and CSF culture, cranial ultrasound and an EEG.

The management involves supportive care, control of the seizures and correction or elimination of the underlying defect. Anticonvulsants commonly used include phenobarbitone (phenobarbital), diazepam and phenytoin.

2.9 Low birth weight

Low birth weight (i.e. <2.5 kg) may result from prema-

Table 12 Types and aetiology of neonatal convulsions

Seizure type*	Aetiology
Focal seizure	Localised structural abnormality, infection, haemorrhage
Multifocal clonic	Hypoglycaemia, hypocalcaemia, hypo/hypernatraemia, HIE, drug withdrawal
Tonic	HIE, diffuse brain injury, haemorrhage, kernicterus
Myoclonic	Multiple causes; usually associated with a poor prognosis
Subtle seizures	Drug withdrawal, HIE, haemorrhage, infection

*Infection, inborn errors of metabolism and kernicterus may manifest any type of seizure.

Table 13 Complications of prematurity

System	Effects
Respiratory	Surfactant deficiency disease
	Apnoea
	Bronchopulmonary dysplasia
Cardiovascular	Persistent ductus arteriosus
Gastrointestinal	Poor feeding (requiring nasogastric feeding)
	Parenteral nutrition
Bone marrow	Anaemia of prematurity
Neurological	Peri/intraventricular haemorrhage
Multisystem	
Fluid balance	Salt and water loss
Biochemical	Hypoglycaemia
	Hypocalcaemia
Infection	Septicaemia
Jaundice	Unconjugated jaundice

Fig. 12 Periventricular haemorrhage: grade II and IV lesions.

turity or intrauterine growth retardation (IUGR, i.e. small for gestational age). These two conditions have different causes, clinical features and outcome.

Prematurity

Prematurity is more common in poor socioeconomic groups and follows premature rupture of membranes, infection, multiple pregnancy and maternal disease (e.g. diabetes, pregnancy-induced hypertension). In many cases, no direct cause for the early delivery can be identified. Premature infants develop problems primarily related to the immaturity of their organs (Table 13).

Infants that are small for gestational age

Intrauterine growth retardation (IUGR) can be symmetrical, when the head circumference and weight are both small and on similar centiles, and asymmetrical, when the head size is appropriate for gestation (i.e. head growth is spared). As shown in Box 7 the symmetrical IUGR is usually caused by congenital abnormalities and infection, whereas asymmetrical retardation is often a consequence of maternal disease.

> **BOX 7**
> **Causes of IUGR**
>
> | Symmetrical | Asymmetrical |
> | --- | --- |
> | Congenital malformations | Toxaemia |
> | Chromosomal abnormality | Smoking |
> | Congenital infection | Maternal disease |

Clinical problems of low-birth-weight infants

Infants with IUGR are often 'stressed' as a result of chronic intrauterine malnutrition or hypoxic–ischaemic injury to vital organs. They may show signs of neurological injury owing to periventricular haemorrhage shortly after birth, and evidence of cerebral injury, with periventricular leucomalacia, during the first few weeks. Passage of meconium ante- or perinatally is common, increasing the risk of meconium aspiration. Hypoglycaemia arises because of reduced glycogen stores in these growth-retarded infants.

Periventricular haemorrhage

Periventricular haemorrhage is a serious complication of the preterm infant (Fig. 12). The haemorrhage originates in the subependymal germinal matrix, which is present until 32 weeks of gestation. Major periventricular haemorrhage with expansion of the ventricular system and intracerebral extension is often fatal. Less severe cases result in hydrocephalus through obstruction of the ventricular system by blood clot, arachnoiditis and venous infarction of the periventricular cerebral tissue.

Periventricular leucomalacia

Periventricular leucomalacia (PVL) describes cystic necrosis of periventricular white matter as a result of hypoxic–ischaemic injury. The injury resulting in PVL may occur before birth, but the risk is greatest for preterm infants with severe respiratory problems requiring prolonged ventilation. Because of the proximity of the corticospinal tracts, spastic diplegia is a common complication of PVL. The cystic changes can be detected and followed up on sequential cranial ultrasound scans.

Necrotising enterocolitis

Necrotising enterocolitis (NEC) is a condition of uncertain aetiology, possibly infection, which results in intestinal wall necrosis and perforation. NEC occurs mainly in sick preterm infants but can also arise in healthy fullterm infants. It presents with abdominal distension, bile-stained vomiting and blood-stained loose stools. The diagnosis is confirmed by a plain X-ray of the abdomen, which shows dilated loops of bowel, thickened bowel walls, intramural gas and pneumoperitoneum if perforation has occurred. Treatment is initially conservative, consisting of withholding feeding and giving systemic antibiotics. Surgery is indicated if bowel infarction and perforation are suspected. Severe disease is often fatal; survivors may continue to have problems as a result of intra-abdominal adhesions, strictures and, in those who have had extensive resection, malabsorption because of a short bowel syndrome.

Outcome of the low-birth-weight infant

The outcome of preterm infants has improved dramatically in recent years. Outcome is primarily dependent on the severity of prematurity, respiratory complications and periventricular haemorrhage. Infants born before 26 weeks of gestation require ventilation for several weeks. Those who develop large periventricular haemorrhages with cerebral involvement have the worst outcome, with a mortality greater than 50% and neurological complications in about 25% of survivors.

The mortality is increased further in infants who have severe IUGR. Those who survive have an increased risk of poor postnatal growth and further neurological abnormalities. The overall outcome is dependent on the underlying cause for the prematurity and IUGR and is worst for infants with increasing prematurity and earlier onset of poor head and body growth in utero.

Self-assessment: questions

Multiple choice questions

1. The following statements are true:
   a. Perinatal mortality refers to neonatal deaths in the first 28 days of life
   b. Infection is the most important cause of neonatal mortality
   c. The incidence of prematurity has not changed for several decades
   d. Multiple pregnancies have decreased in recent years
   e. Maternal smoking is associated with increased risk of prematurity

2. During pregnancy:
   a. Low maternal α-fetoprotein indicates an increased risk of neural tube defects
   b. Polyhydramnios may be associated with fetal abnormalities
   c. Uncontrolled diabetes results in small-for-dates infants
   d. Maternal steroid therapy effectively reduces the severity of surfactant deficiency disease
   e. All mothers are screened for syphilis during pregnancy

3. With regard to the examination of the newborn after birth:
   a. Only newborn infants with a medical problem are routinely examined
   b. The femoral pulses are commonly not palpable in newborn infants
   c. A respiratory rate greater than 60 breaths per minutes is normal
   d. Petechiae on the face and neck suggest a clotting deficiency
   e. Bilateral limb oedema is a feature of Turner syndrome

4. With regard to congenital abnormalities:
   a. Down syndrome is the most common chromosomal disorder
   b. Sacral agenesis is associated with maternal alcohol ingestion
   c. Maternal infection is associated with congenital anomalies
   d. Trisomy 18 is usually fatal
   e. Infants with Pierre–Robin sequence may suffer respiratory difficulties

5. The following statements describe congenital dislocation of the hips (CDH):
   a. CDH is more common in boys
   b. Suspicion of dislocated hips is an indication for X-ray examination of the hips
   c. Breech deliveries are associated with an increased risk of dislocated hips
   d. Dislocated hips may be corrected by using double nappies
   e. Routine examination will successfully identify all infants with congenital dislocation of the hips

6. With regard to congenital abnormalities:
   a. Infants with cleft palate require immediate surgery to facilitate feeding
   b. The risk of recurrence in future pregnancies following birth of a child with congenital cleft palate is significant
   c. A subaponeurotic haemorrhage is of no significance
   d. Congenital malformations are usually isolated defects
   e. A single palmar (Simian) crease is always indicative of Down syndrome

7. Birth asphyxia in the newborn:
   a. Is an important cause of cerebral palsy
   b. Is diagnosed on the basis of the Apgar score
   c. Usually results from an underlying fetal abnormality
   d. Indicates a need for immediate intubation and mechanical ventilation
   e. May be associated with several seizure types

8. In congenital abnormalities of the upper gastrointestinal tract:
   a. Oesophageal atresia is usually diagnosed antenatally
   b. Oesophageal atresia may present with cyanosis soon after birth
   c. Diagnosis of oesophageal atresia may be confirmed by ultrasound examination after birth
   d. Oesophageal atresia is not usually associated with a fistula
   e. Jejunal atresia is characteristic of Down syndrome

9. In respiratory distress in the newborn:
   a. Pneumonia can be differentiated from surfactant deficiency by the appearance on chest X-ray film
   b. *Pneumococcus pneumoniae* is the most important cause of neonatal pneumonia
   c. Pneumonia can be prevented by maternal antibiotic therapy
   d. Pulmonary hypertension may occur following meconium aspiration
   e. Prompt aspiration of the airway at birth reduces the risk of significant meconium aspiration

10. In respiratory distress in the newborn:
    a. Meconium aspiration is more common in the small-for-dates infant

b. Surfactant deficiency disease is particularly severe in small-for-dates infants
c. The severity of surfactant deficiency disease is reduced by surfactant replacement
d. Ventilation by face mask increases the respiratory distress in those with diaphragmatic hernia
e. Transient tachypnoea of the newborn (TTN) results in respiratory distress that always resolves within 4 hours from birth

11. The following statements are true:
a. The correct management of an infant who has bile-stained vomiting but is otherwise well is to withhold feeds and observe
b. The likeliest diagnosis in an infant who develops bile-stained vomiting and bloody stools is necrotising enterocolitis (NEC)
c. The risk of NEC is greater with an indwelling umbilical arterial catheter
d. Gastroschisis is rarely associated with other abnormalities
e. The most serious problem in infants with renal agenesis after birth is respiratory failure

12. The following statements describe infections in the perinatal period:
a. Admission of a newborn infant to the special care baby unit is not a significant risk factor for infection
b. Infections in the newborn consistently present with fever
c. Treatment of infection in newborn infants should await the results of investigations
d. Congenital infections often have similar clinical features
e. Most childhood HIV infection occurs after birth

13. With regard to jaundice in the newborn period:
a. Jaundice is unusual in premature infants compared with those born at term
b. Neonatal jaundice should always be investigated
c. Physiological jaundice appears during the first 24 hours after birth
d. Jaundice is uncommon in breast fed infants
e. Conjugated hyperbilirubinaemia is always pathological

14. With regard to jaundice in the newborn period:
a. Pale stools in a jaundiced infant suggest haemolytic disease
b. Phototherapy effectively reduces jaundice by reducing the severity of haemolysis
c. Exchange transfusion is rarely used for the treatment of neonatal jaundice
d. Exchange transfusion is indicated for severe conjugated hyperbilirubinaemia
e. Preterm infants are at increased risk of kernicterus

Short notes

Write short notes on the following:

1. Temperature control in the premature infant
2. Hypoglycaemia in the newborn.

Viva voce question

You have been asked to review a newborn infant who is dysmorphic. Outline the key points in your management.

Self-assessment: answers

Multiple choice answers

1. a. **False**. The perinatal mortality rate refers to deaths after 24 weeks' gestation to the first 6 days of life per 1000 total births.
    b. **False**. Congenital malformation and prematurity account for more than 80% of neonatal deaths.
    c. **True**. The incidence of births before 37 completed weeks of gestation has been about 7% since the 1960s.
    d. **False**. The introduction of assisted conception techniques has resulted in a great increase in multiple pregnancies.
    e. **False**. Maternal smoking is associated with fetal growth retardation but not prematurity.

2. a. **False**. Raised maternal α-fetoprotein levels suggest a neural tube defect while low maternal α-fetoprotein may be associated with an increased risk of Down syndrome.
    b. **True**. Polyhydramnios may be associated with fetal intestinal obstruction or neuromuscular disease.
    c. **False**. Infants are usually large, above the 90th centile.
    d. **True**. Maternal steroid therapy during the 24 hours before delivery induces fetal lung maturation, and reduces the severity of surfactant deficiency disease, and the incidence and severity of intraventricular haemorrhage (IVH).
    e. **True**. It is routine to screen for rubella, hepatitis and syphilis at booking in the antenatal clinic; in some countries, but not in the UK, screening of the mother for toxoplasma is also performed.

3. a. **False**. It is normal practice for all newborn infants to be examined at least once after birth and before discharge from hospital.
    b. **False**. Femoral pulses should be palpable; absent femoral pulses indicate coarctation of the aorta.
    c. **False**. A newborn infant commonly has a respiratory rate of 30–50 breaths per minute; a rate of greater than 60 per minute suggests respiratory distress.
    d. **False**. Petechiae over the face and neck after birth are usually caused by birth trauma, particularly if the delivery was difficult, prolonged or by breech.
    e. **True**. A characteristic feature of Turner syndrome (XO).

4. a. **True**. Down syndrome occurs in about 1 in 700 children.
    b. **False**. Sacral agenesis characteristically occurs in infants of diabetic mothers, resulting in a patulous anus and urinary incontinence.
    c. **True**. Maternal infection with toxoplasmosis, cytomegalovirus, rubella, syphilis and other infection (TORCHS) can all result in fetal abnormalities.
    d. **True**. Infants with trisomy 18 (Edwards syndrome) characteristically have clenched fingers, low set ears, micrognathia and die soon after birth.
    e. **True**. The Pierre–Robin sequence includes cleft palate, micrognathia and posterior position of the tongue, which causes respiratory obstruction; nursing the infant in the prone position helps, but occasionally a nasopharyngeal airway or fixing of the tongue by suture may be required.

5. a. **False**. It is more common in girls.
    b. **False**. X-ray examination should not be performed during the first few months; ultrasound examination is preferred to exclude dislocated hips.
    c. **True**. A positive family history, breech delivery and postural abnormalities indicate an increased risk of CDH.
    d. **False**. Dislocated hips should be treated by splinting in abduction using a pelvic harness; double nappies are not effective.
    e. **False**. Despite routine examination, congenital dislocation of the hips can still be missed until later through poor examination technique and, in some cases, manifests some weeks after birth.

6. a. **False**. Most infants will feed successfully, though occasionally a dental plate may be used to assist with sucking; increasing the size of the opening of the teat or the use of special teats (e.g. Haberman teats) may also facilitate feeding. The lip is repaired at 0 to 3 months of age and the palate at about 8 months of age.
    b. **True**. The recurrence risk is about 2.5%.
    c. **False**. Cephalhaematoma is of no significance but a subaponeurotic haemorrhage, which is not limited by cranial sutures, can cause significant hypovolaemia.
    d. **False**. One defect should always prompt the search for others.
    e. **False**. Can be an isolated finding of no significance (provided the remainder of the examination is entirely normal).

7. a. **True**. Cerebral palsy (CP) is defined as a non-progressive disorder of motor function caused by antenatal or perinatal cerebral injury; 20% of cases of CP are caused by perinatal asphyxia.

b. **False**. The Apgar score is a convenient, simple way of describing an infant's condition at birth; the diagnosis of birth asphyxia is based on evidence of fetal distress, the presence of a metabolic acidosis and the condition of the infant at birth.

c. **False**. In most cases of birth asphyxia the fetus is normal; occasionally there is an underlying neuromuscular, metabolic or infectious disease.

d. **False**. Many asphyxiated infants will establish spontaneous respirations after stimulation; intubation is warranted when respiratory depression is associated with bradycardia.

e. **True**. These may take the form of tonic–clonic seizures, limb or facial twitching, subtle seizures (abnormal sucking movements and apnoeic spells).

8. a. **False**. Polyhydramnios and abnormal echogenicity on antenatal ultrasound scan should raise the suspicion of intestinal obstruction including oesophageal atresia.

b. **True**. If not recognised antenatally, oesophageal atresia causes respiratory difficulty and cyanosis, particularly after feeding.

c. **False**. The diagnosis is confirmed by passing a nasogastric tube and showing that the tube is held up in the oesophagus, as visualised with a chest X-ray.

d. **False**. In 85%, oesophageal atresia is associated with a fistula between the distal oesophagus and the trachea.

e. **False**. It is duodenal atresia.

9. a. **False**. Pneumonia and surfactant deficiency may have an identical appearance on a chest X-ray, i.e. a ground glass appearance and air bronchogram.

b. **False**. Group B streptococcal infection is the commonest cause of neonatal pneumonia.

c. **True**. Antibiotic treatment of the mother during labour effectively reduces the risk of congenital pneumonia.

d. **True**. Significant pulmonary hypertension often complicates severe meconium aspiration; treatment includes pulmonary vasodilators such as tolazoline or prostacyclin. Recently nitric oxide has been reported to be effective in this condition.

e. **True**. This is the single most important measure to reduce the severity of aspiration.

10. a. **True**. Infants who are small for gestational age are more likely to suffer intrapartum asphyxia and hence meconium aspiration.

b. **False**. Surfactant deficiency disease occurs in immature infants but is less likely to occur in small-for-gestational age infants because lung maturation is enhanced in this condition.

c. **True**. Exogenous intratracheal surfactant reduces the severity of surfactant deficiency disease, reducing the mortality of preterm infants in this condition by about 40%.

d. **True**. This forces air into the bowel lying within the chest and further compresses the underdeveloped lung(s).

e. **False**. TTN is caused by retained lung fluid; in many cases it will resolve within 4 hours, and certainly by 24 hours.

11. a. **False**. Bile-stained vomiting is the cardinal sign of intestinal obstruction and may be intermittent if the cause is malrotation and volvulus of the bowel. Therefore, all cases should be urgently investigated as a delay in diagnosis may result in vascular impairment and ischaemia of the bowel.

b. **True**. Bile-stained vomiting suggests bowel stasis caused by obstruction or ileus, and blood-stained stools are indicative of mucosal sloughing, both features of NEC.

c. **True**. Especially in neonates with cyanotic congenital heart disease, hypoxia, acidosis and sepsis.

d. **True**. Whereas exomphalos is commonly associated with chromosomal and other malformations, gastroschisis is usually an isolated defect and, therefore, has a better prognosis.

e. **True**. Renal agenesis results in no fetal urine production; the resulting oligohydramnios interferes with fetal breathing and causes pulmonary hypoplasia, which is usually fatal.

12. a. **False**. Admission to the special care baby unit significantly increases the risk for nosocomial infections.

b. **False**. Fever is unusual in neonates, even with infections. Hypothermia is more likely together with non-specific signs, including a change in behaviour, poor feeding, vomiting and apnoea.

c. **False**. Successful outcome following perinatal infections depends on prompt treatment, which should not be delayed until the results of the investigation are made available.

d. **True**. Congenital infections have common clinical features, such as a low birth weight, jaundice, hepatosplenomegaly, petechiae owing to thrombocytopenia, and cranial and ophthalmic complications.

e. **False**. Most children acquire HIV at the time of birth; treatment of the mother with zidovudine during the last trimester may prevent neonatal infection.

13. a. **False**. Jaundice occurs in more than half of newborn infants.

b. **False**. Most neonatal jaudice is mild;

investigation or treatment is indicated when jaundice appears during the first 24 hours, increases rapidly or persists for more than 10 days.

c. **False**. Jaundice in the first 24 hours is likely to be caused by haemolysis, especially related to blood group incompatibility; physiological jaundice commonly occurs at 48 to 72 hours of age and resolves by 7 to 10 days.

d. **False**. Breast fed infants are more likely to become jaundiced and this may persist for 2 to 3 weeks.

e. **True**. Conjugated hyperbilirubinaemia is always pathological and requires investigation.

14. a. **False**. Pale stools in a jaundiced baby are indicative of conjugated hyperbilirubinaemia resulting from hepatitis or biliary tract obstruction.

b. **False**. Phototherapy effectively converts unconjugated bilirubin to a non-toxic photoisomer; it does not affect the haemolytic process.

c. **True**. Most jaundiced infants do not require treatment; phototherapy is effective for moderate jaundice whereas exchange transfusion is indicated in severe haemolytic disease and in sick preterm infants.

d. **False**. Conjugated bilirubin is not neurotoxic and is not an indication for exchange transfusion.

e. **True**. Preterm infants, particularly if acidotic or hypoxic, are especially susceptible to bilirubin encephalopathy, commonly called kernicterus.

Short notes answers

1. Smaller infants have less subcutaneous insulation, greater relative surface area and a greater problem with heat loss. A cold infant is more likely to develop:

- poor peripheral perfusion and a metabolic acidosis
- increased respiratory distress and hypoxia
- surfactant deficiency disease through insufficient surfactant
- hypoglycaemia
- excess utilisation of calories and weight loss.

Hence, rigorous measures must be taken to prevent heat loss. All newborns, and especially premature babies, should be placed in a (pre) warm environment immediately after birth. They should be dried using warm towels and wrapped in a second, warm dry towel to avoid unnecessary exposure. They should not be placed on cold, wet surfaces nor exposed to a draught. Premature and low-birth-weight infants should be transferred to a prewarmed incubator with warmed, humidified air/oxygen. Very-low-birth-weight infants will require an overhead heater and/or space blankets. Those with exposed mucosae/organs (e.g. gastroschisis, exomphalos, ectopia vesicae) must be wrapped in clean, plastic film. All infusion products should be prewarmed. Finally, the ambient temperature of the neonatal unit must be higher than normal at all times.

2. Hypoglycaemia in the newborn is defined as a blood glucose of <1.7 mmol/l in the term infant and <1.1 mmol/l in preterms in the first week of life. It is caused by:

- exhaustive utilisation of glycogen stores
- hyperinsulinism
- other diseases.

Depleted stores of glycogen can occur in:

- small-for-dates and premature infants
- birth asphyxia, acidosis
- hypothermia
- 'stress': septicaemia, cardiac failure or arrest, meconium aspiration, necrotising enterocolitis, intraventricular haemorrhage
- underfeeding, starvation.

Hyperinsulinism is seen in:

- infants of diabetic mothers
- haemolytic disease of newborn (HDN).

There are also a number of other diseases that cause hypoglycaemia:

- hypothyroidism
- Beckwith–Wiedemann syndrome
- glycogen storage disease
- galactosaemia
- tyrosinaemia
- aminoacidopathies.

Symptoms. Newborns revert to metabolism of proteins (gluconeogenesis) and, later, fatty acids as a source of energy and may, therefore, be asymptomatic but hypoglycaemic for 1–3 hours. Symptoms and signs include increased jitteriness, convulsions and apnoeic spells, pallor, tachy- or bradycardia, hypotension, respiratory distress and increased lethargy.

Prevention. Blood glucose 'stix' should be performed routinely and at frequent intervals in all at-risk infants before they become symptomatic. If levels are low, the result must be confirmed by estimation of blood glucose in a laboratory. At-risk infants such as those born to diabetic mothers, small-for-dates and very-low-birth weight infants should be fed every 2–4 hours.

Treatment. Asymptomatic infants should be given the next full strength feed, preferably by the oral or nasogastric route. The glucose 'stix' should be checked 1 hour later and normal feeds continued if the glucose has returned to normal. If glucose is still low, oral feeds have not been established or the baby is symptomatic, then a single dose of 0.5 g/kg 10% dextrose should be given intravenously followed by a dextrose infusion at 60 ml/kg per day. Rarely, 15–20% dextrose and glucagon is required.

Viva voce answer

You should introduce yourself to the mother, explaining that you have come to examine her child. Proceed to perform a thorough examination, taking extra care in the assessment of the three 'Hs' – the head, hands and heart – where dysmorphic features are most likely to be noted. Note the shape of the head and measure the head circumference; note the size of the fontanelles; the hairline; shape, size and position of the eyes, nose, mouth and ears; the presence of a protruding tongue, epicanthic folds and Brushfield spots; and feel for a cleft palate. Examine the iris and retina with the ophthalmoscope to exclude colobomata. Note the length of the neck and redundant tissue at the nape. Document the shape, position (and number) of all four limbs and digits. Assess the baby's cry, suck and feeding, general tone and posture, while noting any abnormal movements. Look for abnormally shaped or positioned nipples, an abnormal chest and abdomen and the presence of umbilical/inguinal herniae. Examine the external genitalia for ambiguity, hypospadias and undescended testes. Assess for signs of congenital heart disease including the absence of femoral pulses. Weigh the infant unclothed and plot on the appropriate centile chart (see Fig. 5 and Table 8).

Re-clothe and resettle the baby before sitting down to talk to the parents. Explain your preliminary findings at this point, your concerns (if any) and the reasons why you feel further assessment/investigation is required. You should explain the rationale behind any tests that you may propose. Proceed to investigate as indicated by the signs on examination, but a cranial ultrasound scan, an echocardiogram, renal ultrasound and karyotype are generally essential in those with major dysmorphic features. An appropriate length of time should be spent with the family to discuss the results, and a sympathetic but realistic view of the prognosis/likelihood of future problems given. Repeated discussions with the family, organisation of genetic counselling and support groups are paramount.

The respiratory system

Key points

You should have an understanding of:

- The normal anatomy and physiology of the respiratory system together with an elementary knowledge of the pathophysiology of the major respiratory disorders
- How to perform an accurate examination of the respiratory system with the appropriate interpretation of the clinical signs
- The accurate interpretation of a chest radiograph
- The important features of both upper and lower respiratory tract infections
- The prevention and treatment of acute and chronic asthma
- The multisystem nature of cystic fibrosis and the principles of its management.

3.1 Introduction

Acute respiratory tract infections and asthma form a major part of paediatric practice. Because of the frequency of respiratory illnesses in children, problems related to this system are common in medical examinations at all levels. An understanding of basic respiratory physiology helps in the correct interpretation of symptoms and physical signs and in the attainment of an age-appropriate differential diagnosis.

3.2 Anatomy, physiology and radiology

Normal anatomy

The nasal passages, pharynx and ears are examined as part of the respiratory tract. The trachea is supported by a series of incomplete cartilage hoops and divides into two bronchi. The right main bronchus is more vertical than the left and it, therefore, offers an easier passage for aspirated foreign bodies. The right lung has three lobes (upper, middle and lower) separated by the horizontal and oblique fissures, respectively. The left lung has two major lobes (upper and lower) separated by an oblique fissure, though the upper lobe is itself divided into upper and lingular lobes. Both lungs project low down behind the dome of the diaphragm and peak behind the clavicles.

Normal physiology

The extrathoracic components of the respiratory tree tend to collapse inwards during inspiration and open during expiration. Therefore, if the extrathoracic airway

is compromised, the obstruction is first evident during inspiration and, as the airway narrows further, obstruction occurs during both phases of breathing (bi-directional).

The intrathoracic airways are actively opened during inspiration by the action of the respiratory muscles. In addition, surfactant reduces the surface tension of the alveoli, thereby reducing the effort necessary to keep the alveoli open during inspiration. During expiration, the airways tend to collapse owing to the natural elasticity or compliance of the lung. Therefore, partial obstruction to the intrathoracic airways causes earlier closure of the airways during expiration and results in 'air-trapping' with eventual overinflation of the lung.

Radiology

In children most chest X-rays are performed in the antero-posterior (AP) position rather than PA views as performed in adults. Figure 13 shows the normal radiological landmarks. It is important to ensure that the film is not rotated (i.e. the ends of the clavicles are equidistant from the midline) and that the course of the trachea is not deviated. The right hemidiaphragm is usually positioned slightly higher than the left. A marked difference in height suggests volume loss on that side, usually caused by lobar collapse. 'Flattened' hemidiaphragms suggest hyperinflation of the lungs. Unilateral hyperinflation associated with increased radiolucency ('blackness of the lung') suggests air trapping and is most commonly seen with ipsilateral foreign bodies.

Parenchymal lung disease in the lower lobes causes loss of definition of the ipsilateral hemidiaphragm. Right middle lobe or left lingular disease causes loss of definition of the right and left cardiac borders, respectively.

The thymus may drape itself over either side of the cardiac contour and, as there is a sharp cut-off at the lower border, may produce a 'sail sign' on the right side. It may also mimic consolidation of the lung.

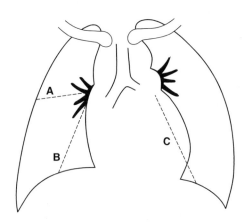

Fig. 13 Normal radiographic landmarks. The right bronchus is wider and more vertical, the right hilum is lower and the right hemidiaphragm is higher. A, right horizontal fissure; B, right oblique fissure; C, left oblique fissure.

3.3 Clinical assessment

Symptoms and signs

Unlike adults, children rarely complain about chest pain or dyspnoea. The respiratory symptoms and signs most commonly encountered result from the local effects of the underlying condition:

- cough
- stridor
- wheeze.

Generalised effects of respiratory disorders may also be seen, for example:

- failure to thrive
- short stature
- poor exercise tolerance
- daytime somnolence.

Cough

The aetiology of a cough may be diagnosed by considering its nature, diurnal variation, chronicity and associated signs (Box 8). An acute onset of a cough is usually associated with an upper respiratory tract infection, although inhalation of a foreign body is a possibility. A predominantly nocturnal chronic cough is characteristic of asthma, as is exercise- or laughter-induced coughing. Coughing associated with feeding in babies may indicate recurrent aspiration of milk or gastro-oesophageal reflux. Small children may have a productive cough but sputum is usually swallowed. Productive coughs are encountered in lower respiratory tract infections or disorders resulting from chronic inflammation. Blood-stained productive coughing is a feature of bronchiectasis. Certain infections may cause characteristic coughing episodes, typified by the paroxysms of coughing seen in whooping cough (pertussis).

BOX 8
Causes of cough

Acute	Chronic
Upper respiratory tract infection	Asthma
	Postnasal drip
Bronchiolitis	Gastro-oesophageal reflux
Pneumonia	aspiration
Foreign body	Cystic fibrosis

Stridor

Stridor is an alteration in the breathing quality of the child. Many parents describe it as 'noisy breathing' or 'a frightening sound' when their child cannot catch their breath. Stridor implies obstruction to the extrathoracic airway and usually involves the upper airways. It is usually more pronounced on inspiration when the airways tend to narrow as a part of normal physiology. The intensity of the stridor does not indicate the degree of severity though severe narrowing will cause stridor during both inspiration and expiration. Indeed, stridor may be soft, as in acute bacterial epiglottitis; it is coarse and loud in acute viral laryngotracheobronchitis (croup). It may be present at birth as a result of a structural anomaly or vocal cord palsy or may develop soon after, as in congenital laryngeal stridor (congenital laryngomalacia). In this condition, stridor increases with increased activity, crying and when lying in the supine position. Initially the soft cartilage of the larynx collapses especially during inspiration, but the stridor resolves as the cartilage calcifies as the infant grows.

Wheeze

Wheeze is a breath sound that is usually produced by air passing through partially fluid-filled narrowed intrathoracic airways. It is often audible to parents, who think their child is 'chesty'. It is present when the airways, especially the bronchioles, are narrowed as a result of infection, inflammation or reversible airways constriction. Wheezing in asthma is classically expiratory.

Other symptoms

Children with a respiratory problem may also present with symptoms related to chronic respiratory insufficiency including poor growth, short stature, delayed puberty, difficulty in sleeping owing to nocturnal cough, and daytime sleepiness. Chest pain is usually pleuritic in nature and is, therefore, worse on deep inspiration.

Respiratory examination

The examination should begin with an assessment of the child's general health and growth and should always include plotting their growth parameters on an appropriate centile chart. Many chronic respiratory disorders will slow growth and physical development. As with all paediatric examinations, the maximum amount of information is derived from observing the child. Observation of the child will identify whether the child is distressed at rest, propped forward to aid the use of accessory muscles, craning the neck to straighten it as a reflex effort to overcome obstruction, or dribbling because of dysphagia associated with serious upper airways obstruction (e.g. epiglottitis).

Cyanosis

Inspect the lips and the tongue for central cyanosis. This arises when the percentage of desaturated haemoglobin increases, and may be caused by acute or chronic respiratory failure and intrapulmonary shunting of desaturated blood through underaerated parts of the lung (ventilation–perfusion mismatch). In chronic respiratory failure, the child may become polycythaemic, manifest as a plethoric appearance, because of the increased circulating erythrocyte mass and haemoglobin concentration.

Clubbing

Nail clubbing results from cardiac, gastrointestinal and respiratory causes. The last include **cystic fibrosis**, **bronchiectasis** and other suppurative lung disorders such as an **empyema**. **Fibrosing alveolitis** is a rare paediatric cause.

Chest wall

The chest wall must be inspected from both the front and lateral aspects. The overall shape is noted including the presence of scars. From the lateral aspect, it is possible to assess whether there has been chronic hyperinflation causing a 'barrel chest' appearance as seen in chronic asthma. Harrison's sulcus is a depression along the length of the 9th ribs bilaterally that develops through the exaggerated action of the diaphragm during respiration. It is an acquired abnormality indicative of long-standing chronic respiratory insufficiency. Developmental anomalies of the chest such as pectus excavatum (depressed sternum) or pectus carinatum (pigeon chest) may also be noted.

Work of respiration

The work of respiration is an important subjective observation. Difficulty in breathing will usually cause tachypnoea and tachycardia. In young children, a respiratory rate of more than 40 breaths per minute is predictive of a lower respiratory tract infection. Chest wall recession (suprasternal, sternal, intercostal and subcostal) indicates increased work of breathing. Recession may be marked in situations of severe respiratory compromise except where there is coexisting lung hyperinflation, when this important clinical sign may be 'masked'. Increased work of respiration in the young infant may manifest as 'grunting', a reflex forced expiratory sound, and nasal flaring. In the older child, the use of accessory muscles including the sternomastoid may be noted. Speech may be difficult if the work of respiration is increased acutely. The equivalent in infants is difficulty in feeding.

Pulse

Changes in both the rate and nature of the pulse are important signs of respiratory distress. Bounding pulses may indicate carbon dioxide retention, whereas significant airways obstruction may be accompanied by pulsus paradoxus. The latter is an exaggerated version of the normal diminution of pulse volume on inspiration. While this may be measured as a reduction in the systolic blood pressure of more than 10 mmHg on inspiration, clinically it is often suspected purely by the examination of the radial pulse.

Palpation and percussion

Expansion of zones of the lungs is assessed by palpation. Palpable wheezing may be felt at the same time. Percussion is difficult to elicit in the infant or small child. However, dullness to percussion may indicate a lobar collapse, consolidation or pleural effusion.

Auscultation

Auscultation may be misleading in small children. Severe lung disease may not be accompanied by an abnormal examination on auscultation. The proximity of the main bronchi may mislead the unwary to diagnose bronchial breathing where none is present, or to confuse transmitted sounds from the upper airways with those emanating from lower airways. Wheezing is generally easy to identify, whereas both inspiratory and expiratory crepitations may be heard in many lung disorders. None are pathognomonic in relation to the aetiology of the lung disease. Routine application of whispering pectriloquoy is unhelpful in the majority of patients.

Upper airways

The ears, nose and pharynx should be examined (except if severe upper airways obstruction is suspected). Nasal inflammation with mucus production may accompany respiratory tract disease, particularly infection or asthma.

Abdominal palpation

Hepatomegaly may accompany lung disease. This may indicate heart failure in the infant with pulmonary oedema and, more commonly, follows downward displacement of the liver resulting from lung hyperexpansion. This is often encountered in infants with acute bronchiolitis.

Peak flow measurements

Peak flow measurements are only reliable in the acute situation if the child has been used to performing them prior to the acute illness (Fig. 14). Children below the age of 5 years rarely perform peak flow measurements effectively so the technique must be carefully monitored if the results are to be believed.

Oximetry

Oximetry is a valuable measurement of oxygenation. It does not record hypercarbia or hyperoxia and is sub-

a

b

Disposable mouthpiece

Disposable mouthpiece

Fig. 14 Peak flow meters. (a) Young children (5–7 years). (b) Children aged 7 years and over.

ject to movement artefact. Oxygenation is measured at skin or mucosal level and erroneously low readings may be obtained when the peripheral perfusion is poor.

Assessment of regular medication

In children receiving regular medication, it is vital to check the type, dose and nature of the medication and method of administration before altering management. Many medications, particularly anti-asthma medication, are given incorrectly or suboptimally.

3.4 Infections

Respiratory tract infections are very common and are responsible for a significant morbidity in all paediatric age groups. The majority of cases have a viral aetiology, presenting and being treated in primary care.

Upper respiratory tract infections

The nose and pharynx are the most common sites of infection. The classic triad of symptoms includes **fever**, **rhinorrhoea** and a **painful throat**. Many viruses are implicated and include rhinoviruses, influenzae viruses and coxsackieviruses. Antibiotics are of no benefit and therapy should be directed at ensuring an adequate fluid intake, appropriate analgesia and antipyretic measures to reduce the possibility of febrile convulsions. Common sequelae include secondary bacterial infection and spread of infection via the short eustachian tube to the middle ear, causing otitis media.

Otitis media

Otitis media is common in the preschool child. Many cases are viral although bacterial agents including *Streptococcus* and *Haemophilus* species occur. The child is usually systemically unwell with a pronounced fever. Clinical signs include a bulging reddened tympanic membrane, which may perforate releasing pus. Auroscopic examination is particularly uncomfortable. Many cases will resolve spontaneously although antibiotics are usually prescribed. This practice may have reduced previously common complications such as mastoiditis and meningitis.

Tonsillopharyngitis

Tonsillopharyngitis is accompanied by pharyngeal erythema and purulent discharge from the tonsils. *Streptococcus pyogenes* and viruses are the usual cause. Early use of penicillin has been partly responsible for the reduction in the incidence of rheumatic fever and poststreptococcal glomerulonephritis. Recurrent tonsillitis is an indication for tonsillectomy. Occasionally this clinical problem may indicate an immunodeficient state, particularly with immunoglobulin A deficiency.

Laryngotracheobronchitis (croup)

Laryngotracheobronchitis is a viral infection involving parainfluenzae, rhinoviruses and respiratory syncytial viruses (RSV). A prodromal period occurs prior to the onset of a harsh barking cough and coarse stridor. The child may become tired and irritable but is not usually systemically unwell. Although usually self-limiting, severe attacks especially in children with underlying laryngeal narrowing may result in severe obstruction requiring intubation to maintain a patent airway. The clinical course often fluctuates, with nocturnal exacerbations of stridor and cough. Croup can be frighteningly unpredictable and the assessment of severity and need for hospital admission should be based on several factors including:

- age of the patient (young infants have narrower airways)
- underlying predisposing pathology
- severity of stridor
- degree of fatigue of the child
- effort of breathing and signs of respiratory distress
- ability of parents to seek urgent medical help (is a telephone available?)
- certainty of diagnosis – exclusion of epiglottitis/tracheitis/foreign body.

Although the majority of patients will improve spontaneously, simple therapies such as humidity or inhaled steroids have been advocated.

Epiglottitis

Epiglottitis, an acute bacterial infection usually with *Haemophilus influenzae* type b, is now rare as a result of Hib vaccination. Although superficially resembling severe croup, epiglottitis presents suddenly with high fever, absence of a prodrome, soft stridor and often dysphagia. The child appears toxic, is most comfortable sitting upright with an extended neck, is often drooling and has signs of respiratory distress including a soft stridor, tachypnoea and marked suprasternal recession. There is a serious risk of total upper airway obstruction if the child becomes upset following examination of the airway. Treatment centres on the maintenance of an adequate airway. Oxygen and nebulised adrenaline by face mask with the child sitting on a parent's lap in quiet surroundings not far from resuscitation equipment is ideal. This usually allows enough time for the most experienced physician with skills in paediatric intubation to arrive and perform tracheal intubation, preferably under controlled conditions in theatre. Intensive supportive care is generally required for about 2–4 days before the epiglottic swelling subsides sufficiently for extubation to be attempted. Intravenous antibiotics, particularly third-generation cephalosporins, have largely superseded the use of chloramphenicol in this condition.

Lower respiratory tract infections

Bronchiolitis

Bronchiolitis is usually caused by RSV although, occasionally, other viral agents may be responsible. It is common during winter months and largely affects those infants below the age of 1 year. Children with predisposing cardiorespiratory abnormalities such as chronic lung disease and cystic fibrosis are more severely affected. The diagnosis is made on clinical grounds, though RSV can be identified within a few hours by rapid immunofluorescence on a specimen of nasopharyngeal aspirate (NPA).

Clinical features
Infants may present with apnoea, though the majority also have mild fever, a dry staccato 'spluttering' cough, marked tachypnoea, recession and intermittent cyanosis. Widespread inspiratory crepitations and occasional wheezes may be heard. Feeds are often refused and dehydration may ensue. Partial bronchiolar obstruction causes hyperinflation, which, in turn, may depress the liver resulting in apparent hepatomegaly.

Chest radiograph
Bilateral hyperinflation with variable, patchy areas of atelectasis is seen.

Management
Management involves general supportive care including oxygen and adequate hydration, often necessitating intravenous fluids. Antibiotics are of no benefit unless a secondary bacterial infection develops. Some infants may need mechanical ventilation. Adjunctive therapies, including inhaled steroids, β_2-adrenoceptor agonists and the guanosine analogue antiviral agent ribavirin have not consistently been shown to improve the outcome. Following bronchiolitis, some infants develop increased bronchial sensitivity and develop recurrent wheezing during other intercurrent infections and on contact with aeroallergens.

Pertussis

Pertussis is a notifiable bacterial infection caused by *Bordetella pertussis* and appears in epidemics. The natural history is biphasic: an early coryzal phase with rhinorrhoea and cough lasts 7–10 days and is followed by the spasmodic phase, which may last for up to 3 months ('100 day cough'). Most cases are diagnosed during this second phase. Paroxysms of coughing typically involve repeated expiratory coughs followed by a inspiratory 'gasping whoop'. The latter may be absent, particularly in small children. The paroxysms may be associated with marked facial suffusion, vomiting, apnoea in infants and syncope owing to hypoxia. The disease is probably mediated by the host's inflammatory response.

Clinical features
Typical coughing spasms are associated with signs of hypoxia, an associated bronchopneumonia or lung collapse. Subconjunctival haemorrhages or peri-orbital petechiae/bruising are evident in those with protracted, severe bouts of coughing.

Chest radiograph
Perihilar bronchial wall thickening together with areas

of segmental collapse and coexisting hyperinflation are common.

Treatment

General supportive care is vital and should include oxygen during a spasm. The severity and frequency of both the spasm and apnoeic episodes may be reduced using inhaled steroids. Erythromycin has been traditionally prescribed to reduce the length of infectivity although it does not alter the course of the disease.

Prophylaxis. A vaccine is routinely available (p. 181).

Pneumonia

Pneumonia may be caused by viral, bacterial and atypical organisms. RSV may be one of the most common viral aetiological agents in infants, whereas bacterial causes include streptococci, staphylococci and *Haemophilus* species. *Mycoplasma* species are common particularly in the older child. In addition to these common infecting organisms, immunocompromised children may develop pneumonia with other rare, 'atypical' agents.

Clinical features

The respiratory rate is almost always increased. Coughing may not be a feature until later in the illness, when it may become troublesome and productive. Many children swallow their sputum rather than expectorate. Fever is usual while cyanosis is seen in those with extensive pulmonary disease and when ventilation–perfusion mismatch arises. Other signs of respiratory distress or respiratory failure may be associated with extensive consolidation or collapse. It must be emphasised that these clinical signs may be *absent* and normal auscultation does not exclude the diagnosis. Atypical infections may result in minimal signs but the child may be hypoxic with marked radiological abnormalities out of proportion to the apparent degree of illness.

Consolidation is characteristic of pneumonia and may be difficult to differentiate from collapse. Radiographic features of consolidation and collapse are described in Table 14 and Figure 15 and the signs in Table 15.

Pathophysiology

With consolidation, the lung parenchyma is filled with inflammatory exudate. This allows sound to travel more efficiently, hence bronchial breathing and increased tactile vocal fremitus (TVF) and whispering pectriloquoy (WP) develop. Resolution of this appearance ensues with liquefaction and production of sputum. This results in crepitations within the alveoli and small airways. Collapse results from complete obstruction of the airway, with resorption of the air distal to the obstruction. This impedes the passage of sound, thus explaining the above clinical findings. There is subsequent loss of volume in that lung.

Chest radiograph

Increased shadowing occurs either in a widespread pattern (bronchopneumonia) or in an anatomical pattern (lobar pneumonia). Consolidation affecting lower lobes impinges and partially obscures the hemidiaphragm. Middle and lingular lobe disease will partially obscure the heart border. Often a bronchogram is seen, indicating a patent bronchus overlying solid lung tissue. Increased radiographic opacification associated with

Table 14 Radiographic features of consolidation and collapse

	Consolidation	**Collapse**
Lobar opacification	Increased	Dense but contracted
Horizontal fissure	Horizontal	Shifted upwards
Bronchogram	May be visible	None
Lung volume	No loss	Loss
Mediastinal/structural shift	None	To affected side

a

b

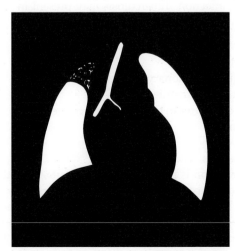

Fig. 15 Radiographic features of pneumonic consolidation and collapse. (a) Consolidation with increased opacification and no loss in lung volume. (b) Increased opacification in collapse is associated with ipsilateral deviation of the trachea and upward shift of the horizontal fissure.

Table 15 Signs of consolidation and collapse

	Consolidation	Collapse
Lung/chest expansion	Reduced lung expansion (ipsilateral)	Reduced chest movement (ipsilateral)
Trachea	Central/no mediastinal shift	Deviated to affected side
Percussion note	Dull	Dull
Tactile vocal fremitus	Increased	Absent
Whispering pectriloquoy	Increased	Absent
Bronchial breathing	Ipsilateral	May or may not be present
Breath sounds	Inspiratory crepitations	Reduced breath sounds

collapse is not accompanied by a bronchogram but loss of lung volume. Pulmonary cysts (**pneumatoceles**) are seen in staphylococcal pneumonia. All pneumonias can cavitate and produce **lung abscesses**. Similarly, pneumonia may stimulate the production of pleural effusions, which may occasionally become infected producing a pus-filled **empyema**. Chronic lower respiratory tract infection following pneumonia or pertussis may result in dilated pus-filled bronchi termed **bronchiectasis**. This complication is more common in those with underlying problems, e.g. immunodeficiency.

Treatment
Supportive care with oxygen therapy to avoid hypoxia and adequate but not excessive hydration is important. Antibiotics may include amoxycillin, cephalosporins and macrolides such as erythromycin; whenever possible, antibiotic therapy should be adjusted according to the results of sputum cultures.

Tuberculosis

Tuberculosis (TB), caused by the acid-fast bacillus *Mycobacterium tuberculosis*, is a relatively uncommon infection in children in the UK but remains a potential and increasing problem in some areas and in at-risk groups. These include Asian immigrant families, lower socio-economic groups and those with immunodeficiencies, particularly cell-mediated immunodeficiency and HIV infection. Tuberculosis may present in one of several ways:

- incidental finding in asymptomatic child
- on screening
- symptomatic pulmonary tuberculosis
- extrapulmonary manifestations
- rarely at birth after in utero transfer (congenital tuberculosis).

Clinical features
Airborne infection is the most common route, with the infective focus becoming established in the periphery of the lung. This focus, also called the **Ghon focus**, then usually involves the regional lymphatics and nodes to form the primary complex. Most patients with TB remain asymptomatic. Others develop fever, lethargy and weight loss. Post-primary spread may occur with rupture of the focus into the airways, causing cough

with productive sputum that is infectious. Failure to produce a primary complex, with rapid spread throughout the lung produces **miliary** TB. Rarely, rupture of the focus into the airways precipitates tuberculous bronchopneumonia. Regional lymphadenopathy may obstruct a bronchus, resulting in a distal bacterial lobar pneumonia that fails to resolve on conventional antibiotics.

Chest radiograph
Evidence of a primary complex may be noted based on a calcified peripheral lesion together with hilar lymphadenopathy. Miliary tuberculosis results in a classical widespread reticulonodular appearance.

Extrapulmonary manifestations
Haematogenous spread is rare. While this is usually rapid, it may occur months after the primary infection. Spread to the central nervous system causes meningitis that, though insidious in onset, is accompanied by a significant mortality and neurological morbidity. Spread to the bones, joints and kidneys is more common than to the peritoneum, tonsils and eyes.

Treatment
Treatment remains controversial but most regimens for pulmonary TB suggest combination therapy including rifampicin, isoniazid and pyrazinamide for 2 months with the two former agents continued for a further 4 months. Alternative regimens are used for extrapulmonary disease.

Screening
Screening using sensitivity to tuberculoprotein is the basis of the Mantoux and Heaf tests. Infection will manifest as a reaction to the protein. A false-negative result may occur if the test is performed very early in the infection or in the presence of a defective immune system. Concurrent steroid therapy will reduce the response. A chest X-ray is necessary in those with a positive response who have not been previously vaccinated.

Pneumocystis carinii *pneumonitis*

Pneumocystis carinii pneumonitis affects those who are immunodeficient through either disease or therapy. Currently, it is the presenting feature of HIV infection in

15–30% of infants. This organism proliferates in the alveoli causing a pneumonitis. Cough with worsening respiratory distress and hypoxia is the main clinical feature, while spreading perihilar infiltrates the radiological hallmark. High-dose cotrimoxazole is used in the acute infection. Lower doses are used as chemoprophylaxis in children at risk, i.e. those receiving immunocytotoxic therapy for acute leukaemia. Pentamidine is used for those who do not respond to cotrimoxazole.

3.5 Asthma

Epidemiology

While the diagnostic category of 'asthma' has broadened and the overall prevalence increased, the actual incidence does seem to be increasing. Asthma is twice as common in boys as in girls and shows geographical and socio-economic variations. However, there is little difference between urban and rural populations. There are several potential precipitating factors, including a genetic predisposition, maternal smoking during pregnancy, parental smoking during infancy, indoor aeroallergens (e.g. cat fur and house dust mite) and viral infections, especially with RSV. Environmental pollutants may precipitate asthmatic episodes but do not seem to be causally linked to the development of childhood asthma.

Pathophysiology

The pathophysiology of asthma is complex. Inflammatory cells including eosinophils are present in the airway lining. These, together with mast cells, are instrumental in producing bronchial hyper-responsiveness to various allergens. They secrete various cytokines such as leukotrienes, which propagate chronic inflammation of the airways associated with hypersecretion of mucus and oedema. Therefore, the asthmatic child has oedematous airways that readily bronchoconstrict to various stimuli.

Acute asthma

Acute asthma is potentially life threatening. Precipitants include allergens and infections. Usually there is a rapid worsening of respiratory function associated with coughing and dyspnoea. Tachypnoea is common and wheezing usually indicates bronchospasm. Clinically, there is a reduction in peak flow caused by airway obstruction and hyperinflation of the lungs. A marked increase in the work of breathing is associated with hypoxia and, eventually, respiratory failure with hypercarbia is established.

Severe life-threatening asthma attacks

Features suggestive of severe life-threatening asthma in children include:

- inability to speak or drink
- cyanosis (hypoxia confirmed by oximetry)
- drowsiness, bounding pulses, tremor/'flap', irritability (caused by hypercarbia)
- palpable pulsus paradoxus
- 'silent chest', indicating insufficient air entry to allow identifiable breath sounds
- inability to produce recordable peak flow (PF) record or PF <33% of usual.

Many attacks may be aborted by appropriate therapy instituted at home using prearranged treatment plans. All acute attacks must be considered as potentially serious with prompt treatment a priority.

Treatment
Treatment comprises:

- reassurance and oxygen therapy
- inhaled β_2-adrenergic agonist therapy by nebuliser, e.g. salbutamol
- commencing oral steroids.

If the child fails to improve:

- inhaled ipratropium (abolishes vagal tone, allowing further bronchodilation)
- repeated inhaled β_2 agonist therapy by nebuliser, e.g. salbutamol
- intravenous hydrocortisone
- intravenous bronchodilators, e.g. aminophylline or salbutamol
- intensive care with respiratory support.

Children suffering acute asthma must be regularly reassessed and monitored to avoid complications such as:

- infection
- pneumothorax
- electrolyte disturbances, including hypokalaemia secondary to bronchodilator therapy.

Chronic asthma

The spectrum of childhood asthma is wide. Some infants cough or are intermittently wheezy only in response to viral illnesses. These children are believed to demonstrate airway hyper-responsiveness. Other have more chronic symptoms. The most common is nocturnal coughing or recurrent wheeze in association with exercise or allergen exposure. Features of note when considering chronic asthma include:

- frequency of acute episodes
- frequency of symptoms such as nocturnal cough
- frequency of use of 'rescue' therapy, e.g. salbutamol
- number of days of missed schooling
- exercise limitation, e.g. inability to compete in sport at school
- slow growth as a result of undercontrolled asthma and/or steroid excess

- presence of chest deformity
- pattern of peak flow measurements, e.g. reduction in early morning values.

Chronic asthma is punctuated with acute episodes. Therapy with β_2-adrenergic agonists remains the mainstay rescue therapy for episodes of wheeze or cough associated with infection, exercise or allergy. However, the frequency of acute attacks may be reduced, together with chronic symptoms, using prophylactic therapy. These are targeted at the underlying airway inflammation rather than just bronchospasm. Several types of prophylactic agent are available, but the most commonly used are inhaled steroids (e.g. budesonide and beclamethasone). Others include sodium cromoglycate, theophyllines and long-acting β_2-adrenergic agonists (e.g. salmeterol). As preventative therapy, these drugs are necessary on a regular basis. In addition, many authorities advocate a reduction in allergen exposure, particularly exposure to the house dust mite, a frequent problem in many asthmatic and non-asthmatic patients. Avoidance of other allergens may be advisable.

In those with allergic disease, upper airway (nasal) inflammation may coexist. This may necessitate the use of topical anti-inflammatory drugs acting on the nasal mucosa, including nasal steroids.

Asthma treatment

Drugs

The variety of potential medications and their delivery systems may appear confusing (Table 16). Indeed failure to improve clinically may not indicate worsening disease or poor compliance but inappropriately delivered treatment. This is particularly common in relation to the types of inhaled therapy.

Most children will be adequately controlled on intermittent bronchodilators either alone or in combination with a prophylactic drug, usually an inhaled steroid. Long-term oral steroids are avoided because of their unwanted side-effects on linear growth.

Table 16 Drugs used in the treatment of asthma

Indications	Drug	Side-effects
Acute bronchospasm	Salbutamol	Tachycardia, agitation
	Terbutaline	Tremor
	Salmeterol	Tachycardia agitation
Prophylaxis Inhaled	Budesonide	Dysphonia
	Beclomethasone	Oral candidosis, adrenal suppression, growth impairment(?)
Inhaled (exercise induced asthma)	Sodium cromoglycate	Very few side-effects
Oral	Theophylline	Risk of toxicity, arrhythmias, affects education, increased sleeping

Delivery devices

The variety of delivery systems is wide. Rescue therapy is usually inhaled. Oral preparations of salbutamol have been largely replaced by the inhaled version for reasons of efficacy and reduced side-effects. However, the oral preparations are often easier to administer to infants. There are four major types of inhaler device. (Fig. 16).

Nebuliser. This is a powered, often portable, pump that delivers a large dose of drug via a face mask.

Large volume spacer. This commonly uses a plastic 'bubble' with a valve that allows slowing of aerosol particles. The particles are inhaled once the child takes an inspiratory breath sufficient to open the valve. The spacer is used with a metered dose inhaler and either a face mask or mouth piece. Multiple doses may be administered.

Metered dose inhaler ('puffer'). This device produces an aerosolised drug and requires a gas propellant. They are difficult to use as actuation and inhalation needs coordination and manual dexterity. The speed of particle release is too rapid for inhalation in most children. Autohalers are metered dose inhalers that are actuated on inspiration in an attempt to aid inhalation and improve drug delivery to the lower airway.

Dry powder devices. These devices (e.g. turbohaler, diskhaler and rotahaler) deliver free drug in the form of a powder that is inhaled and not aerosolised. They allow inhalation at lower inspiratory flow rates. Although the need for coordinated activation and inhalation is less they still require a substantial degree of manual dexterity.

Device use

As a rough guide, the following devices are best used at the following ages:

- Nebuliser: infancy to any age
- Large volume spacer with metered dose inhaler: infancy to any age
- Dry powder devices: 5 years onwards
- Metered dose inhalers including autohalers: 8 years and above.

Inhalation technique

Regardless of the delivery device, it is imperative that the delivery device and inhalation technique are monitored at clinic visits and prior to discharge from hospital for every patient.

The optimal inhalation technique is as follows. The child:

- stands (allows full use of the diaphragm)
- tilts the jaw slightly upwards to ensure maximal oropharyngeal airway
- performs full exhalation
- places the device in the mouth and makes a firm seal with the lips
- activates the device (if metered dose inhaler, actuates after starting inhalation)
- inhales fully and holds breath for 10 seconds.

Fig. 16 Drug delivery in asthma.

If a spacer is used in an infant, the spacer must be tilted to allow the valve to open. The chamber is 'primed' with one puff from the inhaler and at least five breaths must be allowed for each dose actuated.

Prognosis

As asthma is a heterogeneous disorder, the prognosis is variable. Infants with viral infection-associated wheezing (including wheeze post-bronchiolitis) generally have a better prognosis than those with chronic asthma associated with an atopic personal and family history of asthma, eczema and hayfever. In one study, 70% of children 'outgrew' their symptoms by late adolescence, with the remainder suffering variable degrees of recurrent wheeze or cough.

3.6 Cystic fibrosis

Genetics

Cystic fibrosis (CF) is the most common autosomal recessive inherited disorder in the UK with a gene carriage rate of approximately 1 in 25 and an incidence of approximately 1 in 2500. The gene affected in CF has been located on chromosome 7. It spans 27 exons and codes for a 1480 KDa peptide termed the cystic fibrosis transmembrane conductance regulator (CFTR). The protein comprises two areas that span the membrane, two nucleotide-binding areas and a regulatory domain. Several gene mutations have been recognised, the most common being ΔF508 where there is an absence of phenylalanine at position 508 in one of the nucleotide-binding areas.

Pathophysiology

The CFTR controls electrolyte secretion and absorption in various organs. In the sweat gland, absence of this protein affects electrolyte reabsorption, hence the abnormal sweat test. In the lungs, there is decreased chloride secretion and increased sodium reabsorption, resulting in viscous secretions and production of a mucus that is difficult to clear. These secretions become colonised with various bacteria, in particularly those of the *Pseudomonas* species. The host response to this colonisation is chronic inflammation, which is believed to be a major cause of the lung damage. Viscid secretions elsewhere give rise to problems in the gastrointestinal, biliary and gonadal systems.

Clinical presentation

Recurrent respiratory symptoms including chronic cough and wheeze are the classic presentation of CF. Other children may present following recurrent infections such as pneumonia or after an atypical, prolonged or severe episode of acute bronchiolitis. Failure to thrive may pass unnoticed until such an infection occurs or it may be a primary presenting feature of CF. The poor growth is usually the result of a combination of recurrent infection and malabsorption with steatorrhoea. Approximately 10% of patients present in the neonatal period with gastrointestinal disease, particularly meconium ileus, when gastrointestinal obstruction results from thick tenacious meconium and a poorly developed large bowel. Surgical resection of the affected gut or surgical removal of the meconium may be required. Rectal prolapse can occur as a result of the combination of chronic steatorrhoea and insufficient ischiorectal fossa fat failing to support the rectum. Some infants are diagnosed by screening techniques performed because of a family history. Rarer presentations include nasal polyps, heat exhaustion, anaemia, short stature and electrolyte imbalance.

Diagnosis

The sweat test is the gold standard investigation for confirming CF. Several methods may be used but all aim to measure the concentration of electrolytes in sweat, particularly sodium and chloride, when levels exceed 70 mmol. The test requires 100 mg sweat for a valid result but false-positive results may still occur. Other methods of diagnosis including stool enzyme activity are rarely used. The phenomenon of increased transnasal mucosal electrical potential has been advocated as a diagnostic tool. Molecular techniques to search for the most likely gene mutations are now widely employed for diagnostic purposes and can be used antenatally.

Complications of cystic fibrosis

Multiple organ systems are affected in CF. Major effects occur in the respiratory and gastrointestinal systems but there are a number of less common complications (Table 17).

Respiratory effects

The majority of CF sufferers develop chronic bacterial colonisation of their lower respiratory tract, a process encouraged by the combination of viscid secretions and reduced mucociliary clearance. A characteristic pattern of colonisation is usually observed with *Staphylococcus*

Table 17 Less common complications of cystic fibrosis

System	Complication
Respiratory	Pneumothorax
	Haemoptysis
	Cor pulmonale
	Nasal polyps
Endocrine	Diabetes mellitus
	Pubertal delay
	Short stature
Male infertility	Absence of vas deferens
Arthropathy	Vasculitis
Psychosocial problems	

aureus and *Haemophilus influenzae* predominating in the infant and *Pseudomonas* species occurring with advancing age. The subsequent inflammatory host response results in eventual damage to the airways and marks the decline in respiratory function.

Physiotherapy is the mainstay of therapy, with early prolonged use of antibiotics for respiratory infections. Authorities are divided on the need for prophylactic antibiotics in infancy and the use of combination intravenous and nebulised antibiotics when permanent colonisation by *Pseudomonas* sp. ensues. Bronchospasm may coexist as a result of the inflammatory process or follows an allergic response to the fungus *Aspergillus*. Therefore, long-term bronchodilator treatment is usually required. As a result of host inflammatory cell and bacterial death, DNA is released in the mucus. Therapeutic administration of the recombinant DNAase enables this DNA to be enzymatically cleaved resulting in thinner, less viscous mucus. Combined heart–lung transplants are now performed in those with advanced disease.

Chest radiograph
Severe abnormalities are commonplace on X-ray examination, with areas of atelectasis alternating with opacities owing to sputum retention. Generalised bronchial wall thickening, lung overinflation and cyst formation occur as the intrapulmonary damage progresses. Various scoring systems have been devised to allow quantification of these radiographic abnormalities.

Gastrointestinal tract effects

Pancreatic insufficiency is common, leading to malabsorption, loss of fat-soluble vitamins and failure to thrive. Loss of ischiorectal fossa fat may result in rectal prolapse. Thick viscous gut secretions may cause meconium ileus in the neonatal period, presenting as gut obstruction shortly after birth. Antenatal perforation of the gut may occur. Rarely, a similar clinical picture with gastrointestinal obstruction may affect the older child and is termed meconium ileus equivalent. Water-attracting radiographic media (gastrografin) may successfully clear the obstruction, although surgery may be necessary.

Life-long pancreatic enzyme replacement is vital.

Nutritional supplementation is often necessary to ensure growth, particularly as energy requirements of these children are higher than normal. Fat-soluble vitamins should be given routinely to avoid vitamin deficiency states. These include hypophosphataemia and rickets (caused by vitamin D deficiency), cerebellar ataxia and haemolytic anaemia (vitamin E deficiency) and coagulation defects (vitamin K deficiency). The last may, in turn, exacerbate any coagulopathy associated with liver dysfunction. Thick viscous bile may result in gallstones, biliary cirrhosis and hepatic impairment which, if severe, may necessitate liver transplantation.

Prognosis

The prognosis in CF is variable, although generally many more children are living into adulthood. In the USA, studies suggest a median life expectancy of 30 years but the rapid pace of change in the management of CF means that life expectancy is expected to continue to improve.

3.7 Other respiratory disorders

Aspiration syndromes

Aspiration may occur at any age although it is more common during infancy when foodstuffs, particularly milk, are the most commonly aspirated materials. The right main bronchus is the most common site for a foreign body. Acute aspiration presents with a history of choking and coughing. This may settle once the airway receptors have adjusted to the aspiration only to recur if the child changes position. Many aspirations go unrecognised in the acute phase and present with consolidation that fails to improve on adequate therapy. Bronchoscopic removal of the foreign material is necessary, with antibiotic cover to prevent infection.

Clinical features

Acute respiratory distress, wheezing and coughing are not always present. Partial airway obstruction may produce a 'ball-valve' effect leading to progressive overinflation of the affected lung with tracheal and mediastinal shift away from the affected side. Poor air entry will be detected in the affected lung, which is hyper-resonant to percussion.

Radiography

The classic abnormality in aspiration syndromes is overinflation of the affected lung on an expiratory film. An inspiratory film may appear normal if the aspirated material is not radio-opaque. Fluoroscopic screening may be helpful in establishing the diagnosis.

Chronic aspiration

Chronic aspiration may present with recurrent respiratory symptoms or infections. It occurs in those with abnormal anatomical connections, e.g. tracheo-oesophageal fistula (particularly 'H' type), those with poorly coordinated swallowing, e.g. cerebral palsy or those with gastro-oesophageal reflux. The last may be managed medically with a combination of antacids and prokinetic drugs (e.g. cisapride) or surgically by fundoplication. In this procedure, the stomach is surgically wrapped around the base of the oesophagus, thus preventing reflux.

Fibrosing alveolitis

Fibrosing alveolitis is a rare disorder in childhood and may be an immune-mediated process or, in a minority of cases, caused by a genetic predisposition. The clinical features include progressive breathlessness and hypoxia. Widespread reticular shadowing is usually evident on the chest radiograph. Steroids may be beneficial in some patients.

Lymphoid interstitial pneumonitis

Superficially resembling fibrosing alveolitis, lymphoid interstitial pneumonitis (LIP) is a feature of HIV infection, occurring in up to 40% of those vertically infected. The aetiology is uncertain although Epstein–Barr virus has been implicated in some patients. Patients usually present with progressive dyspnoea, persistent coughing, clubbing and occasionally, parotid gland enlargement. Abnormalities on X-ray examination include fine, generalised reticular mottling and these may precede clinical features. Both steroids and zidovudine have been beneficial in some sufferers.

Immune defects and the lung

Recurrent respiratory infections are common in those with immunodeficiency states including the common IgA deficiency and minor defects such IgG subclass deficiency. Defective cell-mediated immunity may predispose to severe viral or fungal infections of the respiratory tract. Similarly, abnormalities of ciliary motility (dyskinesia) predispose to all types of respiratory infection. In Kartagener syndrome, the ciliary defect is associated with recurrent sinusitis, bronchiectasis and situs inversus (including dextrocardia).

Self-assessment: questions

Multiple choice questions

1. Features of bronchiolitis include:
   a. Stridor
   b. Apnoea
   c. Hepatomegaly
   d. Paroxysmal coughing
   e. Wheeze

2. The following clinical findings are seen in lung consolidation:
   a. Ipsilateral bronchial breathing
   b. Absent tactile vocal fremitus (TVF)
   c. Deviation of the trachea away from the affected side
   d. Hyper-resonant percussion note
   e. Absent breath sounds

3. Features suggestive of croup include:
   a. A fever of about 40°C or greater
   b. Wheeze
   c. Dysphagia
   d. Barking cough
   e. Variable stridor

4. Pulmonary tuberculosis in childhood:
   a. Usually follows infection with *Mycobacterium bovis*
   b. Usually causes a severe bronchopneumonia
   c. May present with widespread reticular shadowing on the chest radiograph
   d. Is prevented by the Mantoux injection
   e. May be severe in those with cell-mediated immunodeficiency

5. Pertussis infection:
   a. Causes atelectasis
   b. Is a notifiable infection
   c. Is optimally treated with ribavirin
   d. Is associated with subconjunctival haemorrhage
   e. May result in seizures

6. Features indicative of severe life-threatening asthma include:
   a. Peak flow measurement less than 60% of normal
   b. Severe coughing
   c. Reduced respiratory rate
   d. Absent breath sounds
   e. Irritability

7. Epidemiological factors of importance in asthma include:
   a. Parental smoking
   b. Previous respiratory syncytial virus infection
   c. Rural existence
   d. Affected mother
   e. Allergy to house dust mite

8. An estimate of the chronicity of asthma symptoms involves:
   a. Monitoring diurnal peak flow measurements
   b. Number of school days missed
   c. Frequency of nocturnal cough
   d. Frequency of the use of rescue therapy
   e. Monitoring of height velocity

9. Which of the following inhalation devices is appropriately paired with the correct age for use:
   a. Metered dose inhaler at 2 years of age
   b. Turbohaler at 18 months of age
   c. Diskhaler at 3 years of age
   d. Autohaler at 3 years of age
   e. Spacing device plus metered dose inhaler from birth

10. The following statements are correct:
    a. Chronic undertreated asthma causes pectus excavatum deformity
    b. Chronic asthma is associated with clubbing
    c. Harrison's sulcus is a sign of acute obstructive airways disease
    d. Salbutamol is the ideal choice for prophylaxis of chronic asthma
    e. Barrel chest deformity is associated with chronic asthma

11. Which of the following statements regarding the genetics of cystic fibrosis is correct:
    a. Gene carriage is approximately 1:2500
    b. Inheritance is autosomal recessive
    c. The gene is located on chromosome 6
    d. The gene product is an enzyme
    e. The most common mutation in UK sufferers is ΔF508

12. Recognised clinical presentations of cystic fibrosis include:
    a. Rectal prolapse
    b. Haemorrhoids
    c. Meconium ileus
    d. Diabetes mellitus
    e. Liver failure

13. Complications of cystic fibrosis include:
    a. Haemoptysis
    b. Pneumothorax
    c. Female infertility
    d. Precocious puberty
    e. Cor pulmonale

14. With regard to cystic fibrosis, the following statements are correctly paired:
    a. Vitamin E and rickets
    b. Vitamin K and haemolytic anaemia
    c. Exocrine insufficiency and poor growth
    d. Vitamin A and steatorrhoea
    e. Vitamin D and cerebellar ataxia

15. Correct statements regarding therapy for cystic fibrosis include:
    a. Physiotherapy is only indicated during acute respiratory infections
    b. Pancreatic supplements are needed even in the absence of steatorrhoea
    c. Glucose intolerance usually results in ketoacidosis
    d. Calorie intake must be increased above normal levels
    e. Nebulised antibiotics may be indicated when chronic *Pseudomonas* species colonisation occurs

16. Aspiration in childhood:
    a. Commonly affects the left main bronchus
    b. Is common in neurologically impaired children
    c. May be silent
    d. Is a chronic complication of tracheo-oesophageal fistula
    e. Is best diagnosed on an inspiratory film

17. Kartagener syndrome includes:
    a. Ciliary dysfunction
    b. Dextrocardia
    c. Gastro-oesophageal reflux
    d. IgA deficiency
    e. Clubbing

18. Causes of clubbing include:
    a. Empyema
    b. Cystic fibrosis
    c. Fibrosing alveolitis
    d. Asthma
    e. Lymphoid interstitial pneumonitis

Case histories

Case history 1

A 2-year-old boy undergoing chemotherapy for acute lymphoblastic leukaemia is admitted with a worsening cough and respiratory distress. His oximetric saturations reveal a saturation of 86% in 30% oxygen given by face mask. His mother has been giving him vitamins but has recently run out of cotrimoxazole.

1. List three useful respiratory investigations to aid in the diagnosis and management
2. What is the most likely cause of the boy's symptoms?
3. What treatment is required?

Case history 2

A 2-year-old child is admitted with an acute onset of coughing that started during a birthday party. He had been seen to choke while running around, having taken some peanuts from a bowl. Shortly afterwards, however, his coughing had settled and he had fallen asleep in his mother's arms.

1. List the clinical features which, on examination, may indicate acute aspiration
2. List two useful investigations
3. What is the treatment of choice for this aspiration?

Case history 3

As a general practitioner, you see the parents of a 4-year-old boy who has been suffering with recurrent attacks of wheezing over the last year. He has been reviewed in a specialty clinic and a diagnosis of asthma has been made and a nebuhaler prescribed.

Outline how you would proceed to provide the parents with advice.

Short notes

Write short notes on the following:

1. The management of a 5-year-old girl referred with recurrent wheeze and nocturnal cough who has a strong family history of atopy and allergy
2. The important features of an asthma inhaler device prior to prescribing such a device for an 8-year-old girl
3. Your respiratory system management in a 12-year-old child with severe cystic fibrosis
4. The pathophysiology of cystic fibrosis with regard to the abnormal molecular biology.

Self-assessment: answers

Multiple choice answers

1. a. **False**. This is a feature of croup or other upper airways obstruction.
    b. **True**. It may be the presenting feature in very young infants.
    c. **True**. Usually occurs because of overinflation of the lungs.
    d. **False**. It is more of a feature of pertussis.
    e. **True**. As a result of airway oedema and mucus.

2. a. **True**. This is a classical feature of consolidation.
    b. **False**. TVF is increased.
    c. **False**. Tracheal deviation is a feature of loss of lung volume (i.e. collapse).
    d. **False**. This is a feature of pneumothorax.
    e. **False**. This is a feature of pleural effusion or lung segment collapse.

3. a. **False**. Toxicity and high fever are more likely with bacterial tracheitis or epiglottitis rather than croup.
    b. **False**. This is a feature of lower respiratory tract disorder.
    c. **False**. This is a feature of epiglottitis or foreign body aspiration.
    d. **True**. It is associated with viral prodromal illness.
    e. **True**. Variability is dependent upon humidity, temperature and diurnal variation.

4. a. **False**. The causative organism is *Mycobacterium tuberculosis*.
    b. **False**. It usually causes subclinical infection revealed as a primary complex or Ghon focus on the chest X-ray.
    c. **True**. Miliary TB may present early as a result of rapid spread of infection.
    d. **False**. Mantoux test reveals sensitivity to tuberculoprotein, i.e. evidence of infection.
    e. **True**. The most effective immune response to infection with *M. tuberculosis* is cell mediated and if this is impaired, the host is unable to contain the organism.

5. a. **True**. It causes whooping cough; a secondary pneumonia may ensue.
    b. **True**. There are approximately 30 notifiable diseases. The prime purpose of the notifications system is speed in detecting possible outbreaks and epidemics.
    c. **False**. Ribavirin is occasionally used to treat bronchiolitis.
    d. **True**. Coughing spasms may cause subconjunctival bleeds.
    e. **True**. Hypoxic seizures may occur.

6. a. **False**. Peak flow less than 33% of predicted indicates severe asthma.
    b. **False**. Not an indication of severity.
    c. **False**. Rate is usually elevated unless the patient is semi-comatose.
    d. **True**. The 'silent' chest.
    e. **True**. It suggests carbon dioxide retention as a result of respiratory failure.

7. a. **True**. Asthma is a multifactorial disorder and the environment can act as a trigger point.
    b. **True**. Particularly in those who have had a lower respiratory tract infection in early childhood.
    c. **False**. There is no difference in prevalence between rural and urban areas.
    d. **True**. Multifactorial inheritance may be involved in this condition.
    e. **True**. Among the various triggers are pollution, house dust mites and pollen.

8. a. **True**. The 'morning dip' indicates poorly controlled asthma.
    b. **True**. Those with severe chronic asthma tend to stay away from school and are often unwell at home rather than admitted to hospital.
    c. **True**. This is an important symptom. Asthma may occur solely as a nocturnal phenomenon and in some children cough rather than wheezing is the most prominent symptom.
    d. **True**. Those with chronic asthma are often able to predict an impending attack and seek relief.
    e. **True**. Chronically undertreated asthma causes short stature by reducing height velocity.

9. a. **False**. This device is inappropriate for a 2-year-old unless used with a spacer device.
    b. **False**. Dry powders are only used in those over 4–5 years.
    c. **False**. It requires too much dexterity for this age.
    d. **False**. It is only useful for older ages.
    e. **True**. It is easy to administer and use for all age groups, particularly for the youngest asthmatics.

10. a. **False**. This is a developmental anomaly.
    b. **False**. Clubbing develops in chronic suppurative lung diseases such as cystic fibrosis or chronic interstitial lung disease and is not a feature of reactive airway disease such as asthma.
    c. **False**. This is a chronic sign.
    d. **False**. Salbutamol is a rescue therapy used in the acute phase.
    e. **True**. It is a sign of chronic overinflation.

11. a. **False**. Gene carriage is 1:25 in the UK.
    b. **True**. If both parents are heterozygotes there is a 1 in 4 chance of the offspring being affected.

c. **False**. It is found on chromosome 7.

d. **False**. It is an ion channel (CF transmembrane conductance regulator).

e. **True**. This is a specific trinucleotide deletion that leads to the loss of phenylalanine from the protein encoded by the CF gene.

12. a. **True**. It is a consequence of malabsorption causing fat loss plus steatorrhoea.

b. **False**. This occurs in individuals with raised portal hypertension, e.g. cirrhosis, extrahepatic portal hypertension.

c. **True**. Approximately 10% present in the neonatal period with meconium ileus.

d. **False**. This is a late complication in 2%.

e. **False**. This is another late complication.

13. a. **True**. Progressive bronchiectasis leads to local hypoxia and an increase in the vasculature around the areas of bronchiectasis. These vessels are often dilated and rupture easily resulting in haemoptysis.

b. **True**. Usually adolescents.

c. **False**. Male infertility can occur.

d. **False**. Pubertal delay occurs.

e. **True**. It is the result of pulmonary disease and its effects on pulmonary vasculature.

14. a. **False**. Vitamin E malabsorption is associated with cerebellar ataxia and haemolytic anaemia.

b. **False**. Vitamin K deficiency can cause coagulopathy.

c. **True**. Exocrine insufficiency results in malabsorption.

d. **False**. Vitamin A does not cause steatorrhoea. It is a fat-soluble vitamin and in the presence of steatorrhoea (fat malabsorption) it may not be adequately absorbed.

e. **False**. Vitamin D deficiency may cause rickets.

15. a. **False**. Physiotherapy is necessary from the time of diagnosis.

b. **True**. Varying amounts are necessary to ensure adequate nutrition.

c. **False**. Ketoacidosis is rare.

d. **True**. Calories required are about 120% of normal.

e. **True**. Systemically administered antibiotics may not adequately penetrate the viscid secretions and inhaled antibiotics may be required to attain sufficient antibacterial levels in the affected tissue.

16. a. **False**. It usually affects the right side.

b. **True**. Especially if there is pseudobulbar palsy, resulting in impaired coordination of swallowing.

c. **True**. It is revealed by repeated pneumonias.

d. **True**. Although not the typical presentation,

recurrent aspiration may occur in certain types, notably the 'H' type fistula without oesophageal atresia.

e. **True**. But only if the aspirated material is either radio-opaque or causes infection. Expiratory films are better with foreign bodies and demonstrate unilateral overinflation as a result of airway obstruction.

17. a. **True**. Kartagener is a subset of the immotile cilia syndrome.

b. **True**. It is felt that the normal rotation of the viscera depends on functioning of embryonic cilia. Without ciliary movement, rotation becomes a chance occurrence: 50% have normal rotation and 50% have dextrorotation. Typically, dextrocardia (non-rotation of the heart) is accompanied by situs inversus totalis.

c. **False**. Gut motility, unlike ciliary motility, is unaffected.

d. **False**. Like gastro-oesophageal reflux, IgA deficiency is also associated with chronic lung disease but not with Kartagener syndrome.

e. **False**. Clubbing occurs not as a component of the syndrome but as a result of the bronchiectasis that ensues because of ciliary dyskinesia.

18. a. **True**. The cause of clubbing is unknown, but it is thought to be the result of chronic hypoxia to the nail bed. It is, therefore, a feature of chronic hypoxic diseases such as central cyanotic conditions, chronic suppurative lung disease and conditions where there is arterio-venous shunting such as cirrhosis.

b. **True**. It is probably a result of the chronic suppuration.

c. **True**. Because of chronic hypoxia.

d. **False**. Hypoxia is characterised by acute episodes rather than a chronic state.

e. **True**. As a result of chronic hypoxia.

Case history answers

Case history 1

1. Useful investigations include:

- chest radiograph: this will show perihilar shadowing.
- arterial blood gas: to assess degree of hypoxia and hypocarbia resulting from impaired diffusion associated with hyperventilation, respectively
- bronchoalveolar lavage, to confirm the diagnosis microbiologically.

2. *Pneumocystis carinii* pneumonitis. This immunocompromised child has stopped his antibiotic prophylaxis (cotrimoxazole) given specifically to prevent pneumocystis pneumonia.

3. High-dose cotrimoxazole or, rarely, pentamidine given intravenously. Once the acute infection has been treated, then the child needs to restart prophylaxis with cotrimoxazole taken orally until no longer immunocompromised.

Case history 2

1. Clinical features include:

- any signs of respiratory distress, e.g. tachypnoea
- decreased air entry and reduced expansion on the side of aspiration
- evidence of tracheal deviation and lung collapse distal to any blockage
- crepitations or evidence of infection distal to blockage
- further coughing bouts as child's position changes.

2. Expiratory chest radiograph, fluoroscopy and, very rarely, a bronchogram is necessary.
3. Bronchoscopy for removal of the foreign body and provision of antibiotic cover.

Case history 3

This type of case history leads you through the diagnosis and you will be given examples of these in other chapters. Some questions will, however, expect you to create your own constructs. In these cases a structured answer is expected and should contain the following headlines:

The diagnosis

- explain what asthma is
- explore the possibility of family atopy or other allergies
- discuss possible precipitating factors.

Management

- management of acute episode with the nebuhaler
- if symptoms do not improve the child may require to be seen in casualty and receive aerosolised therapy and be put on steroids
- prophylactic treatment is required if the episodes are frequent
- teach peak flow measurements
- make sure parents and child are aware of how to use the age-appropriate device for drug administration.

Prognosis

- will have intermittent symptoms but there is a good chance that this will improve with age
- can cause life-threatening attacks which require urgent treatment; educate the parents about the symptoms.

Complications of medications

- bronchodilators and steroids
- measure height and weight and maintain follow-up.

Education and compliance

- ensure that the health visitor and specialist asthma nurse are involved, particularly in compliance
- provide monitoring diaries and written educational literature for child and parents.

Short notes answers

1. The following points should be covered:
   a. Take a history to identify precipitating factors for wheeze and cough
   b. Explore the degree of familial atopy and asthma
   c. Discuss the use of skin tests, etc.
   d. Assess any alternative diagnosis, e.g. cystic fibrosis
   e. Assess severity of symptoms and degree of effect on life
   f. Discuss allergen exposure and reduction, e.g. house dust mite, allergy to pets
   g. Measure height, weight and teach peak flow measurement
   h. Examine for evidence of acute or chronic respiratory disease
   i. Demonstrate an age-appropriate device for rescue therapy and prophylaxis (if history suggests that prophylaxis is necessary)
   j. Provide monitoring diaries and written educational literature for child and parents
   k. Construct emergency guidelines and ensure the parents are conversant with these
   l. Involve general practitioner and specialist asthma nurse/health visitor in follow-up, particularly in monitoring compliance.

2. Important features include:

- degree of complexity to operate
- degree of manual dexterity of the child
- degree of effort to inhale particles, i.e. flow rate required to operate device
- single or multiple doses available?
- ease of packing and social acceptability (necessary for compliance).

3. Respiratory management would include:

- ensure adequate physiotherapy on a regular basis
- treat infective exacerbations promptly
- some authorities suggest regular courses of intravenous anti-pseudomonal therapy, e.g. every 3 months
- nebulised anti-pseudomonal therapy if colonised
- treat any tendency to asthma/bronchospasm: many need inhaled steroids
- encourage exercise
- ensure adequate nutrition
- treat fungal infections
- home oxygen therapy if necessary
- consider other therapies, e.g. DNAase.

4. The abnormal gene is a defective chloride channel transmembrane conductance regulator. The most common gene abnormality results in the absence of phenylalanine in one of the nucleotide-binding areas. Decreased chloride secretion with subsequent increased sodium reabsorption higher up in the respiratory tract causes relative dehydration of the respiratory mucus. The mucus is more viscous and more difficult to clear by the mucociliary carpet and becomes secondarily colonised with bacteria. The subsequent anti-inflammatory host response seems to be responsible for the ensuing tissue damage.

The cardiovascular system

Key points

You should have an understanding of:

- The basic anatomy and physiology of the normal heart
- The performance of an adequate cardiovascular examination
- The important acyanotic conditions, especially atrial and ventricular septal defects, aortic and pulmonary stenosis and coarctation of the aorta
- The important cyanotic conditions, especially tetralogy of Fallot and transposition of the great arteries
- The interpretation of the 'cardiac' chest X-ray
- The interpretation of basic electrocardiograms
- How to treat cardiac failure and supraventricular tachycardia; you need only a rudimentary idea of surgical procedures for the correction of congenital cardiac lesions.

4.1 Introduction

Congenital malformations make up the bulk of cardiac disease in childhood and the majority can be diagnosed correctly at the patient's bedside. The heart is a con-

tained structure with a defined pattern of blood flow. A change in its structure or flow results in consistently reproducible abnormal symptoms and signs. When approached logically, examination of the cardiovascular system is straightforward. Coupled with electrocardiography (ECG) and chest X-ray, this is sufficient to make a good 'working' diagnosis in almost all cases.

Normal anatomy

Figure 17 shows the normal position of the heart; it is this that determines the cardiac silhouette on the chest X-ray film. The right border is formed by the right atrium, with the superior and inferior vena cava above and below, respectively. The left border is formed by the left ventricle below, the bulge from the pulmonary trunk in the middle, and the arch of the aorta above. The cardiac landmarks are dictated by the normal position of the heart in the thorax (Fig. 18).

4.2 Clinical assessment

Symptoms

Cardiac disease in childhood consists of structural abnormalities, diseases of the myocardium and arrhythmias. Structural abnormalities are often picked up inci-

Silhouette on X-ray

Position of cardiac valves

Fig. 17 Normal cardiac position and silhouette on X-ray. SVC, superior vena cava; RA, right atrium; RV, right ventricle; PA, pulmonary artery; LV, left ventricle; AA, aortic artery; T, tricuspid valve; M, mitral valve; P, pulmonary valve; A, aortic valve.

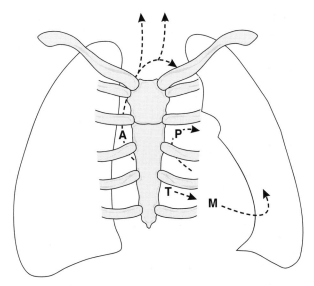

Fig. 18 Normal cardiac landmarks relative to the sternum. A, aortic area, second right intercostal space; P, pulmonary area, second left intercostal space; T, tricuspid area, fourth left intercostal space; M, mitral area, fourth intercostal space, mid-clavicular line.

dentally with the chance finding of a murmur. Others produce abnormal strain on the pumping chambers and result in cardiac failure. Alternatively, congenital abnormalities involving incorrect connection of cardiac structures may result in **right-to-left** shunts and cyanosis.

Heart failure

Symptoms attributable to heart failure can be divided into those caused by 'right heart failure' (RHF) and 'left heart failure' (LHF). RHF results in systemic venous congestion and presents with fluid retention. LHF results in pulmonary venous congestion, which presents with breathlessness and frequent lower respiratory tract infections (LRTI). In children, right and left heart failure are often present simultaneously.

Infants expend a considerable amount of energy during feeds. Those with heart failure become breathless with increased sweating during feeding. They are unable to suck for prolonged periods and repeatedly 'come up for air' during feeds. An increased risk of LRTIs may further exacerbate cardiac failure. Not only do these infants feed poorly, but much of their energy is channelled into maintaining an adequate cardiac output and they, therefore, fail to thrive. Older children with heart failure have little reserve to cope with everyday or additional stress and often deteriorate during exertion or an intercurrent illness.

Cyanosis

As a result of shunting of blood from the right to the left side of the heart, venous blood meant for the pulmonary circulation is rerouted back into the systemic circulation, bypassing the lungs. As a result, there is a drop in the arterial blood oxygen concentration (PO_2)

and tissue hypoxia ensues, clinically manifest as central cyanosis. The body compensates for progessive hypoxia by two mechanisms: an increase in heart rate (tachycardia) in order to increase cardiac output, and an increase in the circulating haemoglobin concentration (polycythaemia). The cardiac reserve is, however, limited and tolerance to exertion is poor. Syncopal episodes may arise in those patients who develop sudden exacerbations of their hypoxic state.

Lower respiratory tract infections

Patients with a history of recurrent LRTI may not always show signs of frank left heart failure but the diagnosis is confirmed by the findings of a murmur, plethora and cardiomegaly on the chest X-ray film and an abnormal ECG.

Arrhythmias

These are usually acute in onset and result in sudden 'palpitations', often associated with breathlessness. The blood pressure may drop during the arrhythmia, resulting in vomiting, 'funny turns' and syncope.

Examination

Start an examination by assessing the child's general state of health. Look for central cyanosis by inspecting the lips and tongue, and for polycythaemia by the presence of a plethoric complexion and conjunctival congestion. Examine the nails for clubbing, anaemia and peripheral cyanosis. Work your way back to the heart, starting first with the pulses, then the blood pressure and finally the precordium.

Pulses

In children, especially infants, the brachial artery is best used for the assessment of the pulse. This provides a good assessment of pulse rate, volume and character. The brachial (as opposed to the radial) artery is the same distance from the heart as the femoral arteries. Hence, with one hand feeling the right brachial pulse, check either femoral pulse for a palpable difference between the two. It is easier to appreciate a **brachio-femoral difference** based on a discrepancy in pulse volume rather than a delay in timing, especially in babies who have a heart rate above 100 beats per minute (Table 18).

Table 18 Change in pulse and blood pressure with age

Age	Pulse (beats/minute)	Mean blood pressure (mmHg)
Neonate	120–160	60
Infant	90–110	75
School age	80–90	90
Teenage	60–80	100

A high volume pulse is often a clue to the presence of a large left-to-right shunt, e.g. a patent ductus arteriosus. An easy way to assess this is to raise the child's arm above the head. The pulse remains easily palpable in those with high volume 'bounding' pulses.

Jugular venous pressure

The jugular venous pressure (JVP) is difficult to assess in infants but can be seen in premature babies and in children aged 2 years or more. The JVP is best seen with the patient lying propped up at 45°, the head turned slightly to the opposite side, and can be accentuated by gentle pressure over the liver (hepatojugular reflux). The JVP is raised in RHF and fluid overload, when the upper level falls during inspiration. However, when the movement of the heart is restricted through pericardial or pulmonary disease (cor pulmonale), the JVP, though elevated, will rise further on inspiration (Kussmaul's sign).

Blood pressure

To measure blood pressure (BP) the cuff size should be two-thirds that of the child's arm. In order not to miss a coarctation of the aorta, it is important to take the BP on both arms and either lower limb. In small babies, an easy method of measuring the systolic BP is to observe the pressure at which the limb turns pink on deflating the cuff ('flush' method). The variation in BP with age is shown in Table 18.

Precordium

Examine the precordium for activity. Place your right hand over the precordium and locate the apical impulse. Normally this is in the fourth intercostal space in the mid-clavicular line. A 'buzzing or whirring' sensation beneath your hand is indicative of transmitted tactile turbulence (a thrill). Using the hypothenar aspect of the hand placed vertically to the left of the sternum, feel for a right ventricular heave, which is suggestive of right ventricular (RV) hypertrophy. A laterally displaced, heaving apical impulse is indicative of left ventricular (LV) hypertrophy.

Heart sounds

Using the bell of the stethoscope, listen over the precordium and initially concentrate on the heart sounds alone (Fig. 19). Listen for the first sound (S1) at the apex and lower left sternal edge (LSE). Concentrate on the second sound (S2). This normally has two components but may, on occasion, be single. The first component results from closure of the aortic valve (A2), the second from closure of the pulmonary valve (P2). On inspiration, there is a fall in the intrathoracic pressure and more blood enters the right heart. This results in a delay in RV emptying and the A2–P2 interval increases. On expira-

Fig. 19 Normal heart sounds: (a) expiration; (b) inspiration (see text for details).

tion, the split narrows and, particularly with a rapid heart rate, S2 may appear to be a single sound. If two components are clearly audible in all phases of respiration, assume there is wide fixed splitting of S2. Next concentrate on the intensity of the sound. Remember to auscultate over both aortic and pulmonary areas: if S2 is louder in the aortic area, then it is the aortic (earlier) component which is accentuated and vice versa. If the child is crying, wait to auscultate when the child pauses for breath.

Added sounds

Third sound
An extra third sound (S3) is said to reproduce the effect of a galloping horse and is often heard in patients with heart failure. You can mimic this effect by drumming three fingers in succession on the table top.

Clicks
Listen for additional sounds in between the two heart sounds. Clicks are momentary high-pitched sounds produced by the sudden opening of a stiff (usually stenotic) heart valve. They are generally produced by the pulmonary and aortic valves at the start of systole, heard immediately after the first heart sound and are invariably followed by a murmur.

Murmurs
Murmurs are sounds of a buzzing, whooshing or whirring nature and are caused by abnormal turbulence within the cardiac chambers or major vessels. Murmurs between S1 and S2 are systolic murmurs and are graded according to a simple system (Table 19). Diastolic murmurs follow S2 and are not graded. The different types of murmur and their common causes are shown in Table 20.

Functional murmurs are present in up to 70% of neonates and 25–50% of older children. They are soft,

Table 19 Grading system for systolic murmurs

Grade	Nature	Thrill
1	Barely audible	None
2	Soft, easily audible	None
3	Loud	None
4	Easily audible	Present
5	Loud, stethoscope barely on chest	Present
6	Heard away from chest wall	Present

Table 20 Murmurs and diagnoses

Murmur	Phonocardiogram	Diagnosis
Ejection systolic		Aortic stenosis, pulmonary stenosis, small ventricular septal defect
Late (ejection) systolic		Coarctation of the aorta, mitral valve prolapse
Pansystolic		Mitral incompetence, tricuspid incompetence, large ventricular septal defect, atrioventricular septal defect
Continuous		Patent ductus arteriosus, collaterals (e.g. with coarctation), prosthetic shunts, arteriovenous fistulae
Early diastolic		Aortic incompetence, pulmonary incompetence
Mid-diastolic		Mitral stenosis

low-pitched sounds grade 1–3/6 and are heard best at the left sternal edge. They are classically not associated with a thrill or other abnormal cardiac signs and have a normal appearance on ECG and chest X-ray examination. They are commonly seen in hyperdynamic situations such as strenuous exercise, intercurrent infection and severe anaemia. Many, particularly those caused by turbulence within veins, are 'positional' and disappear with a change in posture. Some functional murmurs are more specific and include:

- **Still's murmur**: this 'buzzing' ejection systolic murmur (ESM) arises through turbulence in the LV and is heard best at the lower LSE.
- **Pulmonary flow**: 'blowing' ESM, heard best in the pulmonary area; P2 normal.
- **Venous hum**: a continuous murmur at the base of the neck and sternoclavicular junction that varies with position.

Pulmonary sounds

It is important to listen to the lung fields for signs of infection and basal crepitations indicative of heart failure.

Hepatomegaly

Hepatomegaly is a useful sign of heart failure, particularly since it is often difficult to assess jugular venous congestion and pedal oedema in children. Remember that the liver edge is normally palpable in small children 1–2 cm below the costal margin.

Confirmation of cyanosis: nitrogen washout test

The infant is assessed in 100% oxygen, where the nitro-

gen has been 'washed out'. The oxygen saturation and, preferably, the arterial PO_2 are measured before and after 100% oxygen. The PO_2 increases in those children with a respiratory or reversible cause for their cyanosis but remains low when an intracardiac right-to-left shunt is present.

Summary

Table 21 summarises the examination in cardiovascular disease.

4.3 Congenital heart disease

The major acyanotic and cyanotic congenital cardiac diseases (CHD) are listed in Table 22.

Table 21 Summary of cardiovascular examination

Examination	Information obtained
General	Well being/unwell
	Failure to thrive
	Central cyanosis/plethora
	Clubbing
Pulses	Volume and rate
	Brachio-femoral difference
Blood pressure	Upper/lower limb differential
Precordium	Position/activity of apex
	Right ventricular heave
	Thrills
Heart sounds	S1
	S2
Added sounds	S3
	Murmurs
	Clicks
Lung fields	Respiratory rate
	Crepitations
Liver size	Hepatomegaly

Table 22 Major acyanotic and cyanotic congenital heart diseases

	Defects[a]	(%)
Acyanotic		
Abnormal connections	Ventricular septal defect (VSD)	25–30
	Atrial septal defect (ASD)	6–8
	Patent ductus arteriosus (PDA)	6–8
Abnormal valves/vessels	Pulmonary stenosis (PS)	5–7
	Aortic stenosis (AS)	4–7
	Coarctation of the aorta (CoA)	5–7
	Mitral stenosis (MS)	1
	Ebstein's anomaly	1
Cyanotic		
Abnormal connections	Transposition of the great arteries (TGA)	3–5
	Total anomalous pulmonary venous drainage (TAPVD)	1–3
Obstruction to flow	Tricuspid atresia (TA)	1–2
	Pulmonary atresia (PA)	1–3
	Hypoplastic left heart (HyLH)	1–3
	Hypoplastic right heart (HyRH)	1–3
Complex	Tetralogy of Fallot (TOF)	5–7
	Arioventricular septal defect (AVSD)	1–3
	Truncus arteriosus (TA)	1–2
	Double outlet right ventricle	<1
	Single ventricle	<1

[a]Less common lesions are shown in italics.

Frequency of specific congenital heart defects

Almost 1 per cent (8 in 1000) of all newborn babies have some form of CHD. Ventricular septal defect is the most common isolated lesion, but it is also found in association with other cardiac and non-cardiac defects. CHD is a common component of many syndromes (e.g. Noonan, Marfan, Williams) and chromosomal abnormalities (e.g. Turner syndrome, trisomy 21 (Down), 18 and 13). In the majority of CHD, the cause is unknown, though CHD may follow intrauterine exposure to various drugs (e.g. ethanol, phenytoin), and infections (e.g. rubella and toxoplasmosis).

Acyanotic congenital heart disease

Abnormal connections

Atrial septal defect

The more common ostium secundum atrial septal defects (ASDs) are positioned at the site of the fossa ovalis and are generally isolated defects. Ostium primum ASDs are less common and arise in the lower part of the septum, where they can be associated with abnormalities of the atrioventricular valves. The pressure in the right atrium is lower than that in the left atrium. This results in shunting of oxygenated blood from the left to the right atrium, increasing blood flow by two to four times through the right side of the heart and pulmonary artery (Fig. 20).

Symptoms. In early childhood the thick-walled RV is able to cope with this enhanced flow, hence children are asymptomatic at this age. RHF tends to appear during the second or third decade of life. This together with

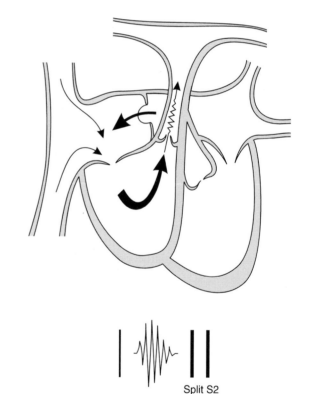

Split S2

ESM in pulmonary area

Fig. 20 Atrial septal defect.

LRTIs and failure to thrive is more likely with primum ASDs.

Signs. Patients are pink with normal pulses and BP. An RV lift may be palpable with established RV hypertrophy. The second heart sound (S2) is widely split in all phases of respiration ('fixed splitting'). This results from the excess volume of blood passing through the pulmonary valve, which delays closure of the valve. A 2–3/6 ESM is heard best at the second left intercostal space, the 'pulmonary area'.

ECG. The 'P' wave may be peaked, indicative of right atrium (RA) enlargement. RV hypertrophy and occasionally RV conduction delay with rSR' in V_1–V_2 is seen.

Chest X-ray. Normal or slight cardiomegaly is seen. There is a prominent pulmonary artery and pulmonary vascularity (plethora).

Complications. It is rare to see complications of ASDs as almost all patients will undergo surgical correction in childhood. If left untreated, complications arise during the third decade and include heart failure, pulmonary hypertension and atrial dysrhythmias. Bacterial endocarditis is extremely rare with an ASD.

Management. Closure is recommended before school entry in all patients. Repair is by direct suturing of small defects and incorporation of an artificial patch (e.g. dacron) in large defects. Non-surgical catheter techniques are currently under review.

Ventricular septal defect

A ventricular septal defect (VSD) is an abnormal interventricular connection. The defect may result from an incomplete fusion of the upper, membranous part of the septum (membranous VSD, 75%) or the lower muscular septum (20%). Membranous VSDs, as a result of their high position, may be associated with defects of the atrioventricular tissues. Muscular VSDs are often multiple. Blood flows under pressure from the left to the right ventricle across the VSD.

The age at presentation and the severity of symptoms depend on the size and, therefore, the degree of left–right shunting through the VSD.

Small VSD (< 0.5 cm²). These may be membranous or muscular.

Symptoms. Small VSDs are generally asymptomatic.

Signs. Patients are pink, with normal pulses and BP. An ESM (or pansystolic murmur, PSM) present at the lower LSE, often with a thrill, is often the only abnormal sign.

ECG and chest X-ray. Both are normal.

Moderate VSD (0.5–1.0 cm²). These are generally membranous.

Symptoms. There are either no symptoms or recurrent chest infections.

Signs. Patients are usually pink, with normal pulses and BP. A thrill at the LSE and an LV impulse may be present. Auscultation confirms a loud P2 heard best in the pulmonary area, and a 2–6/6 PSM heard all over the precordium but best at the LSE (Fig. 21a).

ECG. This shows LV hypertrophy.

Chest X-ray. Examination indicates slight-to-moderate cardiomegaly and plethora.

Large VSD (> 1.0 cm²). These are always membranous.

Symptoms. These are the symptoms of heart failure, e.g. shortness of breath and excessive sweating on exertion or with feeds, recurrent LRTIs and failure to thrive.

Signs. These defects produce a significant left to right shunt and a large volume pulse is usually present. The apical beat is forceful and laterally displaced and a parasternal heave is present, signifying LV and RV hypertrophy, respectively. A thrill at the LSE is common. On auscultation, a loud P2 caused by pulmonary hypertension is often present (Fig. 21a). A third sound (S3) is heard in those in congestive cardiac failuré (CCF). A 2–6/6 PSM all over the precordium but best heard at the lower LSE may be followed by a mid-diastolic murmur (MDM) at the apex caused by excessive flow across the mitral valve. Pulmonary crepitations and hepatomegaly are present in those patients in CCF.

ECG. This shows RV and LV hypertrophy.

Chest X-ray. Cardiomegaly and pulmonary plethora are demonstrated (Fig. 21b).

Complications. Failure to thrive and LRTIs are common with large defects. Bacterial endocarditis generally occurs at the site of least turbulence, on the right of the interventricular wall. The excess pulmonary blood flow, which is under pressure, results in progressive reactive pathological changes in the pulmonary vasculature. Pulmonary arterial resistance increases and pulmonary hypertension develops. If left untreated, the progressive

a

b

Fig. 21 Findings in moderate-sized VSD. (a) Phonocardiogram shows a PSM at the LSE and a loud P2. (b) Chest X-ray film shows cardiomegaly and plethora.

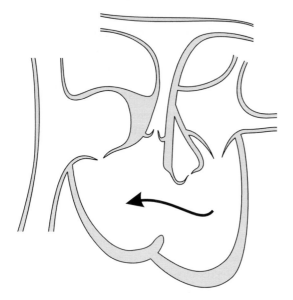

Fig. 22 Ventricular septal defect.

increase in pulmonary resistance can result in shunt reversal. The patient now becomes cyanosed and the shunt murmur disappears. This process is known as **Eisenmenger syndrome**.

Management. Up to 70% of small defects close spontaneously. Those with significant shunts develop heart failure and chest infections. These should be controlled and calorific intake maximised to prevent failure to thrive. Closure of the defect by patch repair under cardiac bypass surgery should be undertaken before school age and certainly before pulmonary hypertension is established.

Patent ductus arteriosus
The ductus arteriosus constricts and closes in response to the rise in PO_2, blood pH and prostacyclin levels after birth. If this mechanism fails or is reversed by prostaglandin E_2, the resulting connection allows blood to flow under pressure from the aorta into the pulmonary arteries. The patent ductus arteriosus (PDA) in the preterm infant is the result of a delay in closure. In a term infant, a PDA is the result of a deficiency in the structural framework of the vessel wall. Therefore, though 100% of premature babies born at 29 weeks of gestation will have a PDA, in the vast majority this closes spontaneously. In contrast, 30% of all term newborns have a persistent connection between the bifurcation of the pulmonary artery and the aortic arch and, in this group, the PDA persists.

Symptoms. There are usually no symptoms and a murmur is noticed incidentally when the PDA is small.

Large defects resulting in a significant left-to-right shunt may present with symptoms of CCF and recurrent chest infections.

Signs. A murmur may be the only abnormal sign in patients with a small shunt. Those with a significant shunt are pink, with large volume, bounding/collapsing pulses. The BP shows a wide pulse pressure. The precordium is hyperdynamic mainly because of an LV impulse at the apex. A thrill is best felt in the left infraclavicular area and second left intercostal space. Large PDAs can result in pulmonary hypertension and may be associated with a loud P2. A continuous 'water-wheel/machinery' murmur (Fig. 23) is best heard at the upper LSE, the left infraclavicular area and back. Signs of CCF include a third heart sound (S3), pulmonary crepitations and hepatomegaly.

ECG. This indicates LV hypertrophy.

Chest X-ray. The film shows moderate cardiomegaly and pulmonary plethora.

Complications. Repeated lower pulmonary infections and CCF may result in failure to thrive. Subacute bacterial endocarditis and pulmonary hypertension are rare complications of a PDA.

Management. The CCF must be treated and conservative measures instituted to close a PDA including fluid restriction, indomethacin and prostacyclin. Obliteration by the implantation of various 'umbrella/coil' devices during cardiac catheterisation is routine, though surgical ligation remains an important method of closure, especially in premature infants.

Abnormal valves and vessels

Pulmonary stenosis
A constricted pulmonary valve ring impedes foward flow of desaturated blood into the lungs, resulting in a volume load on the right ventricle. Pulmonary stenosis (PS) is usually an isolated lesion but can occur with other complex CHD and syndromes (e.g. Noonan).

Symptoms. There are no symptoms although exercise intolerance may occur. RHF is rare.

Signs. Patients with PS are pink, with normal pulses and BP. In mild PS, the precordium is usually normal. An ejection click from the stiff valve, which snaps open, follows the first heart sound. There is wide but variable splitting of S2 because of a delay in P2. A 2–3/6 ESM in the pulmonary area radiates through to the back. In moderate/severe PS, a systolic thrill may be palpable at the upper LSE and a RV heave detectable. Because of the relative immobility of severely stenosed valve cusps, the ejection click is absent and the P2 is soft or inaudible. A 3–4/6 ESM that extends to overlap the S2

Fig. 23 Patent ductus arteriosus. Continuous 'machinery' murmur.

a b

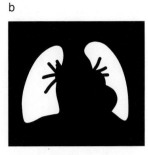

Fig. 24 Findings in pulmonary stenosis. (a) Phonocardiogram shows an ejection click and an ESM in the pulmonary area. (b) Chest X-ray film shows a prominent pulmonary conus and an uplifted apex caused by RV hypertrophy.

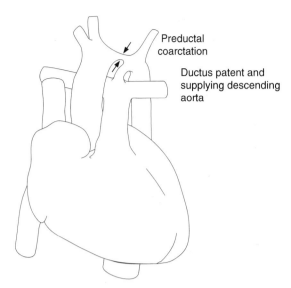

Preductal coarctation

Ductus patent and supplying descending aorta

Fig. 25 Coarctation of the aorta.

is best heard in the pulmonary area, radiating to the back (Fig. 24).

ECG. This shows RV hypertrophy.

Chest X-ray. A prominent pulmonary conus caused by post-stenotic dilatation and an uplifted apex owing to RV hypertrophy are observed.

Complications. PS is remarkably well tolerated and RHF is only seen in severe cases.

Management. Conservative pulmonary valvoplasty by balloon dilatation during cardiac catheter procedures is safe and effective. If necessary, this procedure may be repeated. Dysplastic valves and severe stenosis, especially if associated with calcification, require formal surgical pulmonary valvotomy. Pulmonary valve replacement is rarely necessary in children.

Pulmonary incompetence

Pulmonary incompetence (PI) may be associated with a dysplastic valve and is common after operations on the RV outflow tract. It is well tolerated and patients are generally asymptomatic. A 2–3/6 early diastolic, 'decrescendo' murmur heard in the pulmonary area and radiating down the LSE may be the only abnormality on examination.

Aortic stenosis

In the majority of patients, aortic stenosis (AS) is caused by fusion of the valvular cusps (valvular AS). Subvalvular (subaortic) stenosis is caused by a fibrous shelf below the valve. Supravalvular stenosis is the least common abnormality but may be associated with stenoses of other arteries and is a feature of Williams syndrome (mental retardation, elfin facies, hypercalcaemia). AS results in a restriction to forward blood flow into the aorta from the LV.

Symptoms. There may be no symptoms or exercise intolerance, dizzy spells and syncopal attacks, arrhythmias, angina, LV failure and sudden death.

Signs. The patient is pink, with a low volume pulse. A thrill is palpable in the suprasternal notch, and an LV impulse is present at the apex. The aortic A2 is loud. An opening ejection click is heard with valvular stenosis and may precede an ESM in the aortic area, upper right sternal edge (RSE) and neck.

ECG. This shows LV hypertrophy.

Chest X-ray. Films show a prominent aortic arch and cardiomegaly owing to LV hypertrophy.

Complications. These include angina, arrhythmias, LV failure and sudden death.

Management. Balloon valvoplasty is possible for moderate valvular stenosis. Surgery is required for dysplastic valves and aortic membranes.

Aortic incompetence

Aortic incompetence (AI) is usually associated with a dysplastic and stenotic valve. It produces a large end-systolic volume in the LV. In order to compensate for this extra load, the LV increases in size, producing a prominent apical impulse on examination.

The pulses are classically 'collapsing' in nature. A decrescendo early diastolic murmur is usually audible in the aortic area and along the LSE (i.e. radiates 'backwards' rather than up the aortic arch and into the neck).

Coarctation of the aorta

Coarctation of the aorta (CoA) is a narrowing in the form of a discrete 'shelf' or a long constriction (Fig. 25). The narrowing may occur before (preductal) or after (postductal) the site of origin of the ductus arteriosus. In 95% of patients, the coarctation is postductal, arising just beyond the origin of the left subclavian artery. This results in hypertension in both upper limbs. A preductal constriction preceding the origin of the left subclavian artery results in hypertension in the right upper limb alone. In children with untreated coarctation, collateral arteries generally develop by mid-childhood and augment the blood supply to the lower torso. Coarctation is often associated with a bicuspid aortic valve. It is the most common CHD in Turner syndrome.

Symptoms. In infancy, coarctation is usually preductal and the descending aorta is supplied by the PDA. When the PDA closes, these patients present in a critical condition with severe CCF and poor perfusion to the lower trunk and limbs. Older patients are asymptomatic or develop dyspnoea and weakness after exercise. Those with hypertension may present with headaches, fainting attacks and dizzy spells.

Signs. The pulses in the lower limbs are weak compared with the right (or both) upper limbs, and brachio-femoral difference/delay is present. The BP is raised in the upper limbs and decreased in the legs. The apical impulse may be forceful, but heart sounds are usually normal. A late systolic murmur at the upper LSE radiating to the back and neck is common. Additional, continuous murmurs over the upper back and axillae are produced by turbulence in the collateral vessels.

ECG. LV failure is a late sign.

Chest X-ray. Cardiomegaly and plethora are observed in neonates. Prestenotic dilatation of the arch and LV prominence are seen in older children. Rib notching between the 4th and 8th ribs posteriorly is caused by intercostal collaterals and is only evident in older children, aged 6–7 years or more.

Complications. Hypertension and LHF are common. Coarctation of the aorta is also associated with aneurysms of the descending aorta and collateral vessels. Associated intracranial aneurysms may bleed, producing subarachnoid haemorrhage.

Management. Medical treatment of hypertension is required. Mild lesions are amenable to balloon dilatation. The optimal age for corrective surgery is 2–4 years. Infants presenting acutely in a critical condition require emergency repair of the aorta. A discrete shelf can be excised and an end-to-end anastamosis performed in 40% of patients. Long segment lesions require complex operations involving an additional artificial patch or creation of a repair flap utilising the left subclavian artery.

Cyanotic congenital heart disease

Abnormal connections

Transposition of the great arteries

Transposition of the great arteries (TGA) is the most common cyanotic lesion in neonates. The aorta arises from the RV and the pulmonary artery from the LV. This results in two separate circulations 'in parallel', which is incompatible with life unless there is an additional right-to-left connection (Fig. 26). This is usually a PDA and/or a VSD.

Symptoms. The lesion results in severe cyanosis and tachypnoea in the newborn period. Closure of the PDA results in sudden collapse in those patients where the circulation is almost entirely dependent on the ductus arteriosus. Those with a large VSD are less cyanosed but CCF is now severe.

Signs. Neonates are usually ill and centrally cyanosed with a hyperdynamic precordium, a tachycardia and marked tachypnoea. The S2 is usually single as both the aortic and pulmonary valves close together. Murmurs are absent in those without a VSD.

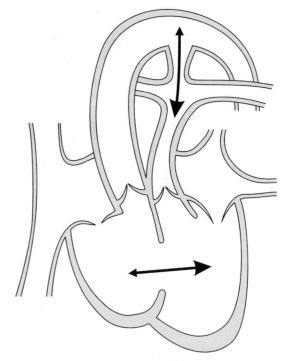

Fig. 26 Transposition of the great arteries. In this example there is mixing, predominantly right to left, at the ventricular level (via VSD) and through the patent ductus arteriosus.

ECG. This is normal or right-sided dominance (no VSD); RV and LV hypertrophy occur with VSD.

Chest X-ray. The film may be normal in the first few days of life or show moderate cardiomegaly and often narrow mediastinum because the aorta and pulmonary artery are lying alongside each other and not at 90° to one another (Fig. 27). This results in a bell-clapper or 'egg-on-side' appearance. Pulmonary plethora is present, especially in TGA with a VSD.

Complications. Patients with TGA are critically ill, in severe CCF and require urgent operative intervention.

Management. This lesion is usually duct dependent and patients are generally unwell at presentation. They require oxygen, urgent treatment for heart failure and prostaglandin E_2 by infusion in order to re-open the ductus. Perforation of the atrial septum by a Rashkind balloon septostomy allows mixing at atrial level and buys time before a definitive procedure is performed. Ideally, the great arteries (and coronaries) are reconnected to their appropriate ventricle ('switch operation'). This procedure is not possible after the first few months of life, when redirection of blood flow to the 'correct' ventricles can be established by means of an intra-atrial baffle or rerouting operation, based on the Mustard and Senning operations.

Total anomalous pulmonary venous drainage

Total anomalous pulmonary venous drainage (TAPVD) can be either supradiaphragmatic or infradiaphragmatic.

Supradiaphragmatic drainage. The pulmonary veins

a

b

Fig. 27 Chest radiograph in transposition of the great arteries. (a) In the absence of a VSD, there is cardiomegaly, a narrow mediastinum and mild pulmonary plethora. (b) With a VSD there is cardiomegaly, a narrow mediastinum and marked plethora.

a

b

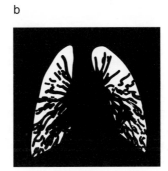

Fig. 28 Anomalous pulmonary venous drainage on chest X-ray film.
(a) Supradiaphragmatic drainage results in cardiomegaly with a wide mediastinum and moderate pulmonary plethora. (b) Infradiaphragmatic drainage results in a small heart, overexpanded lungs and marked pulmonary plethora.

(PV) do not connect with the left atrium (LA) and return to the RA directly or via large mediastinal veins. Breathlessness is associated with signs of high-output CCF. Murmurs are often absent. Venous return is not obstructed and the mediastinum is congested, casting a wide shadow on X-ray film (cottage loaf/snowman appearance) (Fig. 28a). The ECG shows R axis deviation and RV hypertrophy.

Infradiaphragmatic drainage. The PVs aggregate behind the LA and return to the RA via a circuitous route beneath the diaphragm, where they become obstructed. A patent foramen ovale is required to sustain life. Dyspnoea and recurrent chest infections are common symptoms, whereas cyanosis, tachypnoea, an RV heave and hepatomegaly are found on examination. Because of the obstructed venous return, the heart is small on X-ray film (Fig. 28b). Pulmonary congestion results in marked plethora.

Management. Treatment of CCF, followed by surgical repair of the aberrant veins is required.

Obstructive lesions

Tricuspid atresia

Tricuspid atresia (TA) prevents foward flow through the tricuspid valve and blood shunts right-to-left across the

foramen ovale/ASD. If present, a VSD allows blood to flow from LV to RV and into the lungs. In many patients, the circulation is maintained by the ductus arteriosus and closure of the ductus results in collapse. Cyanosis is associated with a PSM in those with a VSD. LV hypertrophy with left axis deviation (superior axis) on ECG is characteristic of TA.

Emergency re-opening of the ductus using prostaglandin precedes the insertion of a left–right shunt. The latter involves a prosthetic tube that connects the subclavian artery to the ipsilateral pulmonary artery (modified Blalock–Taussig shunt). This procedure may be repeated on the other side before a corrective operation is possible, e.g. RA connected to pulmonary artery via a conduit (Fontain procedure).

Pulmonary atresia

In pulmonary atresia (PA) the atretic pulmonary outflow tract prevents foward flow into the lungs, and pulmonary blood flow is sustained by a PDA or VSD. Infants without a VSD collapse as the PDA closes, or present with severe cyanosis, tachypnoea and single S2 owing to the absence of the pulmonary component. The heart size is variable and pulmonary oligaemia marked.

Patients with a VSD present with progressive cyanosis and breathlessness. Collateral vessels develop directly from the aorta (at systemic pressure) to supply

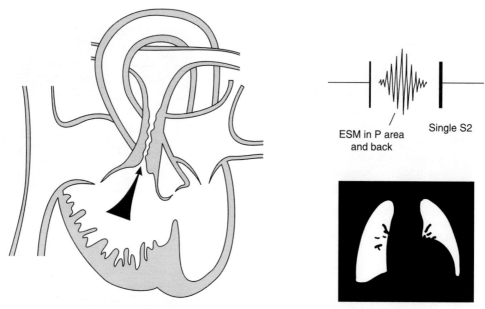

Fig. 29 Findings in Fallot tetralogy. (a) Phonocardiogram shows an ESM in the pulmonary area and a single S2. (b) Chest radiograph shows absent pulmonary conus, RV hypertrophy and oligaemia.

some parts of the lungs, resulting in patchy pulmonary congestion. Patients have signs of CCF and continuous murmurs over the back (owing to collateral vessels).

Management. Palliative Blalock–Taussig shunt(s) are necessary before a 'corrective' procedure (e.g Fontain operation) is feasible.

Hypoplastic left heart syndrome

Hypoplastic left heart syndrome is the most common cardiac cause of death in neonates. The main left pumping chamber is severely underdeveloped, resulting in CCF in the first few weeks of life. Until recently, this was a uniformly lethal condition, though a three-stage (Norwood) corrective procedure is showing promising results.

Complex congenital heart disease

Tetralogy of Fallot

Tetralogy of Fallot (TOF) is the commonest cyanotic CHD of childhood. It has four features:

- RV outflow tract (RVOT) obstruction
- RV hypertrophy (resulting from obstruction)
- a large VSD beneath the aortic outlet
- the aorta straddles both the left as well as the right ventricle (so called 'overriding' aorta).

As a result, desaturated blood entering the right heart is shunted back into the systemic circulation (i.e. right to left). Twenty per cent of patients with TOF have a right-sided aortic arch; a few may have complete absence of the pulmonary valve.

Symptoms. A common symptom is breathlessness on exertion. To obtain symptomatic relief when dyspnoea arises, infants and toddlers will lie down whereas older children assume a squatting position.

Paroxysmal hypercyanotic episodes ('blue spells') classically arise in young children aged 2 years or less, following defaecation, crying or feeding. They are characterised by increasing irritability, prolonged crying, rapid deep respiratory movements and a dramatic exacerbation of cyanosis.

Signs. Cyanosis may not be obvious at birth. At this age, the RV outflow obstruction is usually not severe and the RV is accustomed to dealing with relatively high pressures. Cyanosis becomes evident with increasing activity, often when crawling commences around 10 months of age. As a result of the progressive hypoxaemia, compensatory polycythaemia develops. An RV heave at the LSE and a systolic thrill at the upper LSE are felt in 50% of patients. The S2 is single since the pulmonary component is absent or faint. The loud ESM at the upper LSE arises through turbulence caused by the infundibular stenosis. During hypercyanotic spells, there is a significant increase in RVOT obstruction, blood flow through the outflow decreases and the murmur disappears. The large VSD produces little turbulence and, therefore, does not produce a murmur.

ECG. This shows right axis deviation and RV hypertrophy.

Chest X-ray. Films show a small pulmonary conus with RV hypertrophy; this results in a boot-shaped heart (*coeur en sabot*). In addition there is pulmonary oligaemia (Fig. 29).

Complications. Progressive cyanosis is associated with failure to thrive. Hypercyanotic spells may be associated with syncopal attacks. Cerebral ischaemia and thromboses usually occur in the first 2 years of life, whereas cerebral abscesses develop in older children. Bacterial endocarditis and CCF are rare.

Management. Attempts to improve weight gain are

essential. An adequate haemoglobin should be maintained, especially in those patients with severe cyanosis and those with hypercyanotic spells. The latter require emergency treatment. The child should be placed in a knee-to-chest position ('simulated squatting') and given oxygen. Intravenous morphine may reduce the RVOT obstruction and is the first drug of choice, followed by sodium bicarbonate and intravenous propranolol. These children should be maintained on regular oral propranolol until surgery. A palliative, Blalock–Taussig shunt improves pulmonary blood flow. It is employed in severely cyanosed infants aged less than 6 months, those who are medically unfit for a major procedure and those with hypercyanotic spells. The definitive repair involves total reconstruction of the RV outflow tract and closure of the VSD. It can be performed without a prior Blalock–Taussig shunt in relatively healthy infants aged more than 6 months and with favourable anatomy. Following a previous successful shunt, repair is usually carried out between the ages of 2–4 years. The operative mortality is about 5–10%.

Atrioventricular septal defect

In the atrioventricular septal defect (AVSD), the central portion of the heart (the 'endocardial cushion') fails to develop, resulting in a large defect straddling both the atria and ventricles and a single large (and incompetent) atrioventricular (A–V) valve. The predominant flow is from LV to RA and, therefore, back to the lungs (Fig. 30). Dyspnoea, CCF and failure to thrive are marked. A sys-

tolic thrill and PSM at the LSE are caused by A–V valve incompetence. The ECG reveals a superior axis and RV hypertrophy, whereas cardiomegaly and pulmonary plethora are seen on X-ray film. Pulmonary hypertension develops rapidly, and aggressive treatment of heart failure is necessary prior to surgical repair before 6–10 months of age. AVSD is classically associated with Down syndrome.

Summary

Table 23 on page 76 summarises the findings in cyanotic congenital heart disease.

4.4 Abnormalities of rhythm

An electrocardiogram is a recording of the electrical activity of the heart on a moving strip of paper. Abnormalities may be within normal variation or may be indicative of disease (Table 24).

Normal variations

Sinus arrhythmia. A normal accentuation of the heart rate with inspiration and the decrease with expiration.

Ectopic beats. These are common and disappear with exercise.

Bradycardias. Sinus bradycardia (<60 beats per

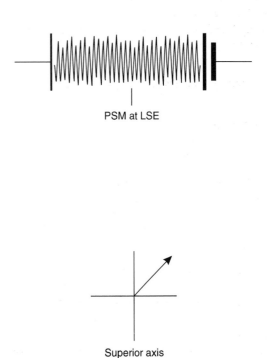

PSM at LSE

Superior axis

Fig. 30 Atrioventricular septal defect.

Table 23 Cyanotic CHD: clinical, ECG and chest X-ray findings

Lesion	Murmur	ECG	Chest X-ray
Presenting with CCF in the neonatal period			
Transposition of the great arteries (TGA) (with VSD)	PSM	RV + LV hypertrophy	Egg-shaped cardiomegaly, marked plethora
Pulmonary atresia (PA) (with VSD)	PSM	RV hypertrophy	Moderate cardiomegaly, moderate plethora
Total anomalous pulmonary venous drainage (TAPVD) (obstructed)	–	RV hypertrophy	Small heart, plethora
Hypoplastic right heart	–	RV hypertrophy	Cardiomegaly, plethora
Presenting without CCF in the neonatal period			
TGA (no VSD)	–	RV dominance	Egg-shaped cardiomegaly, moderate plethora
PA (no VSD)	–	LV dominance	Cardiomegaly, oligaemia
Tricuspid atresia (TA)	± PSM	Superior axis	Moderate cardiomegaly, oligaemia
Presenting with CCF in infancy			
Atrioventricular septal defect (AVSD)	PSM	RV hypertrophy, superior axis	Cardiomegaly, plethora
TAPVD (unobstructed)	–	RV hypertrophy	Cottage loaf cardiomegaly, plethora
Presenting without CCF in infancy			
Fallot's tetralogy	ESM	RV hypertrophy	Boot-shaped cardiomegaly, oligaemia

Table 24 Common ECG abnormalities

ECG finding	Diagnosis
Peaked p wave	Right atrial hypertrophy
Broad, notched p waves	Left atrial hypertrophy
Tall R in V_1, deep S in V_6, R axis deviation	Right ventricular hypertrophy
Tall R in V_6, deep S in V_1, L axis deviation	Left ventricular hypertrophy
Broad QRS (>0.1 s)	Bundle branch block
Flat QRS, T waves	Pericarditis
Long Q–T, depressed S–T, T wave	Hypokalaemia
Long P–R, wide QRS, peaked T wave	Hyperkalaemia
Long Q–T	Hypocalcaemia
Short Q–T	Hypercalcaemia
Bradycardia, small complexes, flat T wave	Hypothyroidism
Tachycardia, atrial fibrillation	Hyperthyroidism
Short Q–T, flat S–T, T waves, coupled beats	Digoxin toxicity

minute (bpm)) is a common finding in fit teenagers and during deep sleep.

Bradyarrhythmias

Heart block

First-degree block

In first-degree block the P–R interval is prolonged compared with the expected norm for age. Causes include TGA, Ebstein's anomaly, digitalis, myocarditis and rheumatic carditis.

Second-degree block

The occasional p wave is not conducted to the ventricle. This may be consistent (Mobitz type I) or associated with progressive lengthening of the P–R interval until an action potential is not conducted (Wenckebach phenomenon).

Third-degree block

Complete heart block occurs when there is no association between the atrial (p) waves and ventricular depolarisation (QRS). If the AV node takes over as the pacemaker, the heart rate is around 60 bpm and the QRS retains a normal appearance. With an alternative ventricular pacemaker, the heart rate is 40 bpm or less and the QRS is wide and bizarre in shape.

Bradycardias

Pathological bradycardias are associated with raised intracranial pressure (in conjunction with hypertension), hypothyroidism and occasionally myocarditis.

Tachyarrhythmias

Supraventricular tachyarrhythmias

Supraventricular tachycardia (SVT) involves a heart rate of about 180–300 bpm (Fig. 31). Patients may be asymptomatic, though they usually experience sweating, listlessness, lethargy, dizziness and may become short of breath during an attack. Older children may report palpitations. Severe episodes may precipitate heart failure.

The p waves are absent on the ECG but the QRS complexes appear normal (Fig. 32). SVTs result from an underlying Wolff–Parkinson–White syndrome (WPW) in 10% of patients and can only be diagnosed on a resting ECG. Abnormal conduction along an aberrant atrioventricular pathway bypasses the AV node and depolarises the ventricles earlier and via a different direction than the norm. This results in a shortened P–R interval (<0.12 s), an initial 'aberrant' depolarisation (producing the slurred δ wave), followed by normal

Fig. 31 ECG showing supraventricular tachycardia.

Fig. 32 The QRS complex; (a) Normal appearance; (b) in Wolff-Parkinson-White syndrome with a slurred δ wave and wide QRS.

Table 25 Symptoms and signs of cardiac failure

Symptoms	Signs
Poor feeding	Cold, clammy peripheries
Poor weight gain	Tachycardia
Cold sweats	Weak, thready pulse
Breathlessness	Gallop rhythm
	Tachypnoea
	Wheezes and crepitations
	Hepatomegaly
	Periorbital, pedal, sacral oedema

ventricular conduction (resulting in a QRS superimposed on the δ wave).

Control of the SVT may be achieved by increasing the vagal (parasympathetic) stimulation to the heart by carotid sinus massage, valsalva manoeuvre and, in infants, an ice pack applied to the face. Adenosine is effective but short acting. Digoxin and beta blockers may be necessary in refractory cases.

Ventricular tachycardia

Ventricular tachycardia (VT) is rare but may be associated with severe aortic stenosis and postcardiac arrest situations. VT results in a loss of cardiac output and necessitates emergency procedures to re-establish sinus rhythm, including intravenous lignocaine and cardioversion.

4.5 Heart failure and acquired cardiac disease

Congestive cardiac failure

Congestive cardiac failure (CCF) is a clinical syndrome in which the heart is unable to pump enough blood to meet the body's needs and is unable to 'clear' venous return. The symptoms and signs have already been discussed earlier in this chapter and are summarised in Table 25.

Diagnosis
ECG. There are no ECG changes diagnostic of CCF.

Chest X-ray. Cardiomegaly, with or without pulmonary plethora, is a cardinal feature of CCF on the chest X-ray film.

Echocardiogram. The echocardiogram uses ultrasound waves to investigate the action of the heart as it beats. It demonstrates dilatation of the ventricular chambers, poor contractility of the ventricular walls and a reduction in the volume of blood expelled with each contraction (i.e. the ejection fraction). The echocardiogram is also extremely useful in establishing the cause for the CCF (Box 9).

BOX 9
Causes of congestive heart failure

In neonates
Congenital heart disease: critical aortic stenosis; preductal coarctation; large VSD, PDA, AVSD; hypoplastic left heart; duct-dependent lesions, TGA
Arrhythmias: SVT
Systemic disease: septicaemia, severe anaemia

In infants
Congenital heart disease: VSD, AVSD, PDA
Myocarditis
Cardiomyopathy
Systemic disease: septicaemia, severe anaemia, hypoxia, acidosis

In children
Congenital heart disease: AS, PS, CoA, MS, PDA, VSD, TAPVD
Myocarditis
Cardiomyopathy
Hypertension
Systemic disease: septicaemia, severe anaemia, hypoxia, acidosis, hypertension, thyrotoxicosis

Abbreviations are defined in Table 22

General management

The patient should be propped upright and humidified oxygen delivered by face mask. Attention should be paid to ensuring an adequate calorie intake and avoidance of excess salt. An accurate fluid balance and daily measurement of body weight are mandatory. An underlying or exacerbating cause such as anaemia, infection, hypertension, arrhythmia and thyrotoxicosis should be treated.

Drug treatment

Diuretics. These alleviate cardiac failure by reducing fluid afterload on the heart. A loop diuretic, and in particular **frusemide**, is the drug of choice. They can be supplemented by an aldosterone antagonist (e.g. spironolactone) which is potassium saving.

Inotropic drugs. These improve cardiac contractility and function. Digitalis glycosides including digoxin are used, often with a diuretic, and should only be commenced after checking a baseline ECG and serum electrolytes. They can be administered intravenously in critically ill children but are best taken by mouth, when a loading dose is given over 12–18 hours, followed by a maintenance dose. A shortening of the Q–T interval and sagging of the S–T segment and T wave are often observed with therapeutic doses. Digoxin toxicity results in a prolongation of the P–R interval, sinus bradycardia, A–V block and supraventricular and, occasionally, ventricular ectopics, bigeminy and tachyarrhythmias. Toxicity is enhanced in patients with renal dysfunction, hypothyroidism, acidosis, severe hypoxia, hypokalaemia, hypercalcaemia and with verapamil and amiodarone.

Dopamine and dobutamine. These inotropic drugs are given by intravenous infusion in situations when cardiac function is severely compromised. Unlike dopamine, dobutamine is virtually cardioselective and does not compromise renal circulation and function when used in high doses.

Afterload reduction. This can be achieved by reducing the systemic vascular resistance by venous or arterial dilatation, or both. Venodilators including nitroglycerides and nitrates reduce venous congestion without improving cardiac contractility. Hydralazine acts by dilating the arteriolar bed and also produces a tachycardia. Enzyme inhibitors such as captopril reduce the systemic resistance by the inhibition of angiotensin II. Like hydralazine and combined venoarteriolar dilators (e.g. nitroprusside), it may cause hypotension.

Myocarditis

Myocarditis is rare but usually follows a viral infection, especially with coxsackievirus B. It is a manifestation of rheumatic fever, diphtheria and some drugs (e.g. cytotoxics). Children who develop myocarditis may have a preceding viral illness and then present with signs of congestive heart failure. Cardiomegaly, pulmonary plethora and occasionally bilateral pulmonary effusions are evident on a chest X-ray film. The ECG shows S–T segment and T wave depression.

Pericarditis

Pericarditis in childhood is related to either infection or chemicals and is associated with myocarditis. Patients often develop a fever, heart failure and retrosternal pain. The last is exacerbated on lying flat and improves on leaning forward, thereby allowing the chest cage to fall away from the inflamed pericardium. A 'scratching' friction rub may be audible on examination and, if a pericardial effusion is present, the heart sounds may appear muffled and distant. Pulsus paradoxus is detected on measuring the BP. 'Globular' cardiomegaly on the chest X-ray film is suggestive of an effusion, whereas low voltage complexes throughout and S–T elevation in the chest leads are typical ECG changes in this condition. Treatment should include adequate rest, oxygen, anti-inflammatory agents such as non-steroidal analgesics and steroids. Penicillin is added with rheumatic fever. Large effusions may cause acute heart failure ('tamponade') and require cardiocentesis.

Bacterial endocarditis

Bacterial endocarditis is inflammation of the lining of the heart cavity and valves. It can be acute or subacute.

Acute endocarditis

This is often caused by *Staphylococcus aureus* and occurs de novo in young infants with septicaemia but without pre-existing disease of the heart. The patients develop severe cardiac failure and the condition is fatal in more than 50% of patients.

Subacute endocarditis

Subacute endocarditis (SABE) occurs in children who have an underlying cardiovascular abnormality, usually comprising a structural defect with a significant pressure gradient within the heart. Although most children with congenital heart disease are at risk for SABE, this complication is particularly common in those with a VSD and aortic stenosis. Children with indwelling central venous catheters and intracardiac prosthetic materials are particularly at risk. Infection follows a bacteraemia, which may be triggered by dental or surgical procedures. In patients with dental caries, a bacteraemia may follow vigorous chewing or brushing of the teeth. Vegetations develop and may fragment, resulting in emboli travelling to the brain, spleen, kidneys and lungs. The causative organisms commonly include *Streptococcus viridans* (*albus*), β-haemolytic streptococci, *Staphylococcus aureus* and enterococci.

Clinical manifestations

The patient presents with a fever, anorexia and general malaise. Examination confirms a raised temperature, a 'new' or additional murmur, splenomegaly in 70% of patients and evidence of microembolic disease. The last includes skin petechiae and haematuria. Finger clubbing, tender spots on the ends of the fingers (Osler's nodes), haemorrhages over the palms and soles (Janeway lesions) and splinter haemorrhages are rare in children with SABE. Pulmonary and central nervous system emboli are usually seen in patients with left-sided cardiac lesions and those with cyanotic CHD.

Investigations

Confirmation of the organism is difficult and requires **repeated blood cultures**, e.g. four to six over the space of 24–48 hours. Arterial rather than venous cultures may provide a better yield. Echocardiography may confirm intracardiac and mural vegetations if >2 mm in diameter.

Management

Heart failure requires urgent treatment. Intravenous high-dose penicillin and gentamicin should be commenced, pending the results of blood cultures. Antibiotics are continued for 4 weeks and adjusted according to in vitro results on bacterial sensitivity. Antibiotic treatment is successful in 80–90% of all patients, though the prognosis varies with the infecting organism. Recovery occurs in 90% of patients with *Streptococcus viridans* infection and 50% with *Staphylococcus aureus* infection. Operative intervention may be required for infected prostheses.

Prevention of SABE

Good dental hygiene is of paramount importance. Anti-bacterial prophylaxis is required prior to all dental procedures, major surgery and surgery on the upper airways, and instrumentation of the gastrointestinal and genitourinary tracts. All patients with CHD are at risk of SABE, except those with a secundum ASD and successfully repaired ASD, PDA or VSD. At-risk patients should receive amoxycillin (or clindamycin if allergic to penicillin) 1 hour before the procedure. In addition, those with acquired valvular heart disease, hypertrophic cardiomyopathy, previous SABE and intracardiac prostheses are at particularly high risk of SABE and an aminoglycoside (usually gentamicin) is added to amoxycillin (altered to vancomycin if allergic to penicillin).

Self-assessment: questions

Multiple choice questions

1. The following describe the cardiac silhouette on X-ray:
   a. The right heart border is formed mainly by the right atrium
   b. The left border is formed mainly by the left atrium
   c. The left atrial appendage is prominent in children
   d. The thymic shadow may obscure the upper cardiac margins
   e. A right-sided aortic arch is always associated with other congenital heart defects

2. The following statements are correct:
   a. Breathlessness is a manifestation of left heart failure
   b. Infants with congestive cardiac failure become more breathless on crying
   c. Cyanosis decreases on crying
   d. A good indicator of central cyanosis in infants is circumoral cyanosis
   e. A liver that is palpable 1 cm below the costal margin suggests right heart failure

3. The following statements are true:
   a. Radio-femoral delay is a reliable sign of coarctation of the aorta in neonates
   b. A thrill is always indicative of a pathological murmur
   c. A parasternal lift suggests left ventricular hypertrophy
   d. A murmur originating from turbulence across the mitral valve is best heard at the left sternal edge
   e. The aortic component of the S2 follows the pulmonary component

4. The following statements are true:
   a. Congenital heart disease occurs approximately once in every 100 live births
   b. Ventricular septal defect is the most common cardiac lesion in Down syndrome
   c. Coarctation of the aorta may be associated with hypertension
   d. Pulmonary stenosis requires surgical repair in almost all patients
   e. The nitrogen washout test amounts to placing a child in 100% oxygen

5. The following congenital heart defects are examples of left-to-right shunts:
   a. Ventricular septal defect
   b. Tetralogy of Fallot
   c. Coarctation of the aorta
   d. Patent ductus arteriosus
   e. Aorto-pulmonary window

6. The following complications are associated with left-to-right shunts:
   a. Lower respiratory tract infections
   b. Bacterial endocarditis
   c. Central cyanosis
   d. Syncopal attacks
   e. Systemic hypertension

7. Congenital cardiac lesions that may result in failure to thrive include:
   a. Aortic stenosis
   b. Large ventricular septal defect
   c. Isolated, small muscular ventricular septal defect
   d. Atrial septal defects
   e. Moderate pulmonary stenosis

8. In congenital heart disease, poorly palpable femoral pulses may be caused by:
   a. Hypercyanotic spells
   b. Coarctation of the aorta
   c. Arteritis
   d. Patent ductus arteriosus
   e. Aortic stenosis

9. Blood flows predominantly from left to right in the following conditions:
   a. Atrial septal defect
   b. Fallot's tetralogy
   c. Ventricular septal defect
   d. Tricuspid atresia
   e. Duct-dependent congenital heart lesions

10. Common complications of Tetralogy of Fallot include:
    a. Failure to thrive
    b. Bacterial endocarditis
    c. Cerebral abcesses
    d. Cerebral thrombosis
    e. Congestive cardiac failure

11. Cyanotic conditions usually presenting with symptoms at birth include:
    a. Pulmonary stenosis
    b. Tetralogy of Fallot
    c. Transposition of the great arteries with pulmonary stenosis
    d. Pulmonary atresia
    e. Tricuspid atresia

12. The following operations may be used in cyanotic CHD:
    a. Senning procedure

b. Rashkind balloon septostomy
c. Aortic flap repair
d. Blalock–Taussig shunt
e. Fontain procedure

13. The following are serious abnormalities:
    a. Ventricular ectopics
    b. Sinus arrhythmia
    c. Atrial ectopic beats
    d. Complete A–V dissociation
    e. Bradycardia during sleep

14. Supraventricular tachycardia:
    a. Can cause CCF in utero, resulting in hydrops fetalis
    b. Usually produces a heart rate of 120 bpm
    c. Is not usually associated with any symptoms
    d. Is increased by parasympathetic stimulation
    e. Can be treated using digoxin and propranolol

15. The following associations are correct:
    a. Wide QRS and short P–R interval in Wolff–Parkinson–White syndrome
    b. Short Q–T, raised S–T in hypokalaemia
    c. Slow sinus rhythm and low voltage complexes with hypothyroidism
    d. Coupled beats, S–T and T wave depression with digoxin toxicity
    e. Short Q–T and hypocalcaemia

16. The following associations are correct:
    a. Progressive prolongation of the P–R interval in Wenckebach block
    b. Ventricular tachycardia and increased blood pressure
    c. Flat QRS and T waves with pericarditis
    d. Atrial fibrillation and hyperthyroidism
    e. Tall R wave in V_1, deep S in V_6 in left ventricular hypertrophy

17. Congestive cardiac failure (CCF) in childhood:
    a. Is rarely a manifestation of congenital heart disease
    b. Has particularly obvious symptoms during feeds in neonates
    c. Generally produces cardiomegaly and oligaemia as seen on the chest X-ray film
    d. May be the presenting abnormality in children with myocarditis
    e. Can be controlled with diuretics and digoxin in most cases

18. First-line agents in the management of CCF include:
    a. Frusemide (furosemide)
    b. Oxygen
    c. Morphine

d. Propranolol
e. Digoxin

19. Myocardial damage is associated with the following:
    a. Coxsackievirus B infection
    b. Beta-haemolytic streptococcal infection
    c. Uraemia
    d. Diphtheria
    e. Cytotoxic agents, especially anthracyclines

20. The manifestations of a pericardial effusion include:
    a. Pulmonary plethora on chest X-ray
    b. A fall in the jugular venous pressure on inspiration
    c. Pulsatile, tender hepatomegaly
    d. Pedal oedema but no ascites
    e. Globular cardiomegaly on chest X-ray

Case histories

Case history 1

A 9-month-old infant presents with lethargy and failure to thrive. He had been admitted twice in the previous 3 months with chest infections. His mother had not noted any colour changes but was certain she could feel a 'vibration' beneath the chest wall.

How would you proceed to establish a diagnosis?

Case history 2

An infant was well for the first 7 days of life after which he became acutely unwell. He refused all feeds, was listless and breathless. On examination he was poorly perfused, tachycardic and tachypnoeic. A blood gas taken with the child in 100% oxygen showed a PO_2 of 4.5 kPa.

How would you manage this child?

Case history 3

A 5-year-old girl known to have a small VSD, presents with fever of 10 days' duration. On examination she appears unwell and pale. Pedal oedema, a 3/6 pansystolic murmur heard best at the lower left sternal edge and basal pulmonary crepitations are detected. The splenic tip is just palpable.

What is the most likely diagnosis and how would you investigate this child?

Case history 4

A 2-year-old girl, previously operated on for Fallot's tetralogy when 10 days old, presents to the local district general hospital. You note a history of progressive lethargy over the past few weeks as well as episodic attacks involving facial pallor and diminished exercise tolerance. The little girl looks cyanosed, has a left-sided intercostal scar and a loud ejection systolic murmur in the pulmonary area.

1. What additional questions would you ask her parents?
2. What additional steps may you take to obtain further information?
3. What operation was performed on day 10 of life?

You organise some tests, which show a haemoglobin of 16.5 g/dl, haematocrit of 57%, oxygen saturation of 82% in air and marked oligaemia on the chest X-ray film.

4. What is the explanation for these results?

You admit the child for observation. During the next 24 hours the nurses reported that she remained lively although she frequently became more 'blue' and had to stop and lie down whilst playing. On one occasion she became very pale and drowsy but responded to loud vocal stimulation.

5. What clinical complication should be considered at this point?
6. What is the physiological explanation for the intermittent decrease in oxygen saturations?
7. Why does the patient lie down whilst playing?
8. What further investigation is indicated?

You have organised transfer to the tertiary centre for next week but are called to see the child as an emergency on the second night. You find that she is unrousable, extremely pale, with weak pulses and no audible murmurs.

9. What is the explanation for this acute deterioration?
10. What action would you take?

Short notes

Write short notes on the following:

1. Criteria to decide whether a heart murmur is likely to be functional (innocent) or related to an underlying structural abnormality
2. The natural history of a moderately sized ventricular septal defect that is left unrepaired
3. The management of heart failure
4. The causes of cardiomyopathy.

Viva voce question

What is the rationale for antibiotics as prophylaxis against bacterial endocarditis in children with congenital heart disease?

Self-assessment: answers

Multiple choice answers

1. a. **True**. The right atrial border with a short section of superior vena cava above and inferior vena cava below.
    b. **False**. It is the left ventricle.
    c. **False**. This is inconspicuous in children.
    d. **True**. Classically it appears as an overlying 'sail' shadow.
    e. **False**. This can be associated with CHD (e.g. Fallot's tetralogy) but is also a normal variant.

2. a. **True**. Other symptoms are lethargy, excessive sweating and poor feeding.
    b. **True**. Crying, like feeding, increases the work of the heart.
    c. **False**. Cyanosis, like breathlessness, increases on crying.
    d. **False**. Central cyanosis is manifest by a bluish discoloration of the lips and mucous membranes.
    e. **False**. This is a common finding in normal children.

3. a. **False**. Brachial rather than radial artery should be used. In neonates, the heart rate is too rapid to detect 'delay' and a difference in pulse volume and BP is more important.
    b. **True**. Innocent murmurs are not accompanied by a thrill.
    c. **False**. It suggests right ventricular hypertrophy.
    d. **False**. Mitral murmurs are best heard over the apical impulse.
    e. **False**. Closure of the pulmonary valve is delayed compared with the aortic valve so that A2 preceeds P2.

4. a. **True**. It is roughly 8 in 1000 live births.
    b. **False**. Atrioventricular septal defects (AVSD).
    c. **True**. It affects both limbs or the right upper limb.
    d. **False**. Many are mild requiring no intervention; the majority can be improved by balloon valvoplasty.
    e. **True**. Nitrogen is effectively 'washed out' in an environment consisting of 100% oxygen.

5. a. **True**. Blood flows from left to right ventricle.
    b. **False**. Right-to-left flow, resulting in cyanosis.
    c. **False**. No shunt present with simple coarctation.
    d. **True**.
    e. **True**. This is a connection between the aorta and pulmonary trunk.

6. a. **True**. Infections occur secondary to increased pulmonary plethora.
    b. **True**. Endocarditis may complicate VSDs where left-to-right shunts exist.
    c. **False**. Central cyanosis is associated with right-to-left shunt.
    d. **False**. Right-to-left shunts and arrhythmias give rise to syncopal attacks.
    e. **False**. Though pulmonary hypertension is a late feature of severe left-to-right shunting.

7. a. **False**. Aortic stenosis is asymptomatic or presents with exercise intolerance, arrhythmias and, occasionally, sudden death.
    b. **True**. Large VSDs present with heart failure in infancy resulting in failure to thrive.
    c. **False**. It only occurs with large, multiple lesions.
    d. **False**. ASDs generally produce minimal haemodynamic constraints on the heart and are, therefore, not usually associated with failure to thrive.
    e. **False**. Though it may occur with critical pulmonary stenosis.

8. a. **True**. In Tetralogy of Fallot.
    b. **True**. This is the classical association.
    c. **True**. Arteritis involving the lower aorta and distal branches will result in poorly palpable femoral pulses.
    d. **False**. PDA gives rise to bounding pulses.
    e. **False**. Femoral pulses are generally palpable with aortic stenosis.

9. a. **True**. Almost always occurs.
    b. **False**. This is a cyanotic condition: therefore, deoxygenated blood must bypass the lungs by shunting right to left across the VSD.
    c. **True**. Except if pulmonary hypertension develops with shunt reversal (Eisenmenger syndrome).
    d. **False**. This is cyanotic CHD.
    e. **False**. These are cyanotic conditions with right-to-left shunting at atrial level (tricuspid, pulmonary atresia) or ventricular level (TGA).

10. a. **True**. As with most cyanotic conditions.
    b. **True**. Occurs in unoperated patients on the right ventricular infundibulum or valves; after correction, patients will require antibiotic prophylaxis for dental and certain surgical procedures.
    c. **True**. From septic emboli secondary to endocarditis.
    d. **True**. Secondary to polycythaemia.
    e. **False**. Heart failure is not usually a feature of Tetralogy of Fallot.

11. a. **False**. This is an acyanotic condition.
    b. **False**. These develop symptoms later in life.
    c. **True**. This presents with cyanosis, heart failure and sudden collapse in the newborn period.
    d. **True**. Presents with cyanosis in the newborn.
    e. **True**. Presents with cyanosis in the newborn.

12. a. **True**. For transposition of the great arteries.
    b. **True**. It is used for duct-dependent lesions.
    c. **False**. This is used to repair coarctation.
    d. **True**. This improves blood flow to the lungs.
    e. **True**. This connects the right atrium to the pulmonary arteries.

13. a. **True**. Ventricular ectopics, especially when they occur in runs, are associated with significantly decreased cardiac output.
    b. **False**. This is a normal finding.
    c. **False**. Atrial ectopics are usually isolated phenomena and are not associated with altered cardiac function.
    d. **True**. This is third-degree heart block.
    e. **False**. This is a normal finding.

14. a. **True**. It is a relatively common cause of hydrops fetalis.
    b. **False**. The heart rate is more than 180 bpm.
    c. **False**. Symptoms include breathlessness, tiredness, syncope, palpitations.
    d. **False**. This will slow an SVT.
    e. **True**. As well as verapamil and flecainide.

15. a. **True**. Together with a delta wave, these are classical features of the WPW syndrome.
    b. **False**. Long Q–T and depressed S–T occur in hyperkalaemia.
    c. **True**. Classical ECG findings in hypothyroidism.
    d. **True**. As well as other dysrrhythmias.
    e. **False**. Hypocalcaemia is associated with a long Q–T.

16. a. **True**. In Wenckebach secondary block, the P–R interval increases progressively until a QRS potential does not materialise and a beat is dropped.
    b. **False**. There is a loss in cardiac output and BP falls.
    c. **True**. Small voltage complexes are typical of pericarditis.
    d. **True**. Hyperthyroidism is associated with rapid arrhythmias including atrial fibrillation.
    e. **False**. These occur in RV hypertrophy; LV hypertrophy produces tall R in V_6 (>20 mm), deep S in V_1 (>20 mm).

17. a. **False**. CCF is common in many cyanotic, duct-dependent conditions and those involving an excessive left-to-right shunt (e.g. VSD).
    b. **True**. This is when they are required to exert maximum effort.
    c. **False**. It produces cardiomegaly and pulmonary plethora.
    d. **True**. Sometimes with associated arrhythmias.
    e. **True**. Though angiotensin-converting enzyme (ACE) inhibitors may be used as well.

18. a. **True**. Frusemide primarily reduces afterload on the heart.
    b. **True**.
    c. **False**. However, it may be used with caution in those in severe distress (NB: it may cause respiratory depression).
    d. **False**. It may precipitate CCF.
    e. **True**. Although still available, its use in childhood is becoming less popular.

19. a. **True**. The virus causes infective myocarditis.
    b. **True**. It gives rise to rheumatic fever.
    c. **True**. This causes chemical myocarditis.
    d. **True**. Toxic myocardiopathy occurs in 15% of patients with diphtheria and is responsible for around 55% of deaths, usually because of secondary arrhythmias.
    e. **True**. Anthracyclines (e.g. doxorubicin, daunorubicin) can result in dose-dependent myocardial damage, loss of myocardial cells and progressive cardiomyopathy.

20. a. **True**. Plethora is secondary to restriction to venous return from the lungs.
    b. **False**. There is a rise in the JVP on inspiration.
    c. **True**. It is caused by restriction to venous return and subsequent venous congestion in the lower body.
    d. **False**. Both pedal oedema and ascites occur.
    e. **True**. Uniform cardiomegaly is typical of a pericardial effusion on X-ray.

Case history answers

Case history 1

The history is suggestive of an acyanotic congenital cardiac defect that is associated with increased pulmonary blood flow and a significant left-to-right shunt. The first stage would be to complete a thorough history and examination, concentrating on symptoms and signs of heart failure and looking for bounding pulses, precordial heaves, a thrill, murmur, pulmonary crepitations and hepatomegaly. An ECG should be ordered to look for signs of ventricular hypertrophy, and a chest X-ray to establish whether the child has cardiomegaly and pulmonary plethora. A provisional diagnosis can now be made. This should be confirmed by echocardiography, which should reveal both the structural abnormality and the extent of the intracardiac shunt. Further information regarding the abnormality and shunt, as well as intracardiac pressures and oxygen saturation can be ascertained during cardiac angiography, using catheter techniques. The last is particulary useful when investigating a patient prior to the consideration for corrective cardiac surgery.

Case history 2

The history is highly suggestive of a duct-dependent congenital heart condition; the collapse has been precipitated by closure of the ductus arteriosus resulting in cyanosis and serious compromise of the cardiac output. The possible diagnoses at this age would include transposition of the great arteries, tricuspid and pulmonary atresias and complex congenital heart disease.

Regardless of the diagnosis, the infant is severely hypoxic and shocked. Therefore, the management should include resuscitation with oxygen and fluids in order to re-establish a reasonable BP. An attempt should be made to re-open the duct with prostaglandin E_2 and respiratory support should be considered. An ECG and chest X-ray should be ordered, a referral to a paediatric cardiac centre organised and arrangements made for an urgent echocardiogram.

Case history 3

This child has probably developed subacute bacterial endocarditis. Embolic signs of SABE including lesions on the hands (splinter haemorrhages, Janeway spots), retina (Roth spots) and kidneys (haematuria) should be looked for. She requires immediate admission to hospital, treatment of the heart failure and urgent investigation. It is important to confirm the microbiological diagnosis and repeated blood cultures should be taken, preferably during a temperature 'spike'. Arterial rather than venous samples are more likely to provide positive cultures. An ECG is required to exclude associated arrhythmias, a chest X-ray to assess cardiomegaly and plethora, and an echocardiogram to look for intracardiac vegetations, assess cardiac damage (e.g. heart valves) and ventricular function.

Case history 4

1. You need to know whether she has had any faints or squats while playing. You require the precise details of the original operation. You need to know if she is on any regular medication. You require details of the tertiary cardiac centre, her consultant, etc.
2. Contact the tertiary centre for all relevant details.
3. A left sided Blalock–Taussig (B–T) shunt.
4. Progressive hypoxia has resulted in a compensatory increase in circulating red cells, resulting in polycythaemia with an increased haemoglobin. The X-ray examination confirms poor blood flow into the lungs, suggesting that the

patient is outgrowing her palliative B–T shunt, which is no longer adequate.
5. The patient is having hypercyanotic spells.
6. Progressive right ventricular outlet tract (RVOT) obstruction has resulted in right ventricular hypertrophy and a progressive rise in RV pressure. Eventually the RV pressure has equalled, and later surpassed, the LV pressure and blood is now shunting from right to left across the ventricular septal defect (VSD) along the reversed pressure gradient. As a consequence, deoxygenated blood is passing directly into the systemic circulation and bypassing the lungs. Acute exacerbations in the RVOT obstruction lead to sudden cyanotic spells, which manifest as acute pallor/dusky attacks.
7. Hypercyanotic spells are associated with profound hypoxia, which prohibits physical exertion. In some cases, the situation is severe enough to result in syncope. Squatting or lying down increases the systemic vascular resistance and, therefore, increases the LV pressure. This action also decreases venous return to the right heart and, in so doing, may decrease the shunt across the VSD and reduce the degree of cyanosis.
8. This story should prompt a further re-evaluation of the patient with an echocardiography and, possibly, cardiac angiography with a view to planning an urgent corrective surgical procedure.
9. Total obstruction of the RVOT has resulted in no blood flow across the pulmonary infundibulum and valvular area and, hence, the disappearance of the murmur. This has led to profound hypoxia, culminating in syncope.
10. Such severe attacks may be aborted with intravenous morphine and propranolol, which reduce the muscular obstruction in the RVOT. The patient should be given oxygen, stabilised and urgently transfered to the tertiary centre.

Short notes answers

1. The criteria can be divided into the following areas.
   History. An innocent murmur would have complete absence of symptoms. Symptoms indicative of an abnormality include:

   - breathlessness
   - excessive fatigue, malaise
   - poor exercise tolerance, poor feeding
   - colour changes
   - recurrent chest infections
   - failure to thrive
   - palpitations.

   Examination. In an innocent murmur there would be no clinical signs apart from the murmur. The murmur:

- would be systolic, normal heart sounds
- would be soft, occasionally shrill; never >3/6; no thrill
- would have little radiation
- would be heard over precordium and/or neck (not back)
- changes with position of the head and neck
- decreases on lying down and with pressure on the ipsilateral jugular vein
- may be exacerbated by exertion.

Investigations. ECG, chest X-ray, echocardiogram examinations are all normal in an innocent murmur.

Follow-up. No abnormal symptoms/signs develop. The murmur often disappears with time.

2. A moderate VSD is associated with a left-to-right shunt. This increases pulmonary blood flow. If unrepaired, this results in the establishment of pulmonary arterial hypertension over a period of years. During this time, the child is likely to develop several lower respiratory tract infections and worsening heart failure. The excessive energy expenditure in maintaining cardiac output results in failure to thrive. Depending on the severity of the shunt, irreversible pulmonary hypertension will develop by the second or third decade of life. This will eventually lead to systemic and suprasystemic pressures in the right ventricle and the left-to-right shunt reverses (Eisenmenger syndrome). The patient would become cyanosed and the condition is no longer operable. Death from pulmonary hypertension and heart failure is inevitable.

3. The management of cardiac failure includes the following (NB: measures appropriate to an intensive setting are shown in italics):

General advice

- improve calorie intake
- avoid excessive salt in diet
- sit/sleep upright
- treat infections.

Improve oxygenation

- correct anaemia
- *give oxygen.*

Inotropic support

- digoxin
- *dopamine, dobutamine.*

Load reduction

- diuretics: frusemide (furosemide), spironolactone
- vasodilators: hydralazine, *nitrates, nitroprusside.*

4. The causes of cardiomyopathy include:

- idiopathic
- postinfection (especially viral)
- drugs (e.g. cytotoxics)
- inborn errors of metabolism (e.g. glycogen storage disease).

Viva voce answer

Children with a structural abnormality of the heart, an endocardial scar or intracardiac prosthetic material are at risk of developing bacterial overgrowth at the abnormal site. This takes the form of adherent vegetations, which may result in local damage and valvular dysfunction and carries the risk of distant embolic disease. The risk of bacterial organisms 'lodging' onto these sites is particularly great during a bacteraemic episode. Therefore, any procedure known to result in bacteraemia, such as dental procedures, gastrointestinal, urogenital and other surgical procedures, should be covered with antibiotics. In so doing, organisms released into the circulation are killed before establishing a focus of endocarditis. The organisms involved are usually staphylococcal, streptococcal and coliform species and, therefore, prophylaxis generally involves a penicillin and an aminoglycoside.

The digestive system

Key points

You should know about:

- The common symptoms of gastrointestinal disease in childhood, its pathogenesis and management
- The presentations of common infections of the gastrointestinal tract
- Assessment for dehydration in a child with diarrhoea and how to carry out rehydration
- Chronic gastrointestinal disorders that can lead to malabsorption and failure to thrive.
- Infections that can affect the liver

5.1 Introduction

Normal features and assessment

The normal function of the gastrointestinal tract is dependent on the balance achieved by the normal motility of the gut, the sphincter tone, exocrine secretion, integrity of the absorptive surfaces and humoral control. These functions begin in utero when amniotic fluid is swallowed by the fetus. The gut undergoes rapid maturation at birth as it adjusts to the onset of intermittent oral feeding and colonisation by microflora. The coordinated swallowing movements develop in the first couple of months and the infant begins to show an interest in solid foods at about 4 months. The earliest stools after birth consist of meconium. As the baby begins to feed, green-brown transition stools replace meconium. Subsequently, there can be a wide variation in the consistency and frequency of the stools, in part influenced by the kind of food and milk being ingested. A protuberant abdomen is common in infants and toddlers and is related to the lordotic stance adopted at that age. It is common to find a palpable liver (up to 2 cm) and a soft spleen tip. Since the abdominal musculature is underdeveloped at this age, the vertebral column and abdominal aortic pulsations are easily felt. It is also normal to be able to feel stools in the left lower quadrant in the descending and sigmoid colon.

Examination of the gastrointestinal tract

In the examination of the gastrointestinal tract in children, it is important to look for systemic signs of dysfunction. These include anaemia, jaundice, clubbing, dependent oedema, distended veins and state of hydration. Remove all clothes so that the pelvic region is clearly visible, otherwise you can easily miss torsion of the testis or an incarcerated hernia! Inspection of the abdomen is often a clue to the presence of organ enlargement or a mass, with the umbilicus often pushed away from the distending mass. A child's abdomen is soft, and vigorous palpation can miss a soft but enlarged liver or spleen. It is better to start palpating

with the edge of the index finger, lower down in the right inguinal fossa and dipping the extended fingers during expiration. Children do not localise pain very well and careful examination is required to identify regions of tenderness or guarding. Hernial orifices, the scrotum and anal regions must be examined and, when required, a per rectal examination is performed.

5.2 Abdominal pain

Acute abdominal pain

In children, the acute abdomen is a common problem. A carefully elicited history and physical examination is often sufficient to distinguish surgical from medical conditions. Most of the conditions mentioned in Figure 33 are described elsewhere in the book and will not be discussed further.

Recurrent abdominal pain

Recurrent abdominal pain is a common problem affecting 10% of children. No cause is found in 90% of children and in the rest a urinary bacterial infection or constipation is often the cause. It is essential to identify those with an organic condition promptly. This enables specific management of physical disease and confident counselling of those with a functional problem. In most cases, a careful history and examination may arrive at a diagnosis. The periodicity of the complaint, localisation of pain to the periumbilical or hypochondrial regions, absence of coexistent symptoms and intervening good health suggest the absence of an organic cause. Usually a blood count and urinalysis are sufficient in the way of investigation. Those with more severe symptoms should be seen during an attack and may require further investigations, as outlined in Table 26.

5.3 Vomiting

Vomiting is a common symptom of childhood. While the cause is often benign, it can cause a great deal of distress. The aetiology is age related. Healthy infants often **posset** or regurgitate feeds. This may happen many times a day and the infant is usually content though possibly hungry. This may be quite distressing to the parent, as apart from all other considerations, it makes all the clothes and furniture smell of vomit. Vomiting is coordinated by the medullary vomiting centre, which is influenced by the chemoreceptor trigger zone and higher CNS centres. Therefore, many systemic conditions may precipitate vomiting. These include causes of raised intracranial pressure, inborn errors of metabolism, systemic acidosis, medications and chemotherapy. Infections, either systemic or localised (otitis media, cystitis), can also present initially with vomiting. The com-

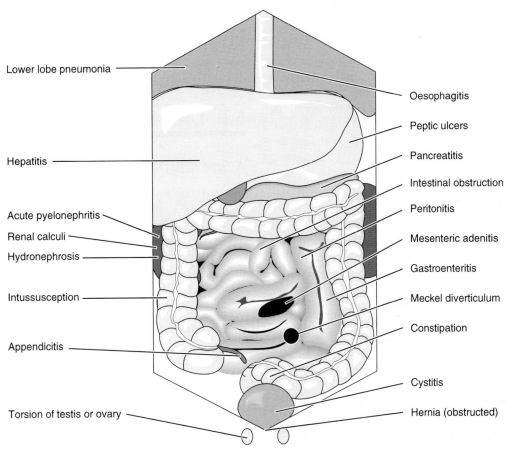

Lower lobe pneumonia

Hepatitis

Acute pyelonephritis

Renal calculi

Hydronephrosis

Intussusception

Appendicitis

Torsion of testis or ovary

Oesophagitis

Peptic ulcers

Pancreatitis

Intestinal obstruction

Peritonitis

Mesenteric adenitis

Gastroenteritis

Meckel diverticulum

Constipation

Cystitis

Hernia (obstructed)

Fig. 33 Causes of acute abdominal pain.

Table 26 Causes of recurrent abdominal pain in children

Disorder	Characteristics	Identifying features
Lactose intolerance	Bloating, flatulence, diarrhoea	Lactose breath hydrogen test, reducing substances in stool
Parasite infection	Diarrhoea, bloating	Stool evaluation, test for *giardia* sp.
Excessive fructose or sorbitol ingestion	Bloating, diarrhoea	Large intake of fruit, fruit juices or sorbitol-containing sweets
Hernia	Dull abdominal wall pain	Physical examination, computed tomography (CT) scan
Cholecystitis	Right upper quadrant pain	Ultrasound of the abdomen
Cholelithiasis	May worsen with meals	Ultrasound of the abdomen
Pancreatitis	Persistent boring pain, may radiate to the back	Serum amylase, lipase, ultrasound
Acid peptic disease	Pain related to meals relieved with antacids	Endoscopy, upper GI contrast X-rays, pH study
Abdominal migraine	Nausea, family history	History
Abdominal epilepsy	May have prodrome	EEG
Acute intermittent porphyria	Severe pain precipitated by drugs, infection, fasting	Urine porphyrins
Lead poisoning	Constipation, anaemia	Serum lead level, haemoglobin
Henoch Schönlein purpura	Systemic symptoms	Clinical diagnosis, urinalysis
Sickle crisis	Anaemia	Haematological evaluation
Gilbert syndrome	Jaundice	Serum bilirubin
Diabetic ketoacidosis	Acidosis, dehydration	Blood sugar, ketones

mon gastrointestinal causes of vomiting include infections, obstruction or motility problems.

Gastro-oesophageal reflux

When the lower oesophageal sphincter is not competent, excessive and passive reflux of the gastric contents may cause significant symptoms. Vomiting or regurgitation has its onset usually within the first week of life and abates by the age of 2 years as the child attains a more upright posture. Bleeding from the associated oesophagitis results in iron-deficiency anaemia and, rarely, haematemesis. Aspiration pneumonia occurs in infancy and can lead to chronic coughing, wheezing and recurrent pneumonia in childhood. In mild cases, a diagnosis is often made by a response to therapy. More complex cases are confirmed by barium oesophagography under fluoroscopic control, endoscopy, gastric scintiscans or by continuous monitoring of the distal oesophagus pH. In most children, simple measures are often effective. Appropriate management includes increased time spent in a baby chair, nursing in the prone position with the head-end elevated, thickening of feeds, antacids, addition of an alginate preparation (e.g. Gaviscon), prokinetic agents (e.g. cisapride) and, if indicated by pH studies, a histamine H_2 receptor antagonist or omeprazole. Where there is danger of an oesophageal stricture forming, surgical intervention in the form of a fundoplication may be necessary.

5.4 Constipation

The definition of constipation is relative. Many children may only have a soft stool once every 2–3 days, which is passed without difficulty. Only when the stool is hard and there is difficulty in passing the stool should a diagnosis of constipation be made. A nursing infant may have infrequent stools. True constipation in the neonatal period is usually secondary to Hirschsprung disease, neurological or spinal disease, intestinal obstruction, drugs or hypothyroidism. In the majority of children, constipation is functional in origin. Ineffective colonic peristalsis, also seen with opiate use and hypothyroidism, will result in defective rectal filling. The resultant stasis leads to the excessive drying of stool and a failure to initiate reflexes from the rectum that normally trigger evacuation. This process is controlled by pressor receptors in the rectal muscles. Consequently, disorders of the spine and of the nerves and muscles that coordinate the action of the rectal muscles and control the anal sphincter may contribute to faecal retention. Constipation tends to be self-perpetuating. Hard and large stools in the rectum become more painful and difficult to evacuate especially if compounded by the presence of an anal fissure. Distension of the rectum and colon decreases the sensitivity of the defecation reflex and the effectiveness of peristalsis. Finally, watery colonic contents may percolate around hard stool and be passed unperceived by the child. This involuntary **encopresis** or soiling may be mistaken for diarrhoea. While constipation by itself causes no long-term systemic effects, it can have a marked emotional effect on the family. In those with functional problems, treatment is divided into four phases: education about the problem; disimpaction, usually with a phosphate enema or stool softeners; prevention of re-accumulation of stools, usually achieved with dietary control and laxatives; and recon-

ditioning to normal bowel habits. The last may have to wait until an anal fissure has healed and needs to be positively reinforced by using star charts or small rewards.

5.5 Diarrhoea

Acute diarrhoea

Acute diarrhoeal illnesses superimposed on malnutrition lead to 10 million to 15 million deaths annually in children worldwide. In the developed world, gastroenteritis is common and usually mild but should not be underestimated. The common aetiological agents and their basic pathogenetic mechanisms are described in Table 27. The mechanisms of diarrhoea differ with the infective agent. The organism may:

- invade the mucosa causing inflammation of the lamina
- produce cytotoxins that disrupt cell function and protein synthesis
- secrete an enterotoxin that alters cellular salt and water balance yet leaves the cell morphology undisturbed
- adhere to the mucosal surface disrupting normal cell function.

About 75% of fluid ingested, which includes the gastric, pancreaticobiliary and intestinal secretions, is reabsorbed by the small intestine and about 24% by the large intestine. Primary absorption of water in the small intestine is done in the **tip** cells of the microvilli. This is an active process using sodium–glucose and sodium–amino acid transporters. Sodium and chloride ions are exchanged actively for hydrogen and bicarbonate ions, maintaining both electroneutrality and pH homeostasis. An active intracellular pump then pumps the excess sodium into the blood stream and the chloride back into the lumen.

Osmotic diarrhoea
As shown in Figure 34 rotavirus invades and destroys the mature villi tip cells. This leads to an increased migration of immature cells from the crypt that are unable to carry on the absorptive process and an **osmotic** diarrhoea results. The cells are restored in 48–72 hours and the diarrhoea resolves. Pathogens like *Giardia* and enteroadhesive *Escherichia coli* can adhere to the brush border, blunting the microvilli and decreasing their absorptive capacity, while invasive pathogens can destroy the villi cells causing an inflammatory exudate.

Secretory diarrhoea
Secretory diarrhoeas occur with enterotoxin-producing organisms. Figure 34 illustrates the binding of cholera

Table 27 Infective causes of acute diarrhoea in childhood

Pathogen	Enterotoxin	Cytotoxin	Invasive	Adhesive	Symptoms	Antimicrobial therapy[a]
Escherichia coli						
Enterotoxicogenic	ST, LT			+	WD	
Enteropathogenic					WD	cotrimoxazole
Enteroinvasive			+++		D	
Enterohaemorrhagic		+++			D	
Enteroadhesive				+++	WD	
Shigella species	Shiga		+++		WD, D	cotrimoxazole, ciprofloxacin
Salmonella species	+	+	++		WD, D	chloramphenicol, cefotaxime
Vibrio cholerae	A and B				WD	doxycycline
Campylobacter jejuni	+		++		WD, D	erythromycin, ciprofloxacin
Clostridium difficile	A and B		++		PMC	metronidazole, vancomycin
Rotavirus		Cytotoxic			WD	–
Entamoeba histolytica			+++		D	metronidazole
Giardia lamblia				+++		metronidazole
Cryptosporidium sp.	?	Cytotoxic				paromomycin[b]

ST, stable toxin; LT, labile toxin; WD, watery diarrhoea; D, blood and mucus, dysentery; PMC, pseudomembranous colitis, bloody diarrhoea, usually antibiotic related.
[a]Only some of the antibiotics that can be used are mentioned. In most instances there are specific indications for using antibiotics, e.g. injudicious use of antibiotics in *Salmonella* infections may actually prolong excretion.
[b]Only for use in those with AIDS.

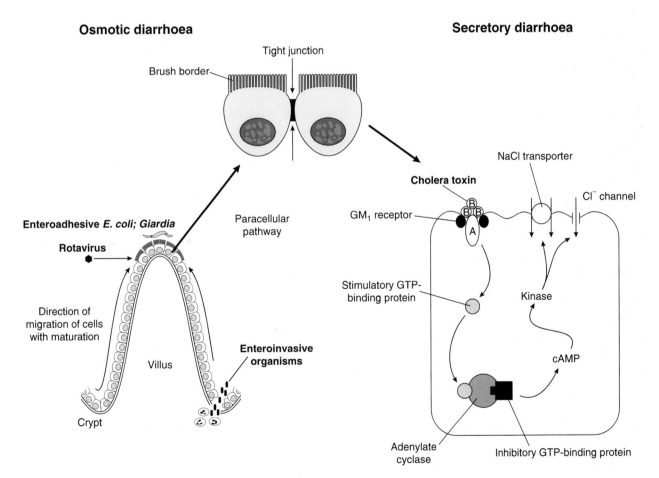

Fig. 34 Mechanisms of acute diarrhoea.

toxin subunit B to the glycolipid (GM₁) receptor. Subunit A penetrates the cell and by increasing cyclic AMP (cAMP), inhibits the sodium/chloride ion pump and stimulates the chloride channel. Since water follows the sodium ion gradient, this results in secretion of water and electrolytes into the intestinal lumen. The toxins produced by enterotoxicogenic *E. coli* behave in a similar fashion.

Table 28 Assessment of dehydration

	Dehydration (loss in body weight, %)		
	Mild (<5%)	Moderate (5–9%)	Severe (>10%)
Heart rate	Normal	Increased	Tachycardia
Blood pressure	Normal	Normal or reduced	Greatly reduced
Skin	Normal	Decreased turgor	Decreased turgor
Fontanelle	Normal	Normal	Sunken
Mucous membrane	Slightly dry	Dry	Dry
Extremities	Perfused	Delayed capillary refill	Cool, mottled
Mental status	Normal	Normal or lethargic	Lethargy, coma
Urine output	Slightly decreased	Decreased	Absent
Thirst	Slightly increased	Increased	Greatly increased

Table 29 Oral rehydration therapy

Composition	UK (mmol/l)	World Health Organization (mmol/l)
Sodium ions	30–50	90
Potassium ions	20	20
Chloride ions	30–50	80
Citrate	10	10
Glucose	200	100
Osmolality	200–265	310

Site of action

In general, enterotoxin-producing agents infect the small intestine, invasive and cytotoxin-producing organisms favour the large intestine while those with enteroadhesive function are seen at both sites.

Dehydration

The result of any of these mechanisms is the net loss of fluid and electrolytes from the body; which is more severe in secretory diarrhoeas. It can place a severe stress in infants who have a higher percentage of body water, a higher metabolic rate and a larger surface-to-volume ratio. The assessment of dehydration relies upon a series of clinical signs that reflect changes in body tissues and circulatory status (Table 28).

In general, mild and moderate dehydration can be corrected using oral rehydration solutions, which contain glucose or sucrose with sodium chloride. Malnourished children often have chronic deficits of electrolytes and depleted energy reserves. The WHO ORS (oral rehydration solution), therefore, has a significantly higher electrolyte content that the solutions commonly used in the UK (Table 29). The solutions vary in composition and often come as powders that require re-constitution. In such cases, careful instructions must be given to the parents to ensure that the solution is made up as recommended. Where such commercial formulations are not available, cheap local ingredients such as boiled rice water with added salt (to taste as salty as tears) can be used. The deficit is generally given over a 4–6 hour period and at that time gradual re-introduction of normal diet can be started, while still providing replacement fluids. In some cases of moderate dehydration and in those with severe dehydration, it is best to use intravenous rehydration. Where the child is in shock, 10–20% of the deficit may be replaced by bolus infusion of crystalloid or colloid solutions. Acidosis may accompany dehydration and while rehydration will correct this to an extent, if it is severe enough to cause air hunger, sodium bicarbonate can be added to the infusion. Serum electrolytes need to be monitored, as dehydration can be associated with hypo- and hypernatraemia. Antibiotics are used only in specific instances (e.g. *Vibrio cholerae*) and **anti-diarrhoeal and anti-emetic agents are not recommended**. In most cases, early feeding will actually enhance the ability of the intestine to regenerate and there is little to recommend the use of dilute or low-lactose-containing formulae on a routine basis to 'decrease the osmotic load'.

Chronic diarrhoea

Persistent diarrhoea in an otherwise thriving child is not an unusual complaint. This so-called **toddler's diarrhoea** occurs between 1 and 5 years of age. Typically, watery stools are produced four to ten times a day and the stool often contains undigested food particles. The child remains otherwise well. The most likely explanation for this is an exaggerated gastrocolic reflex. Therapy is directed at reassuring anxious parents, decreasing the amount of fluid and fruit juice ingested and increasing the fibre and fat content of the diet.

Post-infectious diarrhoea

Post-infectious diarrhoea is caused by brush border damage. This leads to secondary, reversible disaccharidase deficiencies and diarrhoea persists because of secondary cow's milk or lactose intolerance. This may be aggravated in children allergic to cow's milk protein or soy protein substitutes, which are often used in such cases. A change to more easily tolerated foods (such as starch-based compounds) is all that is usually required. Rarely some children may have congenital lactase or sucrase–isomaltase deficiency or galactose–glucose malabsorption; these are characterised by diarrhoea from birth and the children will require life-long abstinence from foods containing the offending sugars.

5.6 Genetic/inflammatory disorders

There are several gastrointestinal disorders of uncertain aetiology that may involve a genetic susceptibility and immune-mediated pathogenesis.

Gluten-sensitive enteropathy (coeliac disease)

Gluten-sensitive enteropathy or coeliac disease (CD) is a permanent inability to tolerate dietary wheat or rye gluten. The incidence is 1 in 2000 in the UK and as high as 1 in 300 in west Ireland; susceptibility is probably inherited. However, the wide range of phenotype from active to silent disease suggests that early dietary and environmental factors play a role as well. CD is an immunologically mediated small-intestinal enteropathy that results in progressive flattening of the villi and malabsorption. The majority of children present before the age of 2 years, with progressive growth failure dating from the time gluten-containing solids were introduced into the diet. Symptoms include greasy, bulky, foul-smelling stools and vomiting. The child becomes irritable, anorexic, anaemic and hypotonic, with a pro-tuberant abdomen. The condition is suspected by the presence of anaemia, which may be microcytic or macrocytic because of iron and folate deficiencies as well as the presence of antigliadin and endomysial antibodies in the serum. Confirmation of the diagnosis is by an intestinal biopsy (Fig. 35) and the therapeutic response to a gluten-free diet. The therapy is with-drawal of wheat, rye, oats and barley, as these contain gluten, and the introduction of rice and maize-based cereals. While some children will tolerate gluten in their diet at a later age, there is concern that those who are not on a gluten-free diet are at an increased risk of developing small bowel malignancies. Dietary restric-tions are, therefore, best recommended lifelong,

Fig. 35 Radiographic position and Crosby capsule for jejunal biopsy.

though compliance may be an issue in the turbulent teens.

Crohn's disease (regional enteritis)

While the aetiology of Crohn's disease remains unknown, there has been a dramatic increase in its prevalence with approximately 10–20 per 100 000 children affected in the UK. While a genetic predisposition is likely, current research is focused around abnormalities in the intestinal mucosal immune system, which is thought to be dysregulated by the faecal stream. The initial lesion is a localised ulcer over a lymphoid follicle. These ulcers then coalesce and inflammation spreads to deeper tissue. Characteristically, there is segmental involvement with 'skip areas' and the bowel wall becomes thickened. Loops of bowel may become adherent and fistulae can develop and progress into chronic abscesses. Later in the course of the disease, deep fissures may form, leading to the classic 'cobblestone' appearance of the mucosa as well as the development of strictures. In children, 50–60% have involvement of the terminal ileum and variable segments of the colon, 30–35% have small bowel involvement only and approximately 10–15% have disease limited to the large bowel. The onset is often insidious and subtle and may lead to a considerable delay in diagnosis. While the manifestations depend on the site of involvement, periumbilical colicky **abdominal pain**, **diarrhoea** with or without blood and **growth failure** are the most common forms of presentation. The intestinal inflammation leads to abdominal pain and diarrhoea, often with rectal bleeding. Diffuse mucosal involvement will result in a protein-losing enteropathy, malabsorption and malnutrition. Occasionally more subtle manifestations such as oropharyngeal disease, perianal skin tags or fissuring may be presenting features. In approximately a quarter of children, extraintestinal manifestations of Crohn's disease and inflammatory bowel disease in general are present. These include intermittent pyrexia, anaemia, arthralgia, uveitis, finger clubbing, and skin manifestations such as erythema nodosum and pyoderma gangrenosum. The clinical diagnosis is confirmed on contrast radiography (Fig. 36) and a mucosal biopsy performed after direct endoscopic visualisation. The presence of skip lesions with narrowing of the lumen and thickening and fissuring (rose-thorn ulcers) of the bowel wall seen on a barium meal are highly suggestive of Crohn's disease. There is currently no cure for Crohn's disease and it follows a waxing–waning course. The goal of therapy is to induce and maintain a remission of active disease and also to correct malnutrition and promote growth. Energetic nutritional programmes based on elemental diets correct the growth failure and induce remission of active disease. Apart from psychosocial and nutritional support, drugs such as corticosteroids, 5-aminosalicylates, metronidazole and immunomodulatory agents are often used for

Fig. 36 Cobblestone appearance of the small intestine on barium radiography in Crohn's disease.

acute episodes. Ultimately, the majority of children will require surgery to deal with complications such as strictures and fistulae.

Ulcerative colitis

As with Crohn's disease, the aetiology of ulcerative colitis remains unknown, though the incidence of disease has not changed appreciably. Current hypotheses include a genetic predisposition with an altered immunological response within the intestinal mucosa. Unlike Crohn's disease, the inflammation is continuous and is usually restricted to the colonic mucosa. Macroscopically, the mucosa is friable and granular and ulceration may be present in association with a bloody mucopurulent exudate. The ulceration is often patchy and may be interspersed with areas of regenerating epithelium, resulting in a pseudopolyp formation. Pancolitis is most common (62%) while disease of the left colon (22%) or rectum (15%) occurs less often. Occasionally there is an inflammatory reaction in the distal ileum, called 'backwash ileitis'. The most common presenting symptom, therefore, is **diarrhoea** mixed with **mucus** and **blood** and accompanied by tenesmus and abdominal pain. Attacks are graded as mild, moderate or severe depending on the stool frequency, abdominal tenderness, fever and the degree of anaemia and hypoalbuminaemia. In 5–10%, the disease may present with fulminating colitis and toxic megacolon. On examination, the only positive findings may be minimal abdominal tenderness, although in severe disease the child may be pyrexial, dehydrated, anaemic and profoundly toxic. Growth retardation is seen in only 20% of those with ulcerative colitis, though other extraintestinal manifestations seen in Crohn's disease are also features of ulcerative colitis. Table 30 lists the common distinguishing features between Crohn's disease and ulcerative colitis. Investigations should include an abdominal roentgenogram to exclude a toxic megacolon (Fig. 37), and stool cultures for infective agents that may mimic ulcerative colitis (e.g. *Shigella, Salmonella* and *Campylobacter* species). Colonoscopy with multiple mucosal biopsy is required to confirm the diagnosis. Childhood disease tends to run a more complicated course than that in adults, with an increased likelihood of pancolonic involvement, proximal extension of initially localised disease and colectomy. Mild disease can often be kept under control with sulfasalazine. Acute attacks are treated with topical corticosteroid preparations, including enemas, foams or suppositories. More extensive disease requires oral or systemic corticosteroids under careful supervision. Extensive refractory colitis may be an indication for immunosuppressant therapy with azathioprine or cyclosporin A. Some children may ultimately require a restorative proctocolectomy with an ileal reservoir.

5.7 Disorders of the liver, pancreas and peritoneum

Infectious hepatitis

An increasing number of hepatotropic viruses are being identified using advanced molecular techniques (Table 31). Many other viruses, such as herpes simplex, cytomegalovirus (CMV), Epstein–Barr virus (EBV), HIV, varicella, enteroviruses, adenovirus and arboviruses can also cause hepatitis as a component of multisystemic disease.

In general, children infected with hepatitis viruses are usually asymptomatic or anicteric. Infection is recognised by the detection of viral antibodies in the serum at a later date. Symptomatic children present with nausea

Table 30 Comparison of Crohn's disease and ulcerative colitis

Characteristic	Crohn's disease	Ulcerative colitis
Rectal bleeding	Occasional	Common
Abdominal mass	Common	Not present
Rectal disease	Occasional	Nearly universal
Ileal involvement	Common	Occasional (backwash ileitis)
Perianal disease	Common	Unusual
Strictures	Common	Unusual
Fistulae	Common	Unusual
Skip lesions	Common	Unusual
Transmural involvement	Common	Unusual
Crypt abscesses	Unusual	Common
Granulomas	Common	Unusual
Risk for colonic cancer	Slightly increased	Greatly increased

Fig. 37 Plain X-ray of the abdomen showing a toxic megacolon in a patient with ulcerative colitis.

Table 31 Hepatic viruses

Virus	Classification	Transmission	Chronicity	Vaccine	Interferon therapy
A (HAV)	Picornavirus	Faeco–oral	No	Yes	No
B (HBV)	Hepadnavirus	Parenteral, perinatal, sexual	Common	Yes	Yes
C (HCV)	Flavivirus-like	Parenteral, rarely perinatal and sexual	Common	No	Yes
D (HDV)[a]	Satellite virus	Parenteral, perinatal, rarely sexual	Common	No	Yes
E (HEV)	Calcivirus	Faeco–oral	No	No	No
F (HFV)	?HBV	?	?	No	No
G (HGV)A–C	Flavivirus-like	Parenteral	Probably	No	No

[a]only occurs with HBV infection.

and vomiting; on examination they are found to be icteric with a tender, enlarged liver. Elevated liver enzymes and serum bilirubin and detection of viral antigen, RNA or antibody confirm the diagnosis. In most cases, supportive care is all that is required (i.e. hydration and analgesia) as the infection runs its course. However, in some children the disease is complicated by acute liver failure. This is characterised by encephalopathy and coagulopathy and fulminant liver failure may ensue. Such critically ill children often have multiorgan failure and require management in an intensive-care unit. The degree of clinical symptoms is a reflection of the intensity of the immune response to the virus. In HBV infection, those with clinical hepatitis usually clear the virus. Carrier status is more commonly seen in younger children, who often have subclinical or anicteric hepatitis.

Chronic hepatitis

Chronic hepatitis is a continuing inflammatory disorder of the liver with a potential to progress to cirrhosis, continue unchanged or resolve with or without treatment. The disease entity is arbitrarily defined into three major pathological categories: chronic persistent, chronic active and the rarer chronic lobular hepatitis. The aetiology includes viral infections (HBV, HCV), autoimmune disease, Wilson's disease, drugs and inflammatory bowel disease. Percutaneous liver biopsy is essential to differentiate between the various conditions. Chronic active hepatitis tends to progress towards cirrhosis and, if associated with HBV infection, carries the risk of hepatocellular carcinoma. Immunosuppressant therapy can provide symptomatic relief and delay the onset of cirrhosis in those with autoimmune chronic hepatitis and α-interferon has been used with a degree of success in chronic carriers of HBV and HCV.

Wilson's disease (hepatolenticular degeneration)

Wilson's disease is an autosomal recessive condition characterised by a defect in the transport and storage of copper. Excess copper is not excreted by the biliary system nor taken up by the copper transport protein caeruloplasmin but is deposited into the tissues instead. Progressive liver damage ensues. Subsequently, with deposition of copper in the basal ganglia, extrapyramidal symptoms may appear and a Kayser–Fleischer ring is seen in the cornea, along with sunflower cataracts. Renal tubular damage and haemolytic anaemia may further complicate matters. Investigations include plasma caeruloplasmin levels (usually low), liver biopsy with copper estimation, and studies of urinary copper excretion. Early diagnosis before irreversible tissue damage occurs allows for a good response to treatment with penicillamine. Genetic counselling and screening should be offered to all siblings.

Cirrhosis

Cirrhosis is the irreversible end stage of liver injury. Pathologically, structurally abnormal nodules surrounded by prominent fibrous tissue replace the liver architecture, and the diagnosis can, therefore, only be confirmed on biopsy. The clinical features are those of chronic hepatocellular failure and portal hypertension. The liver is usually small (enlarged in biliary cirrhosis) and the spleen is often palpable. Collateral veins may be present on the abdomen, with portal blood being deviated via the paraumbilical veins to the umbilicus and radiating from the umbilicus to the systemic circulation. Jaundice and ascites may also be present. Cutaneous features include spider angiomata (naevi), palmar erythema and clubbing. Those with compensated cirrhosis may be asymptomatic. Signs of decompensation include the development of dependent oedema, ascites, hepatic encephalopathy, septicaemia and/or peritonitis and alimentary bleeding from oesophageal or rectal varices secondary to portal hypertension. An aetiological diagnosis must be sought and the histological diagnosis confirmed. Treatment is supportive. Nutritional supplementation should take into account fat malabsorption and resultant vitamin A, D, K and E deficiency. In end-stage cirrhosis, only a liver transplant will be of long-term benefit.

Portal hypertension

Portal hypertension usually presents with intestinal bleeding and splenomegaly. The majority of cases are caused by thrombosis of the portal vein (extrahepatic), either idiopathic or secondary to sepsis of the umbilical vein and portal system in infancy. Hepatic cirrhosis and congenital hepatic fibrosis may also cause portal hypertension. The exact cause needs to be established by selective angiography of the coeliac axis and a liver biopsy. In portal venous thrombosis, long-term management is conservative for as long as possible with ligation of varices where necessary. There is a tendency for bleeding from oesophageal varices to improve with age. Splenorenal shunts are technically difficult and rarely successful before the age of 10 years.

Reye syndrome

Reye syndrome is a relatively rare, heterogeneous condition characterised by an acute derangement of liver and brain function. The principal abnormality is a severe self-limiting disturbance of the hepatic mitochondrial architecture with decreased mitochondrial enzyme activity lasting up to 6 days. The reasons for the mitochondrial dysfunction are unknown. However, the use of aspirin and viral infections have been causally linked. It seems prudent, therefore, to avoid the use of aspirin in children with viral infections. The clinical picture is characterised by refractory vomiting, reduced consciousness and convulsions. Low blood glucose, elevated plasma ammonia, high liver transaminases and prolonged coagulation are the hallmarks of the condition. Management must be within an intensive-care unit with facilities for ventilation and control of raised intracranial pressure. Reye syndrome is associated with a high mortality rate and many survivors are handicapped for life.

Pancreatitis

Viral infections, drugs, biliary microlithiasis and blunt abdominal injuries account for the majority of acute pancreatitis seen in children. It is characterised by abdominal pain, persistent vomiting and fever. The pain is epigastric and does not always radiate to the back. The abdomen may be distended and quite tender and a mass (pancreatic pseudocyst) may be palpable. Diagnosis is based on ultrasonography and raised serum amylase and lipase. Medical management aims to restore fluid–electrolyte homeostasis and relieve pain. The prognosis is excellent in uncomplicated cases but poor in those with acute haemorrhagic pancreatitis.

Peritonitis

Peritonitis can be a result of infectious, autoimmune, chemical or neoplastic processes. Infectious peritonitis is either primary or secondary in origin. Primary peritonitis tends to occur in children with ascites resulting from either nephrotic syndrome or cirrhosis. The causative agents are often encapsulated bacteria such as pneumococci and *Haemophilus influenzae*. The onset may be sudden or insidious and is characterised by fever, abdominal pain and a toxic appearance. Abdominal palpation may reveal rebound tenderness and rigidity with absent bowel sounds. When in doubt, the diagnosis needs to be confirmed by paracentesis and culture of the peritoneal fluid. In primary peritonitis, only a single organism should be isolated. The presence of multiple organisms is suggestive of secondary peritonitis and is an indication for a laparotomy to localise a possible intestinal perforation. The management is primarily antibiotics, fluids and bowel rest (nil orally, nasogastric drainage). Surgery is only required for those in whom a perforated viscus is suspected.

Self-assessment: questions

Multiple choice questions

1. The following describe dental caries:
   a. The commonest site is in the occlusal surfaces of the incisor teeth
   b. Bottle feeds can cause caries of the neck of the teeth
   c. Patients with xerostomia are at a higher risk
   d. Decreasing the frequency rather than the amount of carbohydrate ingested is more important in prevention
   e. It may be prevented by drinking tea

2. Ulceration of the buccal mucosa is classically seen in:
   a. Vincent angina
   b. Herpes simplex infection
   c. Herpangina
   d. Oral candidiasis
   e. Prodromal measles

3. A 4-month-old infant presents with recurrent chest infections and failure to thrive. The possible diagnoses are:
   a. Cricopharyngeal incoordination
   b. Achalasia cardia
   c. Gastro-oesophageal reflux
   d. Tracheoesophageal fistula
   e. Coeliac disease

4. With regard to intestinal polyps:
   a. The majority can be detected on per rectal examination
   b. The commonest presentation is painless rectal bleeding
   c. The polyps seen in Peutz–Jegher syndrome are premalignant
   d. The polyps seen in Gardner syndrome are benign
   e. Non-familial juvenile colonic polyps usually occur as solitary lesions

5. The following are causes of secretory diarrhoea:
   a. *Vibrio cholerae*
   b. Neuroblastoma
   c. Enteropathogenic *Escherichia coli*
   d. Rotavirus
   e. Coeliac disease

6. Features of Crohn's disease include:
   a. Abdominal mass
   b. Non-caseating granulomas
   c. Crypt abscesses
   d. Strictures
   e. Increased risk of colonic cancer

7. Features of ulcerative colitis include:
   a. Rectal bleeding
   b. Abdominal mass
   c. Fistulae
   d. Increased risk of colonic cancer
   e. Involvement of the terminal ileum

8. A 6-year-old child presents with painful, bloody mucus diarrhoea and has bilateral swollen tender knee joints. The differential diagnoses include:
   a. Shigellosis
   b. Ulcerative colitis
   c. Tuberculosis
   d. Crohn's disease
   e. *Campylobacter* infection

9. The following describe hepatic viruses:
   a. B and D are parenterally transmitted
   b. A, C and E are primarily enterally transmitted
   c. B, C, and D can cause chronic infections
   d. B, C and D are associated with an increased risk of hepatocellular cancer
   e. D can only occur in the presence of infection with B

10. With regard to the digestion of carbohydrates:
    a. Disaccharidases are located on the intestinal brush border
    b. Sucrose intolerance is detected by testing the stool with a Clinitest tablet
    c. Monosaccharides are directly absorbed in the duodenum
    d. Disaccharide intolerance is a component of toddler's diarrhoea
    e. Salivary and pancreatic amylases break down starch to glucose and maltose

11. In normal digestive function:
    a. Iron is converted to the ferric form in the stomach
    b. The soluble iron compound is mainly absorbed passively in the duodenum
    c. Malabsorption of D-xylose suggests a proximal intestinal mucosal lesion
    d. Calcium is absorbed actively in the lower intestine
    e. The hormone secretin stimulates secretion of pancreatic enzymes

12. The following describe lipid absorption:
    a. It is dependent on the presence of bile salts
    b. Digestion of triglycerides by lipase begins in the duodenum
    c. Chylomicron formation facilitates absorption by the villi

    d. Medium-chain fatty acids are directly absorbed in the stomach

    e. Unused bile salts are excreted, imparting to the faeces their characteristic colour

13. Complications of the short bowel syndrome include:
    a. Megaloblastic anaemia
    b. Ileal bacterial overgrowth
    c. Gastric hypersecretion
    d. Failure to thrive
    e. Osmotic diarrhoea

Case histories

Case history 1

> A 5-year-old boy is brought to you with a history of three episodes of bloody stools, a month apart.

Discuss your approach to making a diagnosis in this patient.

Case history 2

> A 2-year-old girl presents with a history of passing 10–15 watery stools and has vomited at least four times in the last 24 hours. She appears distressed but otherwise cooperative and drinks thirstily from a glass of fruit juice but then vomits. The nurse informs you that her pulse is 96 beats/minute, temperature 37.9°C and blood pressure 100/60 mmHg.

Discuss the management of this child.

Case history 3

> While on night rounds, you see a child newly diagnosed with ulcerative colitis admitted for colonoscopy the following morning. The parents draw you aside and say that while their son has responded well to the treatment they are unsure of the prognosis.

Explain how you will proceed to tackle this situation.

Short notes

Write short notes on short bowel syndrome.

Self-assessment: answers

Multiple choice answers

1. a. **False**. It usually occurs on the occlusal surfaces of the molar teeth.
   b. **True**. It is also called nursing bottle caries.
   c. **True**. Saliva helps keep the teeth clean!
   d. **True**. Starts at 3–4 months and stops by 2 years.
   e. **True**. Tea contains 100 ppm fluoride, an anti-caries agent.

2. a. **True**.
   b. **True**. It is caused by anaerobic infection of the gingival tissues.
   c. **True**. The causative agent is coxsackievirus A.
   d. **False**. It causes 'thrush', small white flecks.
   e. **False**. Measles causes an enanthem, sandy, grainy flecks on the buccal mucosa called Koplik spots.

3. a. **True**. This is an oesophageal motility disorder that presents with symptoms similar to gastro-oesophageal reflux.
   b. **True**. This is an oesophageal motility disorder with obstruction occurring at the gastro-oesophageal junction.
   c. **True**. The acid contents of the stomach are aspirated into the lungs.
   d. **True**. Only the H type will present at this age.
   e. **False**. Failure to thrive occurs later as gluten-containing solids are introduced and respiratory disease is not a feature.

4. a. **True**.
   b. **True**. Mostly seen during or immediately after a bowel movement.
   c. **False**. This is an autosomal dominant condition with mucocutaneous pigmentation and polyposis. While the polyps themselves are not premalignant, there is an increased risk of intestinal or extraintestinal cancer.
   d. **False**. This is an autosomal dominant condition with multiple intestinal polyps and tumours of the soft tissue and bone, pigmented fundi and extracolonic cancers. The intestinal polyps are premalignant.
   e. **True**. More than half of the children affected have more than one polyp, though multiple polyps are rare.

5. a. **True**. It produces a secretory toxin.
   b. **True**. It is caused by production of vasoactive intestinal peptide (VIP).
   c. **False**. Enterotoxicogenic *E. coli* produces secretory diarrhoea via ST and LT toxins.

d. **False**. Rotavirus produces osmotic diarrhoea.
   e. **False**. Diarrhoea results from malabsorption.

6. a. **True**. Mass results from inflammation and formation of adhesions.
   b. **True**.
   c. **False**. This is a feature of ulcerative colitis.
   d. **True**. Transmural inflammation leads to partial small-bowel obstruction.
   e. **True**. As in all inflammatory bowel disease.

7. a. **True**. Bleeding is often from localised rectal ulceration (proctitis).
   b. **False**. This is a feature of Crohn's disease.
   c. **False**. This is a feature of Crohn's disease.
   d. **True**. This is a feature of all inflammatory bowel disease.
   e. **False**. This is a feature of a Crohn's disease.

8. a. **True**. It is also known as Reiter syndrome.
   b. **True**. Arthritis may become chronic in nature.
   c. **False**. While tuberculous intestinal ulcerations can occur and so can arthritis, they do not occur together.
   d. **True**. Usually pauciarticular with occasional spondylitis.
   e. **True**. It can cause a reactive, self-limiting arthritis.

9. a. **True**.
   b. **False**. C is parenterally transmitted.
   c. **True**.
   d. **False**. While D can only exist in the presence of B, it does not in itself increase the chance of hepatocellular carcinoma.
   e. **True**. D is an incomplete RNA or satellite virus.

10. a. **True**. They occur in the 'tip' cells located on the top of the microvilli.
    b. **False**. Clinitest only detects reducing sugars; sucrose needs to be hydrolysed to be detected by this method (Clinistix method).
    c. **True**. Since they do not need to be broken down.
    d. **False**. This is a probably a motility disorder.
    e. **True**. Glucose is absorbed and maltose is further hydrolysed by glucosidase.

11. a. **False**. It is converted into the soluble ferrous form.
    b. **False**. It is actively absorbed.
    c. **True**. It is a pentose that is minimally metabolised and is almost entirely absorbed by the upper small intestine.

d. **False**. Active absorption occurs in the upper small intestine.

e. **False**. It stimulates secretion of bicarbonate ions and pancreatic fluid.

12. a. **True**. Bile salts form micelles with lipids ensuring the efficient transportation of their hydrolysed products to the absorptive epithelium.

b. **True**. This lipase is secreted by the pancreas into the duodenum.

c. **True**. Chylomicron contains a complex of triglycerides and cholesterol that can be directly transported into the lymph.

d. **False**. Medium-chain triglycerides do not require emulsification or micelle formation and are directly absorbed in the small intestine.

e. **False**. Bile salts are mainly absorbed (enterohepatic circulation); bile pigments provide the characteristic colour.

13. a. **True**. It is caused by folate malabsorption.

b. **True**. This results from stasis.

c. **True**. Hypergastrinaemia occurs but is usually not a clinical problem.

d. **True**. Failure to thrive is caused by a combination of chronic diarrhoea and malabsorption.

e. **True**. The inability to absorb normally secreted intestinal contents through loss of absorptive surface results in osmotic diarrhoea.

Case history answers

Case history 1

In this child we can exclude a bacterial enteritis as this presents acutely. An intussusception is unlikely to be recurrent. There are several possible conditions.

Anal fissure. Is there a history of constipation? Is defecation painful? Is there an anal tag and is an anal fissure visible on inspection? Does the blood coat an otherwise normal stool?

Colonic polyps. Is there a family history of similar problems or bowel cancer (familial polyposis syndrome)? Is there unusual pigmentation of the skin (Peutz–Jegher and Gardner syndrome)? In the majority, a rectal examination is sufficient to detect a polyp, though fibreoptic colonoscopy must be performed to look for other polyps.

Inflammatory bowel disease. Usually ulcerative colitis presents with blood and mucus in the stools. The diagnosis is based on history and confirmed on colonoscopic biopsy.

Meckel diverticulum. This is discussed in Chapter 12.

Henoch–Schönlein purpura. This is discussed in Chapter 11.

Sexual abuse. This is obviously a diagnosis of exclusion. Clues are provided by bruising and tearing around the anal sphincter and the presence of any form of sexually transmitted disease.

Case history 2

The child has mild-to-moderate dehydration. You need to ascertain when she last passed urine. She should be admitted and started on oral rehydration: 150 ml/kg body weight should be prescribed over 24 hours. The first 50 ml/kg should be given alone over the first 4–6 hours. On re-evaluation, the child should have passed urine at this point and be better hydrated. If so, then additional feeds (either milk or solids) are allowed if the child desires it. If dehydration persists, intravenous fluids are required. The fluid should be offered as frequent small feeds and the parent reassured that the vomiting will lessen as the hydration improves. Neither anti-emetics nor anti-diarrhoeals are to be encouraged. A serum urea and packed cell volume (PCV) will confirm the state of hydration. Serum electrolytes need to be checked to confirm that the child has not developed hypo- or hypernatraemia. The stool can be examined for pathogens. In this age group with this kind of a presentation the causative agent is often rotavirus. If the child is well hydrated at 24 hours, the oral rehydration fluid should be continued intermittently with feeds. The parents should be reassured that the diarrhoea will decrease over the next few days. A small number of children are unable to digest milk or milk-containing products immediately after the diarrhoea and may require alternative food products such as lactose-free or soy-based formulae for 2–3 weeks before reintroduction of a normal diet.

Case history 3

An answer can be divided into several parts.

The setting. This is a child with a chronic disease that follows a relapsing pattern with potential serious sequelae. Information like this preferably needs to be discussed in a quiet corner where the parents are comfortable and not on an open ward. It is also beneficial to have a member of the nursing staff present when you talk to the parents so they are able to reinforce what you have said.

Pacing. You need to know first what the parents know about the situation and their understanding of the disease.

Information. Provide the information they require. Do not overburden them with too much information or jargon. Explain in this instance that 90% of patients with ulcerative colitis will experience one or more relapses after initial treatment. Most will lead a normal life despite chronic disease, but about a fifth will be chronically incapacitated. The prognosis is linked to extent of involvement and those with isolated distal colitis have the best outcome. While most will be managed on a combination of medical and supportive measures, a proportion of patients (30%) will require surgery and often a colostomy for the control of symptoms. Explain the symptoms of fulminant colitis and that it is a medical emergency requiring urgent admission. Since there is a risk (though small) of developing a malignancy, regular surveillance of the colonic mucosa needs to be carried out using colonoscopy and biopsy.

Respond to feelings. Be prepared for statements like 'we didn't know that' or 'no-one told us that' as they may well be in a state of denial. If the parents are overtly anxious, you may need to inform the members of the team looking after the child about their doubts and concerns.

Short notes answer

The short bowel syndrome occurs when there is a congenital or acquired loss or shortening of the bowel and a resultant decrease in its absorptive surface. Malabsorption results in vitamin B_{12} deficiency (and hence the megaloblastic anaemia), failure to thrive and an osmotic diarrhoea. An alteration in the intestinal milieu leading to changes in pH results in bacterial overgrowth and occasionally can lead to oversecretion of gastrin. The latter results in gastric hypersecretion.

Neuromuscular disease

Key points

You should be able to:

- Perform a basic examination of the cranial nerves and peripheral nerves
- Appreciate the comprehensive problems associated with handicap
- Recognise and manage infection involving the nervous system
- Recognise different types of headache
- Understand the types and treatment of convulsions
- Assess children with neuromuscular disease.

6.1 Introduction

The average medical student is filled with dread at the prospect of having to examine the nervous system in a child. This is unnecessary; this system, though complex, is concerned with clearly defined functions and a logical, systematic approach will result in a realistic appreciation of the basic problem(s) facing the neurologically abnormal child. Certainly, the undergraduate is not expected to be conversant with rare neurodegenerative conditions, but must be able to discuss the problems relating to cerebral palsy and similar conditions which, ultimately, make up a significant proportion of the paediatric workload.

6.2 Examination

General examination

If the examination is presented as a game, most children will cooperate sufficiently to enable a good assessment of the nervous system. Observation of the child while playing and interacting with parents and siblings is of paramount importance. The head shape should be noted and head circumference measured. Mannerisms, movements and posturing must be observed in the light of the child's chronological age. Particular attention to neurocutaneous stigmata, hepatosplenomegaly and dysmorphic features should form a routine part of the general examination.

The cranial nerves

The first cranial nerve is rarely examined in children and requires the use of standard smelling agents. A cursory assessment is possible by asking direct questions about the child's sense of smell. The II nerve is tested individually by covering one eye and asking the older child to read picture cards (acuity), checking visual fields using an interesting small toy with the child focusing on your nose and fundoscopy. The III, IV and VI nerves are tested together by steadying the head while asking the child to follow a bright object traversing a large 'H' with his eyes. The sensory modality of the Vth nerve is checked by asking the child to close his eyes and say 'yes' every time you touch the three divisions (ophthalmic, maxillary and mandibular). The corneal reflex is unpleasant and limited to comatose children and very small infants. If the motor component of the Vth nerve is intact, the child should be able to push his jaw laterally against your hand. Facial asymmetry with loss of nasolabial folds and drawing of the face to the normal side on smiling/grimacing is indicative of a VIIth palsy. The child should normally be able to bury his eyelashes, blow out the cheeks and open/close the mouth tightly. Weakness throughout one side suggests a VIIth lower motor neurone lesion; preservation of the forehead creases implies an upper motor neurone lesion. The VIIIth nerve is checked by direct questions relating to hearing and a distraction test in children aged 6–18 months. The IX–Xth nerves are functioning normally if the uvula rises symmetrically on asking the child to say 'aagh'. An intact XIth nerve allows the child to raise his shoulders and push his head against resistance. The XIIth nerve is assessed by asking the child to protrude and waggle the tongue from side to side. An accurate examination of the cranial nerves is possible, even in young infants (Table 32).

Motor examination

Initially, it is essential to establish whether the child experiences any pain in any joints or limbs, and the examination must be conducted carefully.

Muscle tone is assessed by observing posture and moving joints through their range of movements. **Hypotonic** neonates assume a frog-leg position, whereas older children are floppy. **Spasticity** is characterised by increased tone that relaxes suddenly (clasp-knife) and is often associated with clonus. **Rigidity** implies constant resistance to passive movement.

Power is appreciated by inviting the child to perform specific functions against resistance and graded from 0–5 (Table 33).

Reflexes are assessed by using a rigid finger in neonates and a small hammer in older children, after

Table 32 Cranial nerve assessment in infants

Nerve	Test
I	Not tested
II	Blinks to bright light; appears to fix/follow (3+ months); fundoscopy
III–VI	Assess highlights on pupils for squint, abnormal position of globe
V	Corneal reflexes; sucking movements
VII	Facial asymmetry especially while crying
VIII	Startles to sound; quietens with soothing; tuneful babbling
IX–X	Gag reflex
XI	Not tested
XII	Tongue movements

Table 33 Grading of muscle power

Power	Observation
0	No power
1	Barely perceptible power
2	Movement with gravity removed (i.e. horizontally)
3	Movement just overcomes gravity
4	Movement against gravity and some resistance
5	Normal power

demonstrating that the exercise is painless. Plantar reflexes are not downgoing until the child is walking.

Mobility and gait (crawling, walking, etc.) must be documented. Abnormal movements include slow twisting movements (**dystonia**), writhing actions (**athetosis**) and rapid involuntary jerks (**chorea**).

Speech is commonly affected in motor disorders including **cerebellar** abnormalities. The latter manifests as staccato speech, hypotonia, pendular nystagmus and reflexes, poor coordination, dysdiadochokinesia and an intention tremor.

Sensory examination

Sensory assessment requires considerable concentration on the part of the child and often proves the most difficult part of the neurological examination. A piece of cotton wool and sterile needle are used to assess **touch** and **pain** sensation. The process must be carefully explained to the child who is then asked to close his eyes and indicate each time there has been contact with the skin. The two sides must be compared simultaneously according to dermatomes. **Vibration** sense is tested with a tuning fork, **temperature** by using warm and cold objects and **joint position** by asking the child to identify positions of the thumbs and big toes with the eyes closed.

6.3 Congenital abnormalities

Neural tube defects

A tuft of hair over the lower back may herald the presence of a minor defect of the spinal processes without any abnormality of nervous tissue, i.e. spina bifida occulta. This is of no consequence and only rarely associated with problems such as a tethered cord (diastematomyelia), syringomyelia or dermoid sinus connecting the skin to the dura. Failure of closure of the neural tube by the 4th week in utero results in **spina bifida**, with exposure of the meninges (meningocoele) and spinal cord (myelomeningocoele) (Fig. 38). The latter is the most serious defect, arising in 0.1% of live births, and may be related to a genetic predisposition, radiation, drugs (e.g. valproic acid) and malnutrition (e.g. folic acid deficiency). Myelomeningocoele is associated with leakage of fetal α fetoprotein. This results in a raised

Fig. 38 Clinical appearance of spina bifida. The figure shows newborn with 'open' thoraco-lumbar myelomeningocoele with patulous anus, flaccid lower limbs, bilateral talipes and also hydrocephalus.

level in the mother's bloodstream. The defects can be demonstrated on antenatal ultrasound scanning. Spina bifida is often associated with an abnormality of the posterior brain (Chiari defect), obstructing the flow of cerebrospinal fluid and resulting in hydrocephalus. This is more likely the higher the lesion, with the surprising exception of high thoracic and cervical lesions, which are often not associated with major neurological deficit and hydrocephalus. Exposed, weeping lesions are at great risk of ascending infection. Lumbar lesions account for 75% of cases: affected infants assume a frog position because of flaccid paresis of the lower limbs and may also have a patulous anus and incontinence of stool and urine. The patulous anus and perineal anaesthesia are evident with lower sacral lesions.

Management

Management requires sympathetic counselling and a multidisciplinary team approach. Supportive care alone may be appropriate for those infants with very large lesions, severe neurological deficit and gross hydrocephalus at birth. With exposed myelomeningocoeles, surgical closure shortly after birth is essential if infection is to be prevented, while the hydrocephalus generally necessitates a ventriculo-peritoneal shunt. Closed lesions may be repaired after a few days. Long-term management involves intensive physiotherapy to the lower limbs, attention to bowel habit and the neurogenic bladder, with intermittent catheterisation to avoid urinary retention and urinary tract infection. Orthopaedic review is required, particularly for any associated kyphoscoliosis, dislocated hips and club feet.

> **BOX 10**
> **Causes of hydrocephalus**
>
> | | Congenital | Acquired |
> |---|---|---|
> | Obstructive causes | Spina bifida | Intraventricular haemorrhage |
> | | Aqueductal stenosis | Meningitis/encephalitis |
> | | Dandy Walker cyst of IVth ventricle | Obstructing tumour |
> | | Chiari malformation of IVth ventricle | |
> | Non-obstructive causes | Choroid plexus papilloma | Intraventricular haemorrhage |
> | | | Meningitis |
> | | | Leukaemic infiltration |

Hydrocephalus

Obstructive (non-communicating) hydrocephalus results from a blockage to cerebrospinal fluid (CSF) flow. Decreased absorption or increased production of CSF fluid causes non-obstructive (communicating) hydrocephalus. Congenital abnormalities of brain development may affect the flow of CSF, whereas intraventricular haemorrhage is the most common cause for acquired obstruction and diminished CSF absorption (Box 10).

Signs and symptoms

Hydrocephalus presents with symptoms and signs of raised intracranial pressure. In neonates this manifests as decreased feeding, vomiting, lethargy, irritability and occasionally convulsions. The fontanelles are wide, tense, convex and connected together by widely open sutures. Distended veins over the scalp, downward displacement of the orbital globes (sun setting), cranial nerve palsies (especially VIth), long tract signs and papilloedema are late signs. The head circumference should be measured daily and plotted on appropriate centile charts. Accurate, serial measurements of the ventricular system are documented on ultrasound, and specific anatomical abnormalities/growths confirmed on CT or MRI of the brain. Symptoms and an excessive increase in head size are indications for drainage of the CSF by lumbar or ventricular tapping until a formal shunt is inserted. An underlying cause for the hydrocephalus such as a congenital cyst must be decompressed as appropriate.

In older children the triad of lethargy, vomiting and headaches often with a diurnal variation (usually worse first thing in the morning), and especially if associated with hypertension and bradycardia, is suggestive of raised intracranial pressure. Cranial nerve palsies (especially VIth, then IIIrd) may be false localising signs, whereas long tract signs and papilloedema develop early compared with infants. Mannitol diuresis and dexamethasone are used to reduce the intracranial pressure in the first instance, while an urgent CT scan will confirm hydrocephalus and may show the primary cause (e.g. a brain tumour). An urgent V–P shunt is required, followed by treatment for the primary lesion (e.g. surgery, radiotherapy). The outcome is largely dependent on the underlying cause. However, children with hydrocephalus have a lower IQ compared with their peers and increased risk of neurodevelopmental, visual and learning problems.

Microcephaly

Microcephaly is defined as a head circumference three standard deviations below the mean for both age and gender. It may be a primary defect or follow an insult that impedes normal brain development (Box 11). A thorough antenatal, perinatal and family history should be obtained. The head circumference should be measured serially, and those of other family members also noted. Many microcephalic children will be developmentally delayed and require supportive treatment, as appropriate.

> **BOX 11**
> **Causes of microcephaly**
>
> **Primary**
> Familial (recessive or dominant)
> Trisomies (18 and 21)
> Deletions (Cri-du-chat, 5p-)
> Certain syndromes (Opitz, de Lange)
>
> **Secondary**
> Hypoxic–ischaemic encephalopathy
> Congenital infection
> Meningitis and encephalitis
> Metabolic (hyperphenylalaninaemia)
> Drugs and alcohol

Craniosynostosis

Craniosynostosis arises when the cranial sutures fuse early, once in every 2000 births, e.g. coronal sutures in Crouzon syndrome, multiple in Apert and Carpenter syndromes. They are commonly associated with marked cosmetic deformity, brain underdevelopment, hydrocephaly and syndactyly of the digits. Management should be directed by a multidisciplinary team.

Neurocutaneous syndromes

Neurocutaneous syndromes are characterised by neurological disorders together with cutaneous stigmata.

Neurofibromatosis (NF) is the most common type, arising in 1 in 4000 of the population. NF-1 is typified by more than five café-au-lait pigmented spots (>5 mm diameter), axillary freckling, neurofibromas (soft and small, or large, pigmented plexiform lesions), Lisch spots in the iris and skeletal deformities. Neurological abnormalities include macrocephaly, hydrocephaly, optic gliomas and CNS hamartomas. An increased incidence of malignant lesions occur in the CNS and elsewhere (e.g. leukaemia, phaeochromocytoma, Wilms tumour). Bilateral acoustic neuromas are typical of NF-2.

Tuberous sclerosis is also an autosomal dominant condition, characterised by hypo- and hyperpigmented skin patches (enhanced under Wood's light), subungual fibromas, facial adenoma sebaceum, and tubers in the retina (phakomata), heart, kidneys and brain. The last often calcify and many of these patients are mentally handicapped and have troublesome epilepsy.

6.4 Handicap

Cerebral palsy

Cerebral palsy describes a disorder of movement that follows a non-progressive insult to the developing brain, including anoxia, infection, haemorrhage, trauma and toxins. Despite the static nature of the insult, clinical signs evolve as the child grows older. Cerebral palsy is commonly associated with disorders of speech, hearing, vision, intellect and seizures. Classification depends on the distribution and type of motor disorder, which, in turn, depends on which part of the brain is primarily affected (Table 34). Those with **spastic cerebral palsy** have increased clasp-knife rigidity and decreased movement in the affected limbs (Fig. 39). The upper motor neurone signs (weakness, increased tone, brisk reflexes) are more marked in the upper limb in **spastic hemiplegia** (bilaterally in **double hemiplegia**). Both lower limbs are affected in **spastic diplegia** and all four in **spastic quadriplegia**, when associated contractures, severe mental retardation and seizures are extremely likely. **Athetoid cerebral palsy** was common following neonatal hyperbilirubinaemia leading to kernicterus. Weakness is associated with marked hypotonia, poor head control and repetitive athetoid movements affecting the limbs and bulbar muscles. Consequently, feeding and speech are often badly affected and these children are at particular risk of

recurrent aspiration pneumonia. Initial investigation is aimed to exclude progressive forms of physical and mental handicap and confirm the extent of damage on imaging (CT or MRI) and electrophysiological studies (EEG). Management requires a dedicated multidisciplinary team with support from educational psychologists and speech, occupational and physiotherapists. Tendon-lengthening procedures to relieve contractures, correction of squints and nystagmus, and hearing aids may improve the quality of life. Baclofen is sometimes useful in cases with severe spasticity.

Neurodegenerative conditions

Neurodegenerative conditions are rare and result from a number of disorders:

- inborn errors of metabolism that result in the accumulation of abnormal metabolites in the brain (e.g. lipidoses, leukodystrophies)

Fig. 39 Clinical manifestations of cerebral palsy. A school-age child with severe cerebral palsy showing generalised 'windswept' deformity due to contractures and marked muscle wasting. The child is still in nappies, requires a nasogastric tube for feeding and is lying on a sheepskin rug to prevent pressure sores.

Table 34 Types of cerebral palsy

Cerebral palsy	Motor distribution	Seizures(%)	Mental handicap (%)
Spastic	Diplegia	<10	<10
	Hemiplegia	25	25
	Quadriplegia	>50	>50
Athetoid	Extrapyramidal	<20	<20

- abnormal mitochondrial function (e.g. Leigh's encephalopathy)
- progressive postinfection syndromes (e.g. subacute sclerosing panencephalitis following measles)
- toxins (e.g. lead, irradiation).

Patients may be relatively normal at birth but deteriorate over a period of months or years until terminal dementia associated with coma is established.

Decreased special senses

Visual impairment

Visual impairment affects up to 0.1% of children. It should be suspected in any child who does not seem to take an interest in their surroundings, preferentially responds to sounds or tactile stimuli and in those with a predisposing abnormality (e.g. cerebral palsy, congenital infection). The causes are legion (Box 12) and every effort should be made to establish a firm diagnosis and instigate the appropriate therapy. Peripatetic teachers and special educational methods are essential if the child is to overcome this severe handicap and achieve their full potential.

BOX 12
Causes of visual impairment

Orbit
Cataracts
Amblyopia
Optic atrophy
Retinopathy of prematurity
Retinal degeneration (retinitis pigmentosa)
Retinal detachment/haemorrhage (trauma, non-accidental injury (NAI))
Coloboma

Central
Hypoxic–ischaemic encephalopathy (cerebral palsy)
Postinfective (meningitis, encephalitis)
Congenital occipital anomalies (encephalocoele)
Hydrocephaly
Tumours
Demyelinating/neurodegenerative diseases

Hearing impairment

Hearing impairment affects 1 in 1000 live birth, and may result from lesions affecting the peripheral auditory apparatus or cerebral cortex (Box 13). Since auditory input is required before language development, hearing loss is often manifest by delayed or unintelligible speech. The distraction test (see viva voce question in Chapter 1) allows a rapid assessment of hearing in young infants who are able to be propped up (>6 months) and still young enough to be taken in by the test (<18 months).

Free field audiometry and auditory-evoked responses are required for older children.

BOX 13
Causes of hearing impairment

Peripheral conductive
Otitis media
Impacted cerumen, foreign body
Perforated tympanic membrane
Disrupted ossicles (trauma)
Bony disruption (craniofacial syndromes)

Peripheral sensorineural
Ototoxics (aminoglycosides, irradiation)
Congenital infections
Excessive noise

Central
Postinfective (viral, meningitis)
Tumours
Demyelinating diseases
Familial/genetic
Certain syndromes (Pendred, Waardenburg, Alport)
Trisomies

6.5 Infections

Bacterial meningitis

Bacterial meningitis is a rapidly progressive, diffuse infection involving the meninges and CSF. Although potentially fatal, it can result in no neurological sequelae if diagnosed early and treated effectively. The microbiological cause of meningitis varies with age group (Box 14). Prior to *Haemophilus influenzae* type b vaccine (Hib), this was the most common infecting organism outside the neonatal period, followed by *Neisseria meningitides* and *Streptococcus pneumoniae*. Patients at particular risk include infants, the immunosuppressed and those with cranial or spinal defects, CSF leak, penetrating trauma and ventricular shunts. Most organisms are acquired by droplet inhalation from close contact with colonised individuals: nasal carriage with *H. influenzae* type b is seen in 5% whereas *N. meningitides* is present in 10% of healthy individuals. Most cases are sporadic (e.g. *N. meningitides* group B), though epidemics occur, especially with *N. meningitides* groups A and C.

Meningitis should always be considered in a child with a fever who has an altered level of consciousness. Although there may be a preceding upper respiratory infection for a few days, the natural history is often rapidly progressive over a few hours. Children may present with fulminating septicaemia, shock and disseminated intravascular coagulation (DIC), especially with meningococcaemia. Indeed, a rapidly evolving purpuric or ecchymotic rash in a toxic child is indicative

BOX 14
Causes of bacterial meningitis

Neonatal period
Group B streptococci
Gram-negative bacilli
Staphylococci
Listeria monocytogenes
Haemophilus influenzae

Children
Haemophilus influenzae
Neisseria meningitides
Streptococcus pneumoniae
Staphylococci
Gram-negative bacilli if immunosuppressed

of meningococcaemia until proven otherwise. Infants are more likely to present with fever, poor feeding, vomiting and drowsiness. Meningism is characterised by irritability, photophobia, neck stiffness, pain on leg extension with the hip flexed (Kernig's sign) and reflex hip flexion when the neck is flexed while supine (Brudzinki's sign). These signs are often absent in infants, who develop signs of raised intracranial pressure with a bulging fontanelle. Focal neurological signs follow vascular occlusion. Convulsions occur in 25% of patients and are less likely with infection with *N. meningitides*. Subdural effusions usually resolve without the need for surgical drainage and, together with resistant organisms or inadequate treatment, may result in a fever persisting beyond 10 days. Hyponatraemia and a hypo-osmolar state occur through inappropriate antidiuretic hormone (ADH) secretion (SIADH).

The diagnosis is confirmed by a lumbar puncture and examination of the CSF, which classically reveals an increase in neutrophils and protein, with a decrease in CSF glucose. A Gram stain may help in the initial identification of the causative organism. In those with raised intracranial pressure or severe cardiorespiratory compromise, the lumbar puncture is preferably delayed. In such cases, blood cultures should be taken and antibiotics started empirically, starting with third-generation cephalosporins, cefotaxime or ceftriaxone, and continuing for 10 days. Where antibiotics have already been given, rapid bacterial antigen detection tests can be applied to the CSF to help to identify the organism.

The advent of *H. influenzae* type b (Hib) vaccine has reduced the incidence of this type of meningitis. Vaccines are available against *N. meningitides* groups A and C but not against the more common group B. Prophylaxis with rifampicin should be prescribed to all close contacts of an index case of *N. meningitides,* and for close contacts below the age of 4 years with *H. influenzae* meningitis. It is not required for contacts of *S. pneumoniae*. Long-term sequelae in survivors include sensorineural deafness (up to 30%), reduced vision, epilepsy, neurodevelopmental delay and retardation.

Viral meningitis

Viral meningitis is usually caused by enteroviruses (80%), arboviruses, herpesviruses and mumps. A non-specific febrile illness generally precedes signs of meningism and convulsions, focal neurological signs and coma may ensure. The CSF contains an increased number of polymorphs but near-normal levels of protein and glucose. Viruses can sometimes be isolated from the CSF, but confirmation is more likely on sequential serum antibody levels. Acyclovir is effective against herpes; otherwise the treatment is supportive and involves control of complications.

Encephalitis

Encephalitis, a diffuse infection of the brain parenchyma, is usually seen with viral agents including enteroviruses (80%), arboviruses, herpes (simplex, varicella), measles, mumps, rubella and HIV, occasionally with toxoplasma, mycobacteria and mycoplasma. The disease is mild and self-limiting (enteroviruses) or severe and rapidly progressive (herpes, mycoplasma). Fever associated with altered consciousness, sometimes seizures, is the hallmark of these conditions. Hallucinations, vomiting, photophobia, neck stiffness and a non-specific erythematous rash develop over a few days and, in the majority, subside as recovery ensues. The CSF shows an increase in white cells but no bacterial organisms. Serological investigation of the CSF and body secretions may confirm the infecting agent. EEG shows a generalised encephalopathic pattern and CT or MRI confirms changes in the grey–white matter. The last characteristically involves the temporal lobes in herpes simplex encephalitis. Treatment includes supportive measures to control complications, including raised intracranial pressure and seizures. Specific anti-microbials are indicated with mycoplasma and TB, whereas acyclovir is the drug of choice with herpes infection.

Brain abscess

Brain abscesses generally occur in early school-age children and follow penetrating trauma, meningitis, septic embolisation (e.g. with Tetralogy of Fallot), and invasive infection in the scalp, skull, ears and ventricular shunts. They usually involve the fronto-parietal lobes, initially presenting with fever, headaches and lethargy followed by seizures, focal neurological signs and coma. Causative agents include *Staphylococcus aureus*, streptococci, Gram-negative bacilli, anaerobes and occasionally fungi. If suspected, the diagnosis is confirmed on CT or MRI scanning. A lumbar puncture is avoided because of the significant risk of precipitating cerebellar herniation (coning). Treatment involves combination antibiotics given intravenously in high dose. Surgical aspiration is required with multilocular or fungal abscesses, and in those complicated by gas formation and pressure effects.

6.6 Seizures and headaches

Epileptic seizures

Seizures occur in 0.5–0.1% of the population and, if febrile seizures are included, affect up to 3–5% of children. They involve episodic involuntary movement, behavioural or sensory activity, often associated with loss of consciousness. Although they are an overt manifestation of abnormal electrical activity in the brain, investigation does not confirm an underlying cause in the majority of cases. Recurrent seizures unrelated to an acute cerebral insult or fever constitutes epilepsy. A detailed history is fundamental in making the diagnosis. The clinical examination is usually unremarkable but must exclude evidence of raised intracranial pressure, hypertension, neurocutaneous stigmata and evidence of a metabolic or storage disorder. Investigation should focus on excluding an underlying metabolic or CNS abnormality and should include an electroencephalogram (EEG). The EEG is a recording of the electrical activity of the brain that may provide useful information on the seizure type, its treatment and prognosis.

Classification of seizures

Epileptic seizures can be divided into partial or generalised types (Table 35).

Simple partial seizures

Simple partial seizures (SPS) involve brief tonic or clonic movements of the face and extremities that may follow an aura but are not associated with impaired consciousness.

Generalised seizures

Absence (generalised) seizures usually affect girls, who experience sudden loss of consciousness for less than 30 seconds, associated with staring and eyelid flickering but no aura or post-ictal state. Typical absences (petit mal) produce 3 per second spike and generalised discharges on the EEG. Atypical absences (complex) are associated with myoclonic movements of the head and extremities and 2 per second discharges on EEG. An adverse outcome is expected in those with

other, tonic–clonic or multiple seizures, a positive family history and low IQ (<90).

Tonic–clonic (generalised) seizures are the most common type of convulsion, commencing with an aura, followed by loss of consciousness, tonic contractures and rhythmic clonic movements in the limbs lasting several minutes. Cyanosis, tongue biting and incontinence of urine are common during the fit, which is followed by a post-ictal phase, generally involving a variable period of sleep.

Myoclonic epilepsy includes a heterogeneous group of conditions characterised by sudden loss of muscle tone, which may result in injury. Some forms are associated with a positive family history and a benign course, whereas others are associated with mental retardation and are refractory to treatment.

Infantile spasms (West's syndrome) usually commence around 3–6 months of age and involve repetitive, symmetrical contractions of the neck, trunk and limbs. The last are mostly flexor spasms producing the characteristic **salaam attacks** but may be interspersed with extensor contractions. Infantile spasms are common just before or after sleep. Up to 20% are idiopathic; the remainder are secondary to hypoxic damage, CNS infection and trauma, neurocutaneous syndromes and storage diseases. Indeed, around 40% of children with infantile spasms have evidence of cerebral palsy and 80% have significant cognitive disability. The EEG is usually chaotic (hypsarrhythmia), and the treatment difficult, especially in non-idiopathic types when the risk of mental retardation is high. Steroids and, more recently, vigabatrin have been shown to be effective.

Multiple seizures are characteristic of the Lennox–Gastaut syndrome. These often include myoclonic seizures associated with tonic activity, atypical absences and infantile spasms. Most children with this syndrome have delayed development with significant motor and cognitive impairment. The condition is often refractory to therapy and only 10% have a reasonable outcome. Occasionally, recourse to surgical resection is necessary (e.g. callostomy for drop attacks).

Management of epilepsy

It is important to establish the type of seizure activity through a detailed history and EEG evidence. Any underlying cause and complications must be controlled and any associated problems addressed (e.g. physical or mental handicap, etc.). A decision must then be taken as to the need for and type of treatment, if any. An expectant approach can be applied for patients with a single, non-febrile seizure in whom there are no abnormal physical signs and a normal EEG. Having established a diagnosis of epilepsy, a single anticonvulsant is started, and the dose built up over a number of weeks until fit control is adequate without drug-related side-effects. Serum anticonvulsant levels can be used as a guide to management. The drug of choice is dependent on the seizure type (Table 36).

Table 35 Types of epileptic seizures

Partial	Generalised
Simple	Absences
Complex	Tonic–clonic
Secondary generalisation	Tonic
	Clonic
	Myotonic
	Atonic
	Infantile spasms

Table 36 Anticonvulsants: indications and side-effects

Anticonvulsant	Seizure type	Side-effects
Benzodiazepine	Myoclonic, status epilepticus Infantile spasms, partial	Sedation, behavioural changes
Carbamazepine	Tonic–clonic, partial	Sedation, liver dysfunction, leucopenia
Ethosuximide	Absences	Rashes, liver dysfunction
Lamotrigine	Tonic–clonic, refractory Myoclonic, absences	Rashes, liver dysfunction, leucopenia, behavioural changes
Paraldehyde	Status epilepticus	Sterile abscesses
Phenobarbitone	Tonic–clonic, partial	Rashes, behavioural changes
Phenytoin	Tonic–clonic, partial, status epilepticus	Rashes, hirsutism, gum hypertrophy
Steroids	Infantile spasms, myoclonic	Weight gain, hypertension, hyperglycaemia
Thiopentone	Status epilepticus	Cardiorespiratory depression, irritant on extravasation
Valproate	Tonic–clonic, absences Myoclonic, partial	Tremor, liver dysfunction
Vigabatrin	Tonic–clonic, refractory Infantile spasms	Sedation, behavioural changes
Ketogenic diet	Tonic–clonic, multiple	

A second drug is added if control is still suboptimal despite maximal doses of the first drug. After a sufficiently long period of control, the initial drug is discontinued.

Cessation of medication can be considered after a 2-year fit-free period in those without risk factors. Weaning should take place over a minimum of 3 months, and up to 70% of these patients will have no further fits. A good outcome is suggested by a single seizure type of short duration and infrequent occurrence, with clear provoking phenomena (e.g. intercurrent illness) and no neurological impairment inbetween seizures. Features indicative of a poor outcome include multiple seizure types, frequent onset, prolonged duration, early onset, absence of provoking phenomena and additional neurological impairment.

Surgery is growing as a viable treatment option for intractable epilepsy, particularly in those with a demonstrable clinical, radiological or electroencephalographic focus.

Non-epileptic seizures

Non-epileptic seizures include those related to a fever or to a CNS insult such as trauma and metabolic derangement. They do not, necessarily, lead to lifetime seizure activity. **Febrile convulsions** are the most common seizures in childhood, usually affecting 4% of children aged 6 months to 6 years, often with a positive family history. They comprise symmetrical, generalised tonic–clonic seizures lasting less than 15 minutes, associated with loss of consciousness and no focal neurological signs. The convulsion is generally triggered with spikes of fever and usually responds to cooling and anti-pyretic measures. Following a febrile convulsion, all children should be examined to exclude a serious underlying infection. If in doubt, a lumbar puncture should be performed. All those with atypical febrile convulsions require investigation with neuroimaging and an EEG. Although there is a slightly increased risk of non-febrile seizure activity later in life in 10% of children, there is no place for routine anticonvulsant therapy in uncomplicated febrile seizures. Adverse factors suggesting continuing seizure activity include complex or atypical initial seizures, a positive family history of epilepsy and preceding neurological abnormality. Treatment involves the administration of rectal diazepam during subsequent convulsions and, where indicated, prophylactic sodium valproate.

Status epilepticus

Constant seizure activity or recurrent fits with no resumption of consciousness persisting beyond 30 minutes constitutes status epilepticus. This is usually seen after prolonged febrile seizures or in patients with preceding neurological or metabolic disease, but also occurs de novo in those without a CNS insult. The excessive convulsive activity causes cerebral hypoglycaemia, lactic acidosis and hypoxia, and results in death in 5% of patients. This medical emergency requires active resuscitation, protection of the airway, correction of the metabolic derangements and anticonvulsants. Intravenous diazepam is the first drug of choice and can be repeated and followed by paraldehyde, phenytoin or phenobarbitone. In refractory cases, general anaesthesia with thiopentone is required.

Seizure-like disorders

A thorough history is essential to differentiate seizures from the non-convulsive disorders listed in Table 37. In particularly difficult cases a period of in-hospital observation combined with an EEG may be necessary.

Table 37 Seizure-like disorders

Preschool children	School children
Breath-holding attacks	Night terrors
Paroxysmal vertigo	Syncopal attacks
Benign myoclonus	Rage attacks
	Narcolepsy
	Munchausen by proxy

Headaches

Tension headaches

Tension headaches are extremely common in school-age children, particularly amongst sensitive, introverted types. They manifest as continuous pressure-like pain usually over the forehead or crown that lasts several minutes or hours. They are generally related to stress and anxiety and are worse toward the end of the day. If prolonged, they may be indicative of serious underlying discord at home or at school, depression and occasionally even child abuse. All children reporting such headaches should have a thorough examination including fundoscopy and blood pressure recording. Reassurance and simple analgesics are usually sufficient treatment.

Migraine

A positive family history of migraine is commonly present in children who present with recurrent, severe, throbbing headaches usually over the eyes, frontal, temporal and occipital areas (often unilaterally). These headaches may be preceded by a visual or sensory aura, are associated with nausea and vomiting and last several hours or days. Abdominal pain is a frequent accompaniment, especially in younger children. Migraine may be precipitated by stress, chocolate, cheese, nuts and meat extracts; it improves with rest in a quiet, dark room and sleep. Rarely, migraine may be associated with transient unilateral weakness (**hemiplegic migraine**), a IIIrd nerve palsy (**ophthalmoplegic migraine**), and vertigo with ataxia (**basilar migraine**). Again, a full examination is mandatory and investigation is usually unnecessary. Analgesics and anti-emetics are required during the acute attack. For those experiencing more than three attacks per month, treatment may be supplemented with prophylaxis in the form of propranolol.

Raised intracranial pressure

Raised intracranial pressure results in headaches that have a diurnal variation, usually worse in the early morning. They are usually accompanied by photophobia, progressive lethargy, nausea and vomiting, and improve after vomiting. Bradycardia, hypertension and papilloedema in the presence of these symptoms suggest raised intracranial pressure and are an indication for an urgent brain scan.

Subarachnoid bleed

A severe, sudden-onset headache associated with an altered level of consciousness and meningism may herald a subarachnoid bleed. The presence of blood and xanthochromia in the CSF necessitates a contrasted CT scan in order to identify a vascular malformation. An arteriogram may be necessary, especially when delicate surgery is contemplated.

6.7 The spinal cord and peripheral nerves

Cord compression

Spinal cord compression may result from tumours within the spinal canal, vertebral collapse and trauma. It presents with lower limb weakness, gait and sphincter disturbances. Back pain may point toward the site of compression and sensory loss in the limbs can localise the block at spinal level. Lower motor neurone signs develop at the site of the lesion, while upper motor neurone signs are seen in neurones arising below the obstruction.

In children where a cervical fracture is suspected, the neck must be immobilised immediately. Cord compression from whatever cause is a medical emergency. The diagnosis is confirmed on radiology and neuroimaging (where MRI excels), and neurosurgical decompression performed as soon as possible. Radiotherapy and/or chemotherapy may be required with spinal tumours, depending on the histology.

Neuropathies

Disorders affecting peripheral neurones may have a congenital, degenerative, postinfectious and toxic aetiology (Box 15).

BOX 15
Causes of peripheral neuronal dysfunction

Congenital	Acquired
Hereditary	Toxic
Peroneal atrophy	Heavy metals
Familial dysautonomia	Organophosphates
Degenerative	Vincristine
Werdnig–Hoffmann	Uraemia
Kugelberg–Welander	Postinfectious
	Guillain–Barré
	Poliomyelitis

Spinal muscular atrophy

Congenital spinal muscular atrophy (SMA) describes a group of progressive, degenerative conditions affecting peripheral nerves. Severe forms (e.g. Werdnig–Hoffmann, SMA type I) present in the neonatal period with marked hypotonia, areflexia and fasciculation, and patients succumb within 2 years from respiratory involvement. Patients with less severe forms (SMA types II/III) may survive into adult life with variable degrees of handicap. The diagnosis is confirmed on muscle and nerve biopsy and where applicable by detection of the abnormal mutation in genetic studies.

Motor–sensory neuropathies

Hereditary motor–sensory neuropathies generally present in late childhood with gait disturbance, foot drop and distal lower limb muscle wasting, producing a champagne glass appearance. Slow velocities on nerve conduction tests confirm the diagnosis. Management involves supportive orthopaedic splints and avoidance of injury to the limbs.

Toxic neuropathies

Toxic neuropathies often involve large nerve fibres (e.g. lead poisoning) and may result in ptosis, constipation and loss of reflexes (e.g. vincristine).

Poliomyelitis

Infection with the polio virus (poliomyelitis) was a common cause of infective motor neurone disease prior to routine vaccination. Up to 95% of infected individuals are asymptomatic or simply develop a mild coryzal illness. A minority develop headache, nausea, vomiting, muscle discomfort and stiffness which resolves (**nonparalytic poliomyelitis**). Asymmetrical muscle, bladder and bowel weakness can occur in **paralytic poliomyelitis**. Milder disorders with involvement of the anterior horn cells causing acute flaccid paralysis, weakness and loss of reflexes can develop after the live attenuated polio vaccine, and infection with echoviruses and coxsackieviruses.

Guillain–Barré syndrome

Guillain–Barré syndrome is a demyelinating disorder that usually follows 10 days after a non-specific illness. The presentation of postinfectious neuronitis is similar to polio although the acute febrile manifestations are less prominent, the flaccid paralysis is symmetrical and sensory involvement can sometimes develop. Weakness progresses slowly from distal to proximal groups, eventually involving bulbar, respiratory and cranial nerves in severe cases. Recovery occurs in reverse pattern and is complete in most patients within 3 weeks. A few patients develop a chronic, relapsing or unremitting polyneuropathy and are left with permanent weakness. The CSF protein level is typically raised while glucose and white cells are normal. Nerve conduction velocity is greatly reduced (motor is greater than sensory). All patients require admission in the acute phase until the disease has stopped progressing. A 5-day course of intravenous immunoglobulin is now standard treatment in the first instance and backed up with plasmapheresis in those with severe or rapidly progressive disease. Physiotherapy is required to mobilise weak muscle groups and artificial ventila-

Fig. 40 Boy with Duchenne muscular dystrophy climbing up himself to stand, (Gower manoeuvre) and showing marked pseudohypertrophy of the calves.

tion is necessary for those with respiratory embarrassment.

6.8 Neuromuscular disorders

Dystrophies

Muscular dystrophies (MD) are genetically determined, progressive disorders involving muscle fibre degeneration. They run a variable course so that children with X-linked recessive **Duchenne MD** are generally wheelchair bound by the end of the first decade and do not survive much beyond three decades. Duchenne MD arises in 1 in 3600 males, presenting with progressive limb weakness and delayed motor milestones. Examination reveals calf pseudohypertrophy, muscle weakness and lumbar lordosis (Fig. 40). Pelvic girdle weakness results in affected boys having to climb up their own limbs in order to stand (Gower sign) and a waddling gait. All patients have a mild degree of intellectual deficit, cardiomyopathy of variable clinical significance and, ultimately, respiratory failure. Investigation reveals a several thousand-fold increase in serum creatinine kinase (also raised in most but not all female carriers), a myopathic EMG but normal nerve conduction. Muscle biopsy and the identification of abnormal **dystrophin** in muscle or an abnormal dystrophin gene in DNA confirms the diagnosis. Physiotherapy and supportive braces are essential to prolong mobility as long as possible, delaying the onset of scoliosis. Recently steroids have been shown to delay the need for a wheelchair, but their use in this condition remains controversial. Surgery may be required for troublesome contractures. Nutrition should be optimised and chest infections treated aggressively. A genetically engineered cure is still awaited.

Boys with **Becker MD** have a similar but milder X-linked disorder and remain ambulatory until early adulthood. Nevertheless, few survive beyond their forties, by which time physical handicap is severe. Other dystrophies are inherited as dominant or recessive traits, and are characterised by weakness in specific muscle distributions, e.g. proximal limbs in **limb girdle dystrophy**, face and distal groups in **myotonic dystrophy** and face plus shoulder girdle in **facioscapulohumeral dystrophy**.

Myopathies

Muscle weakness, wasting and myopathic changes observed with electromyography (EMG) may follow congenital disease (mitochondrial myopathy) or are secondary to endocrine disease (hyper- and hypothyroidism, Cushing syndrome, hyperparathyroidism), electrolyte imbalance (hypo- and hyperkalaemia), and inborn errors of lipid and glycogen storage.

Myasthenia gravis

Myasthenia gravis is seen, transiently, in neonates born to affected mothers. An immune response against the motor end-plate rarely develops in older children, who present with ptosis, facial weakness, difficulty in swallowing and limb weakness. Rapid onset of fatigue is the hallmark of myasthenia. Hence, symptoms are worse toward the end of the day and clinical signs can be enhanced by asking the child to perform repeated exercises. A similar trend is observed on EMG, which, like the clinical signs, can be reversed with a cholinesterase inhibitor (e.g. edrophonium). Treatment entails the use of similar, longer-acting drugs, such as neostigmine.

Self-assessment: questions

Multiple choice questions

1. The following statements describe meningitis:
   a. Meningococci are the most common bacteria to invade the CSF in neonates
   b. *Streptococcus pneumoniae* meningitis is not associated with deafness
   c. Antibiotic prophylaxis is required for all contacts of bacterial meningitis
   d. Viral meningitis is associated with very low glucose levels in the CSF
   e. Viral meningitis usually resolves without long-term complications

2. The management of cerebral palsy may include:
   a. Tendon release operations
   b. Nasogastric feeding
   c. Attention to pressure areas
   d. Control of seizures
   e. Regular chest physiotherapy

3. Abnormalities of the cranial nerves result in the following:
   a. Foot drop with a Xth nerve palsy
   b. Failure of abduction of the eye with a VIth nerve palsy
   c. 'Down and out' position of the globe with a IIIrd nerve palsy
   d. Total facial palsy with an upper motor neurone defect of the VIIth nerve
   e. Deviation of the protruded tongue to the affected side with a XIIth palsy

4. The following features are observed in neurocutaneous syndromes:
   a. Strawberry naevi
   b. Recurrent purpuric spots
   c. Plexiform neurofibromas
   d. Retinal phakomata
   e. Port wine stain

5. The following are indicative of raised intracranial pressure:
   a. Hypotension
   b. Hypertension
   c. Tachycardia
   d. Unilateral papilloedema
   e. Somnolence

6. The following drugs and side-effects are correctly matched:
   a. Phenytoin and gum hypertrophy
   b. Clonazepam and respiratory depression
   c. Sodium valproate and sterile abscesses
   d. Carbamazepine and liver dysfunction
   e. Ethosuximide and hirsutism

7. In Guillain–Barré syndrome:
   a. Sensory deficit does not occur
   b. Signs of recovery within 3 weeks are a good prognostic indicator
   c. Reflexes are lost early but recover rapidly
   d. Respiratory depression is an indication for plasmapheresis
   e. Steroids are the mainstay of treatment

8. The following are causes of peripheral neuropathy:
   a. Organophosphates
   b. Chemotherapeutic agents
   c. Steroids
   d. Carbamazepine
   e. Mercury poisoning

9. The following are characteristics of febrile convulsions:
   a. They affect children aged 6 months to 6 years
   b. They are the most common seizure type observed in childhood
   c. They are mainly observed in boys
   d. They last more than 30 minutes
   e. They result in chronic epilepsy in the majority of children

10. Regarding the intelligence quotient (IQ) in children:
    a. IQ is an extremely precise measurement of intelligence
    b. The IQ score can vary from day to day
    c. The IQ may be low in children with glue ears
    d. An IQ of less than 90 implies severe mental retardation
    e. Children with Down syndrome average an IQ of about 50

Case histories

Case history 1

A 10-year-old boy presents with 'funny turns', whereby he becomes vacant for a few seconds, sometimes associated with flickering of his eyelids. He is bullied at school where, recently, his performance has deteriorated.

How would you determine the diagnosis?

Case history 2

> A 10-year-old boy is admitted to casualty at 23.30 h in a semi-comatose state. Earlier that same day he had returned from a school outing to a nearby pharmaceutical factory. He had complained of tiredness and a headache, had refused supper and had gone to bed at 19.45 h. His parents heard him moaning in bed at 22.50 h and brought him to hospital, where you confirm his altered conscious level and note a few purpuric spots over the lower limbs and torso.

1. What important features would you check on clinical examination?
2. What is the presumptive diagnosis?
3. How would you confirm the diagnosis?
4. What immediate therapeutic steps would you take in casualty?

> Despite the initial management, the conscious level continues to deteriorate such that he is not rousable 1 hour after admission. By this time, he is centrally cyanosed, the blood pressure is 65/35 and the rash has spread over most of his body and is partly confluent over the toes. Some bleeding is noted around the i.v. cannulae insertion sites.

5. What complications have developed?
6. What further investigations are required at this point?

7. What further therapeutic intervention is required at this point?

> The parents are frantically asking what is going on. You leave the resuscitation to your colleagues and take them to one side for a chat.

8. What would you tell them at this point?
9. What community-based precautions are required?

> Despite incipient gangrene of two toes, the patient's condition stabilises and starts to improve over the next 3 days. Although he is lucid and fully orientated on day 10, he remains slightly irritable with a fever of around 38°C.

10. What might explain his condition and how would you investigate the temperature?

Short notes

Outline the key points in the management of status epilepticus

Viva voce question

A 5-year-old boy is brought to casualty in a coma following a fall onto the head from a height. What would you be concerned about and what steps would you take to confirm this? Outline your initial management.

Self-assessment: answers

Multiple choice answers

1. a. **False**. Gram-negative bacilli are most common.
   b. **False**. As with other types of bacterial meningitis.
   c. **False**. It is not necessary with *Streptococcus pneumoniae*.
   d. **False**. CSF glucose is normal or slightly reduced.
   e. **True**. Although persistent neurological deficit is not uncommon if an associated encephalitis is also present, especially with herpes simplex and CMV infections.

2. a. **True**. This will help with contractures.
   b. **True**. This maintains enteral feeds when there is bulbar and pseudobulbar involvement, general debility and weakness.
   c. **True**. Pressure sores develop easily at pressure points in relatively immobile patients.
   d. **True**. Seizures are common complications of cerebral palsy.
   e. **True**. Chest infections are common in the immobile patient.

3. a. **False**. A Xth nerve palsy produces difficulty in swallowing.
   b. **True**. Abduction is primarily limited in the horizontal plane.
   c. **True**. This position is the result of the unopposed, combined action of the IVth (downward) and VIth (lateral) cranial nerves.
   d. **False**. Preservation of the upper division occurs with upper motor neurone defect; total paralysis occurs with lower motor neurone defect.
   e. **True**. It is pushed over by the normal side.

4. a. **False**. Cutaneous manifestations of neurocutaneous syndromes include café au lait spots (neurofibromatosis); adenoma sebaceum, shagreen and hypopigmented patches (tuberous sclerosis); and port wine naevi (Sturge–Weber syndrome).
   b. **False**. See above.
   c. **True**. This is neurofibromatosis type I.
   d. **True**. This occurs in tuberous sclerosis.
   e. **True**. Occurs on the face in Sturge–Weber syndrome.

5. a. **True**. Occurs in end-stage raised intracranial pressure.
   b. **True**. Occurs together with bradycardia.
   c. **False**. Bradycardia is an indication.
   d. **True**. Initially, papilloedema may be unilateral.
   e. **True**. This completes the classical triad with vomiting and headaches.

6. a. **True**. This is a classical side-effect of phenytoin.
   b. **True**. As with all benzodiazepines.
   c. **False**. This occurs with paraldehyde.
   d. **True**. Hence the need to perform regular liver function tests in patients taking carbamazepine.
   e. **False**. This occurs with phenytoin.

7. a. **False**. Sensory nerves may be affected.
   b. **True**. This implies a greater chance of total recovery.
   c. **False**. Weakness improves well before the reflexes.
   d. **True**. Plasmapheresis is indicated with rapidly progressive neuropathy, bulbar and respiratory involvement.
   e. **False**. Intravenous immunoglobulin is the main treatment.

8. a. **True**. These irreversibly inhibit acetylcholinesterases and cause accumulation of acetylcholine at muscarinic and nicotinic synapses.
   b. **True**. Occurs particularly with vincristine.
   c. **False**. Steroids may cause a myopathy.
   d. **False**. Neuropathy is not a recognised complication of carbamazepine.
   e. **True**. As with other heavy metals, e.g. lead.

9. a. **True**. Although febrile convulsions occasionally develop in older children.
   b. **True**. Febrile convulsions affect 3–5% of children.
   c. **False**. They are seen in both sexes.
   d. **False**. They last less than 15 minutes.
   e. **False**. Very few develop epilepsy.

10. a. **False**. It is no more than a good guide.
    b. **True**. IQ assessment depends on a child's well-being, mood and cooperation.
    c. **True**. Most IQ tests are language based and rely on hearing.
    d. **False**. Less than 70 is the value used.
    e. **True**.

Case history answers

Case history 1

Despite the potential psychosomatic element introduced by the bullying, the history is sufficiently suspicious of seizure activity, particularly of generalised absences. A causal relationship to the bullying should be sought, and a drug and family history obtained. Features such as definite loss of consciousness, incontinence, cyanosis and rhythmic, jerky movements of the limbs, as well as 'runs' of these episodes, several times daily including during sleep, point strongly toward epilepsy. A thorough examination is mandatory to exclude signs of raised intracranial pressure, hypertension and neurological and metabolic disease. A period of in-hospital observation may be helpful in distinguishing between organic and psychosomatic symptoms. An EEG is required and performed at rest, with photic stimulation and hyperventilation. In addition, in a child with previously undiagnosed seizure activity, neuroimaging (e.g. CT scan) is indicated.

Case history 2

1. The peripheral and central temperature, pulse rate and volume, blood pressure, state of peripheral perfusion and signs of meningeal irritation, i.e. photophobia, neck stiffness and resistance to extension of the knees while flexing the hips (Kernig's sign). Papilloedema is unlikely at this early stage.
2. Meningococcal septicaemia, probably with meningitis, caused by *Neisseria meningitides* (group A, B or C).
3. Immediate blood cultures and serum for rapid antigen testing. The latter is not always reliable, especially with *N. meningitides* group B. A sample of CSF would be helpful but is contraindicated in a child with a deteriorating conscious level. Scraping of the purpuric lesions for culture can reveal the organism even up to 48 hours later.
4. One, preferably two, large-bore intravenous cannulae should be inserted and the blood cultures taken from the same access site. Plasma-substitute follows immediately (20 ml/kg over $\frac{1}{4}$ hour) and repeated as required, as well as intravenous ceftriaxone.
5. Progressive cardiovascular collapse (shock), associated with respiratory failure owing to pulmonary oedema and possibly cerebral oedema, and disseminated intravascular coagulation. Bleeding into the adrenal glands may account for the deteriorating hypotension (Waterhouse–Friderichsen syndrome). Renal failure is likely to ensue.
6. An urgent blood gas analysis and chest X-ray, electrolyte, urea and creatinine assessment, cross-match and clotting profile, including fibrinogen degradation products, are required.
7. He requires urgent plasma expansion using colloid, fresh frozen plasma and, probably, blood. The introduction of a central line would be extremely important at this stage for the immediate commencement of inotropic support (e.g. dopamine and adrenaline by infusion). In addition, he requires intubation, ventilation and transfer to the intensive-care unit.
8. Explain the nature and severity of their son's condition. You will need to point out the possibility that he may not survive the acute episode and that,

if he does, he may be left with residual sequelae including neurological handicap. You will also need to introduce the need for antibiotic prophylaxis for all close contacts.
9. Hence, the local public health authority must be notified. A thorough investigation into close 'contacts' is indicated. These include all individuals within the same household and friends with whom he may have had close (almost touching) contact for several hours within the preceding 24 hours, including contacts during the school trip. These should be given chemoprophylaxis with rifampicin (children) or ciprofloxacin (adults). There is no indication for mass, 'blind' prophylaxis – indeed, this will encourage the emergence of resistant strains.
10. Provided there is no other obvious focus of infection, the fever may be caused by persisting, low-grade infection in the CSF, a cerebral abscess or subdural collection. It may be related to the antibiotic (or other medication). A full septic screen including blood cultures and CT brain scan followed by a lumbar puncture are necessary.

Short notes answer

The management of status epilepticus involves: (i) control of the fits and (ii) determining and treating any underlying cause, as follows:

a. place child in left lateral position
b. administer oxygen by face mask with oral airway in situ
c. cool child (undress, per rectal paracetamol)
d. give diazepam per rectum while obtaining intravenous access
e. blood sent for glucose, electrolytes, calcium, blood gas and culture
f. correct hypoxia, acidosis, hypoglycaemia, metabolic derangements
g. repeat diazepam i.v., followed by paraldehyde if fits not controlled
h. continuous i.v. phenytoin, benzodiazepine are third-line agents
i. thiopentone with full ventilatory support in refractory cases
j. transfer to intensive-care unit with continuous ECG, EEG monitoring in refractory cases.

Investigation is aimed at excluding infection (septicaemia, meningitis, encephalitis), intracranial pathology (e.g. space-occupying lesion, intractable epileptic focus) and metabolic and neurodegenerative disease. Subsequent treatment will depend on the specific cause.

Viva voce answer

Given that the child is in coma, it is reasonable to assume that he has sustained a significant injury to the brain and/or neck. These could include depressed or multiple skull fractures, major intracranial contusion(s) and haemorrhage(s), as well as fracture(s) of the cervical vertebrae with spinal compression. The neck must be immobilised immediately with an appropriate collar prior to a detailed examination to assess for signs of shock, raised intracranial pressure, focal neurological signs and injuries elsewhere (e.g. limb fractures, pneumothorax, acute abdomen, etc.). If shocked, the child must be resuscitated. Intravenous access is obtained and fluids commenced: initially at 50% of maintenance in view of the risk of raised intracranial pressure and incipient brain oedema. Inotropic support may be required if hypotensive. Comprehensive X-rays of the skull and cervical spine, together with a brain CT scan, are mandatory and must be reviewed with the neurosurgical team. In addition, a cervical MRI scan may be required. Further management will depend on the result of these investigations and may involve neurosurgery for intracranial haematoma and treatment of cerebral oedema with hyperventilation and fluid restriction.

The urinary system

Key points

You should have an understanding of:

- The management of urinary tract infections
- The investigation of a child with proteinuria
- The investigation of a child with haematuria
- The basic symptoms and signs suggestive of renal failure, and have a working overview of its management.

7.1 Introduction

As a result of non-specific symptoms and a paucity of signs, pathology in the urinary system in childhood is often 'forgotten'. However, the routine measurement of blood pressure and a simple urinalysis would alert one to the possibility of renal disease in most cases. Infection is the most common problem involving the urinary tract in childhood and, especially if associated with congenital anomalies and reflux, may result in significant morbidity. A clear understanding of its aetiology, clinical manifestations, investigation and treatment is required in order to prevent long-term complications, including renal failure.

Proteinuria and haematuria are manifestations of the renal tract as well as systemic diseases and are easily confirmed on simple urinalysis. Both require further investigation of renal function. Although rare in childhood, renal failure results in acute and chronic complications that necessitate prompt intervention if morbidity and mortality are to be avoided. Children with end-stage renal failure will require renal-replacement therapy and, ultimately, a percentage will go on to renal transplantation. The undergraduate should be familiar with the indications but not the details of these treatment modalities.

7.2 Symptoms and examination

Symptoms of urinary tract disease

Symptoms are generally absent in young children and a high level of suspicion must be maintained. A **fever** without an obvious focus should raise the possibility of urinary tract infection (UTI). In neonates, prolonged jaundice, vomiting and weight loss are subtle pointers toward a UTI and the urine and renal tracts should be investigated. Older children may complain of pain or a burning sensation on micturition (**dysuria**) and loin and/or abdominal pain. **Frequency** and an alteration in urinary habit, particularly with regression to incontinence, are relatively common presenting complaints. An alteration in **urinary consistency** is rarely volunteered and should be asked for specifically. Offensive smelling,

cloudy urine is suggestive of urinary infection, frothy urine of proteinuria and smokey urine of haematuria. Marked lethargy with a waxy pallor and, at times, itching may suggest uraemia in children with renal failure.

Signs of urinary tract disease

Clinical signs in reno-urinary disease may be conspicuous by their absence. Many **dysmorphic syndromes** are associated with renal anomalies. Some congenital anomalies are specifically indicative of renal disease, e.g. preauricular pits, two instead of three vessels in the umbilical cord, perineal and genital anomalies. **Anaemia** is a common association in children with renal failure and should be looked for. All those with suspected renal disease should have their **blood pressure** measured and **urinalysis** performed. Large kidneys and **renal masses** in the loin can be balloted using both hands. A **distended bladder** is confirmed by finding a firm, rounded mass that is dull to percussion and rises out of the pelvis.

7.3 Congenital abnormalities

Renal agenesis

Bilateral renal agenesis results in complete renal failure antenatally, culminating in oligohydramnios followed by stillbirth. Affected infants have the **Potter facies** with a broad, flat nose, widely spaced eyes, epicanthic folds and low set ears. Severe renal dysplasia and obstructive uropathy may produce a similar appearance. Unilateral agenesis may be suspected with the presence of a single umbilical artery and is compatible with a normal existence, provided there are no other major anomalies of the genitourinary, skeletal, cardiac and gastrointestinal systems.

Maldevelopment

Incomplete upward migration of the embryonic kidney results in an **ectopic** kidney, usually sited in the pelvis. Fusion of the lower poles of each kidney produces a **horseshoe** kidney, whereas underdevelopment of the number of nephrons constitutes **renal hypoplasia**. The last carries a risk of hypertension in early childhood and, if bilateral, renal failure later in life. Renal **dysplasia** describes structurally abnormal nephrons and renal parenchyma and may present with renal masses, hypertension and renal failure.

Polycystic kidney disease

Autosomal dominant polycystic kidney disease

Autosomal dominant polycystic kidney disease is associated with large cystic lesions in the kidneys and liver that increase in size over several decades. Children are generally asymptomatic, although enlarged kidneys may be palpable. Hypertension and renal failure may ensue in adulthood. Subarachnoid haemorrhage may result from associated cerebral aneurysms.

Autosomal recessive polycystic kidney disease

Autosomal recessive polycystic kidney disease may present in the neonatal period through to the teenage years, often with bilateral flank masses. The earlier presenting types are associated with pulmonary hypoplasia and early death. Surviving patients develop multiple cysts of the collecting ducts, progressive renal fibrosis, tubular atrophy and inexorable renal failure. The diagnosis is confirmed on renal ultrasound scanning, intravenous pyelography and renal biopsy.

Hydronephrosis and hydroureters

These are discussed in Chapter 12.

Vesicoureteric reflux

Vesicoureteric reflux (VUR) is a common problem in childhood caused by lower ureteric sphincter incompetence, sometimes as a result of malinsertion of the ureter into the bladder. It is almost invariably present with ureterocoeles and, if severe, results in varying degrees of hydroureter and hydronephrosis. Reflux is graded according to the level to which urine flows retrogradely on voiding (Fig. 41). When associated with recurrent urinary infections, reflux carries a high risk of renal scarring and, eventually, renal failure (**reflux nephropathy**).

7.4 Infections

Pathophysiology of urinary tract infection

Urinary tract infection (UTI) is the most common bacte-

rial infection in childhood, affecting up to 1% of boys and 2% of girls. As many as 25% of those with recurrent UTIs develop renal scarring, especially if VUR is also present. The risk of renal scarring is particularly great in infancy and can, with time, result in hypertension and chronic renal failure. UTI is usually caused by Gram-negative organisms that gain entry via the bloodstream or by retrograde passage from the external genitalia and perineum (Box 16). Children with congenital abnormalities of the renal tracts, reflux, urinary stasis and repeated catheterisation are at a considerably increased risk of UTI (Box 17).

BOX 16
Causes of urinary tract infection

Gram-negative bacteria
Escherichia coli (85%)
Klebsiella spp.
Proteus spp.
Pseudomonas spp.

Gram-positive bacteria
Streptococcus faecalis
Staphylococcus saprophyticus

Viruses: several

Fungi
Candida spp.

BOX 17
Predisposing factors for urinary tract infection

Renal factors	Other factors
Congenital anomalies	Chronic constipation
Vesicoureteric reflux	Sexual abuse
Urinary obstruction and stasis	Immunosuppression
Urinary calculi	Diabetes mellitus
Bladder dysfunction	

Diagnosis of UTI

It is essential to obtain a clean specimen of urine **prior to commencing antibiotics**. A bag specimen is suitable for

Grade I   Grade II   Grade III   Grade IV   Grade V

Fig. 41 Grading of vesicoureteric reflux.

infants after appropriate cleansing of the perineum, whereas a 'clean catch', mid-stream specimen is possible in older children. A suprapubic aspirate should be performed whenever there is a delay in sampling and other methods have failed. Catheter specimens are generally reserved for those with neurogenic bladders. Simple urinalysis may confirm the presence of increased white cells, with or without red cells and protein. In addition, every urine sample should be sent to the laboratory for culture and sensitivity. Dipslide cultures are extremely useful when immediate microbiological services may not be available. The presence of >10⁵ colony-forming units in a voided specimen constitutes significant bacteriuria, whereas any growth in a suprapubic sample is significant. In an ill-looking poorly perfused child a UTI is usually accompanied by a raised white cell count and positive blood cultures.

Management of UTI

Once confirmed, a 7-day course of oral trimethoprim, first-generation cephalosporin or nitrofurantoin will treat common organisms including *E. coli*. A subsequent urine sample should be assessed to ensure eradication of the infection. Infants should be treated aggressively with intravenous antibiotics (e.g. cefotaxime and gentamicin). Following a first infection, infants and those below the age of 4 years should be started on prophylactic trimethoprim as a single night-time dose. This will

prevent recurrences until renal tract investigations can be organised as shown in Figure 42. Ultrasound in order to exclude congenital anomalies, dilatation resulting from obstruction and calculi should be carried out in all patients. A plain abdominal X-ray is useful to exclude spinal abnormalities and detect small calculi. Renal scarring is best evaluated by means of a renal isotope DMSA scan (technetium-labelled 2,3-dimercaptosuccinic acid), 6 weeks after the UTI, especially in preschool and school-age children at risk (Fig. 43a). Isotope renography using DTPA scan (technetium-labelled diethylenetriaminepentaacetic acid), or MAG3 is useful in demonstrating differential renal function, excretion and obstruction (Fig. 43b). A micturating cystogram (MCUG) is necessary to assess ureteric reflux and bladder emptying. It should be performed once the UTI has cleared in all children aged 3 years or less, and in those with renal scarring, a positive family history of reflux nephropathy or other renal anomaly. Serum electrolytes, urea, creatinine and glomerular filtration rate (GFR) are indicated in patients with evidence of renal damage where renal dysfunction is a possibility. An intravenous urography (IVU) assessment is carried out if there is no reflux.

The indications for antibiotic prophylaxis are shown in Table 38. For those whose imaging is normal, follow-up should include urine cultures if symptoms recur. Children in whom VUR is present should continue on prophylactic antibiotics and have their urine checked

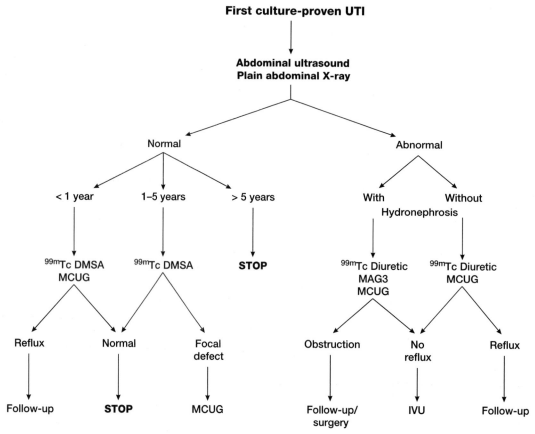

Fig. 42 Protocol for investigation of UTI in children. See text for explanation.

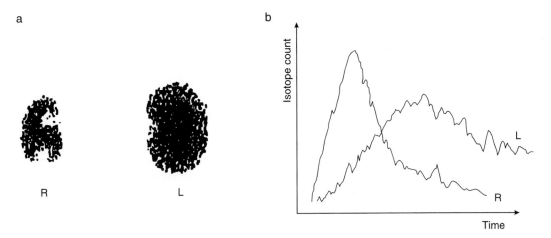

Fig. 43 Renal scans. (a) DMSA scan showing an atrophied right kidney with filling defects representing renal scars. (b) A DTPA excretion curve shows a normal pattern in the right with reduced and delayed excretion in the obstructed left kidney.

Table 38 Indications for antibiotic prophylaxis

First UTI prior to results of ultrasound/DMSA scanning/MCUG
Recurrent UTIs
Reflux
Renal tract anomalies
Renal scars
Compromised renal function

routinely every 3 months. Prophylaxis should continue for the first 4 years, provided renal scarring on DMSA scanning remains absent. For those with renal scars but no VUR, biannual DMSA scans are required. Recurrent breakthrough infections, the persistence of reflux on repeat MCUG, development of scars on DMSA, deteriorating renal function and underlying renal tract anomalies are indications for surgery. All patients with scars should have annual blood pressure measurements, together with urinalysis for proteinuria. The potential risk of a deterioration in renal function during pregnancy must be explained.

Renal abscess

Pyelonephritis with abscess formation is a rare complication of UTI. The toxic, febrile patient presents with bacteriuria, pyuria and haematuria. A painful loin mass is confirmed on ultrasound scanning (and, if necessary, by CT scan). The urine may be sterile in children previously treated with antibiotics. The pus must be drained by means of a nephrostomy tube under direct imaging or surgery, and antibiotics given intravenously for 10 days.

7.5 Proteinuria

Estimation of proteinuria

Protein loss in the urine amounting to not more than 150 mg in 24 hours lies within normal limits and mainly comprises albumin and Tamm–Horsfall mucoprotein. Dipsticks are highly sensitive for albuminuria but less so for other proteins and may result in many false-positive results. If suspected, proteinuria is best quantified in a 24-hour urine collection, but a good estimate is obtained by calculating the urine protein:creatinine ratio (normal <0.5 and <0.2 in infants and older children, respectively). Proteinuria in excess of 1000 mg in 24 hours is almost always pathological, especially when associated with oedema.

Benign proteinuria

Transient proteinuria <1 g in 24 hours (<2+ on dipstick) may arise during exercise and intercurrent febrile illnesses. Increased urinary protein loss on standing (**orthostatic** proteinuria) can be shown to resolve on comparing daytime samples with night-time urine voided in the supine position. Children with postural proteinuria require long-term monitoring of blood pressure, renal function and protein loss.

Pathological proteinuria

Damage to the proximal renal tubules by congenital or acquired disease can result in **tubular proteinuria**, which does not usually exceed 1 g in 24 hours (Box 18). It is generally associated with obvious features of the underlying disease process and other features of tubular dysfunction. In contrast, **glomerular proteinuria** is far more common and may be present in asymptomatic patients. The amount of protein loss varies enormously and may include albumin and low-molecular-weight proteins (selective) or albumin plus large proteins (nonselective).

Nephrotic syndrome

Nephrotic syndrome is typified by proteinuria, hypoproteinaemia, oedema and hyperlipidaemia. It is

---

BOX 18
Non-benign causes of proteinuria

	Acquired	Congenital
Glomerular	Nephrotic syndrome	Nephrotic syndrome
	Glomerulonephritis	
	Toxins (heavy metals)	
	Drugs (captopril, phenytoin)	
Tubular	Tubular necrosis	Tubular acidosis
	Interstitial nephritis	Cystinosis
	Toxins (heavy metals)	Wilson's disease
	Drugs (antibiotics)	Galactosaemia

---

idiopathic in 90% of patients and histopathology will show minimal change disease (85%), focal sclerosis (10%) or mesangial proliferation (5%). The remaining 10% are secondary to glomerulonephritis, malignant tumours (e.g. lymphoma), drugs and toxins. Autosomal recessive **congenital nephrotic syndrome** (Finnish type) is extremely rare and associated with a poor outcome. In all cases, increased glomerular permeability results in protein loss (especially albumin), usually exceeding 2 g per 24 hours (>3+ on dipstick). Oedema develops as the serum albumin falls below 25 g/dl. Hyperlipidaemia is caused by decreased lipid catabolism and increased lipoprotein production in the liver. Serum calcium is low because of loss of albumin-binding capacity. In addition, patients are at an increased risk of infection, partly through loss of complement and protein-bound immunoglobulins. Peritonitis caused by *Strep. pneumoniae* is common and, in view of the masking effect of steroid therapy, may not present with overt signs; as a result, a low threshold of suspicion must be maintained. An increased thrombotic tendency arises because of elevated coagulation factors and reduced fibrinolysis. It is exacerbated by the low plasma oncotic pressure, which results in loss of intravascular fluid to the interstitial space with a subsequent decrease in circulatory volume.

Idiopathic nephrotic syndrome due to **minimal change disease** is characterised by normal appearances on light microscopy but fusion of epithelial cell foot processes on electron microscopy. The majority (95%) are responsive to steroids and the prognosis is excellent. Steroid resistance is seen in up to 50% of those with mesangial proliferation and 80% with focal sclerosis, where progressive disease leading to end-stage renal failure is likely. Minimal change disease usually affects boys (more than girls) aged between 2–6 years, who present with periorbital and peripheral oedema shortly after an unremarkable viral-like upper respiratory infection. Ascites and diminished urine output follow. A few patients with minimal change disease are hypertensive. Urinalysis confirms significant proteinuria (>2 g per 24 hours) and occasionally microscopic haematuria. Creatinine clearance is low because of poor renal perfusion owing to the decreased intravascular volume.

Serum albumin and calcium are both low. As it is likely that there will be a response to steroids, all patients should be started on prednisolone, 2 mg/kg daily in divided doses. Renal biopsy is only indicated in those with atypical features and failure to respond with steroids. Salt restriction is important until the oedema clears. Any suspicion of infection must be treated with systemic Gram-positive and Gram-negative antibiotic cover. Mild oedema can be controlled with chlorothiazide and spironolactone if hypokalaemia develops. Severe oedema requires careful fluid restriction and the combination of frusemide (furosemide) and metolazone, with monitoring of serum electrolytes as there is underlying hypovolaemia despite the obvious oedema. Infusions of 25% albumin are likely to produce only transient improvement.

Clearing of urinary protein occurs within 2 weeks in most patients, and the dose of prednisolone can then be changed to an alternate day regimen and continued for 3–6 months. In those who have had no relapses, steroids can be tailed off rapidly, although corticosteroids must be provided during subsequent illness or surgery in the following 12 months. Persistence of proteinuria after 4 weeks of steroid therapy constitutes **steroid resistance** and is an indication for renal biopsy. Relapses involve recurrence of proteinuria with oedema and are initially treated with steroids in a similar fashion. Cyclophosphamide can be added when steroid toxicity is unacceptable. This drug is also useful in steroid-resistant and frequently relapsing disease and is usually given for 12 weeks, during which time weekly estimates of the white cell count are mandatory. Although many patients will suffer multiple relapses, the nephrotic syndrome generally burns out during the teenage years. A significant risk of end-stage renal failure is present with steroid-resistant disease secondary to focal and segmental glomerulosclerosis.

7.6 Haematuria

Microscopic haematuria describes more than five red cells per high power field in urine and may be present in up to 1% of asymptomatic schoolchildren. Blood in the urine may originate as a result of diseases primarily affecting the kidneys and lower urinary tract, as well as coagulopathies, drugs and exercise (Boxes 19 and 20).

Glomerular causes of haematuria

Glomerulonephritis

Glomerular damage that follows various immunological or toxic insults may result in glomerular bleeding together with loss of protein. In addition, some types of glomerulonephritis can be associated with acute renal failure while others progress to chronic disease with end-stage renal failure.

BOX 19
Renal causes of haematuria

Glomerular
Glomerulonephritis
Recurrent haematuria
Haemolytic uraemic syndrome (HUS)
Henoch–Schönlein purpura
Systemic lupus erythematosus (SLE)

Non-glomerular
Polycystic disease
Congenital anomalies
Infection
Trauma
Tumours
Calculi

BOX 20
Non-renal causes of haematuria

Haematological
Coagulopathies
Thrombocytopenia
Renal vein thrombosis
Sickle cell disease

Non-haematological
Exercise
Drugs

Poststreptococcal glomerulonephritis

The incidence of poststreptococcal glomerulonephritis is declining and it is now a less common cause of haematuria than IgA nephropathy (see below). It affects young children greater than 3 years of age, who present with low-grade fever, lethargy and smokey or red urine, sometimes accompanied by oedema and hypertension. The acute nephritis develops 1–2 weeks after a preceding upper respiratory tract or skin infection caused by group A β-haemolytic streptococci. Urinalysis confirms haematuria, often in the form of casts, as well as proteinuria and increased urinary white cells. Characteristically, investigation reveals a mild anaemia, leucocytosis, decreased C3 levels, haemolytic streptococci on throat swab culture, and positive anti-streptococcal antibodies (e.g. ASOT or DNAase B antigen). Renal biopsy would confirm an increase in glomerular size, mesangial and inflammatory cell proliferation with few, if any, crescents. However, biopsy is only necessary in children with 'non-classical' features, including acute renal failure, nephrotic syndrome, normal C3 levels, no evidence of streptococcal infection and persistence of symptoms beyond 2–3 months. Up to 95% of patients make a full recovery. Treatment is essentially supportive. Complications such as renal failure and hypertension must be controlled. Although penicillin is given for 10 days to clear residual streptococci, it has no effect on the nephritic process.

Membranous glomerulonephritis

Membranous glomerulonephritis is rare in childhood,

affecting those above the age of 10 years. The child presents with a nephrotic syndrome and microscopic haematuria, together with a normal blood pressure and C3 levels. This disease may be associated with systemic lupus erythematosus (SLE), heavy metals and hepatitis B virus (HBV) infection. Biopsy shows diffuse thickening of the glomerular basement membrane (GBM) resulting from IgG and C3 immune-complex deposition without significant cell proliferation. Most cases resolve with control of the nephrotic element using salt restriction and diuretics.

Membranoproliferative glomerulonephritis

Membranoproliferative glomerulonephritis is the most common cause of **chronic** glomerulonephritis. It affects children over the age of 10 years, who present with gross or microscopic haematuria, proteinuria, hypertension and a moderate decrease in C3 levels and renal function. These symptoms persist beyond 2 months, at which point a biopsy will show an increase in mesangial cells with deposition of C3 rather than immunoglobulin in the subendothelial region and crescent formation. The outcome is poor, the severity increasing with increasing number of crescents. Some response may follow renal supportive measures and prednisolone, but the majority develop end-stage renal failure.

Rapidly progressive glomerulonephritis

Although crescents are a feature of several types of glomerulonephritis, they are typical of idiopathic, rapidly progressive crescentic nephritis. Patients present with nephrotic or nephritic features and renal dysfunction, which progresses within a few weeks to end-stage renal failure. Only a small minority respond to immunosuppression with steroids, azathioprine, cyclophosphamide and plasmapheresis.

Infection-related glomerulonephritis

Infection-related glomerulonephritis is caused by damage resulting from the deposition of immune complexes in the glomeruli. It is associated with chronic infection including hepatitis B and C, malaria, syphilis, candidiasis, subacute endocarditis and chronically infected ventriculoperitoneal shunts. Patients develop a nephrotic or nephritic syndrome, often with low C3 levels, which resolves on treatment of the infection.

SLE-related glomerulonephritis

SLE-related glomerulonephritis is one of the most serious complications of this condition. All adolescent girls with SLE and haematuria or proteinuria, with or without renal dysfunction, should undergo renal biopsy. This reveals varying degrees of mesangial and subendothelial deposits, and focal or segmental cellular proliferation with crescent formation and necrosis. Thickening of the capillary wall produces the **wire loop appearance**. Aggressive immunosuppression with multiple agents is usually required to keep the disease under control.

Goodpasture disease

Goodpasture disease involves antibodies against lung and GBM, resulting in pulmonary haemorrhage and a glomerulonephritis similar to rapidly progressive disease with crescents. Patients present with haemoptysis, haematuria, proteinuria and renal failure. Few respond to immunosuppression and plasmapheresis and the mortality from pulmonary haemorrhage is high.

Recurrent haematuria

Some conditions are characterised by recurrent haematuria that may be gross or microscopic. The latter may follow a brief latent period of 1–3 days after a non-specific viral illness and recurs with subsequent infections. Mild proteinuria is common, but complications such as hypertension, oedema and renal failure are unusual. Blood tests and renal imaging are normal. The diagnosis is confirmed on renal biopsy. A normal biopsy characterises **idiopathic haematuria**, which carries a good prognosis. Predominant IgA mesangial deposits are seen in **IgA (Berger) nephropathy**, 30% of which develop complications and require immunosuppressant therapy. **Alport syndrome** is an X-linked dominant nephritis associated with sensorineural deafness that presents with haematuria and mild proteinuria. Biopsy shows splitting of the GBM, sometimes with sclerosis and fibrosis; if these are present renal failure in the second to third decade can be expected.

Henoch–Schönlein purpura

Henoch–Schönlein purpura is discussed in Chapter 11.

Haemolytic uraemic syndrome

Haemolytic uraemic syndrome (HUS) is the commonest cause of acute renal failure in preschool children. Most cases follow 7 days after gastrointestinal (sometimes upper respiratory) infections, often with verotoxin-producing *E. coli*. (0157:H7) or rarely other bacterial or viral agents. Thickening of the glomerular capillaries and fibrin deposition may result in glomerular sclerosis and cortical necrosis. Damage to red cells as they pass through the abnormal renal vasculature results in microangiopathic haemolytic anaemia. Similarly, platelet damage and consumption in intrarenal clot formation result in thrombocytopenia. Patients present with oliguria together with severe lethargy and marked pallor, sometimes with petechiae. Investigation confirms a haemoglobin of 5–8 g/dl, platelets <50 × 10⁹ cells/l and elevated white cell count. Blood film analysis shows fragmented cells (Fig. 44) and the Coombs' test is negative. Full-blown disseminated intravascular coagulopathy is unusual. Microscopic haematuria and proteinuria is coupled with raised serum urea and creatinine levels. Ultrasound of the kidneys is helpful in

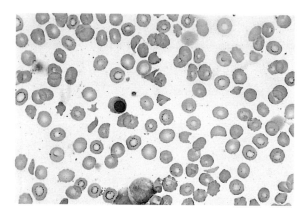

Fig. 44 Blood film in haemolytic uraemic syndrome, showing anaemia with fragmented red blood cells (microangiopathic haemolytic anaemia) and thrombocytopaenia.

excluding renal vein thrombosis but renal biopsy is contraindicated. Management entails aggressive treatment of renal failure with dialysis, control of complications such as hypertension and hyperkalaemia, and careful anticoagulation with heparin. The majority of patients make a full recovery but require long-term follow-up of their blood pressure and renal function.

Tubular causes of haematuria

Haematuria is a feature of urinary infections and tumours, when it is usually microscopic. Macroscopic haematuria may develop from bleeding congenital anomalies such as haemangiomas, cysts and polycystic disease. In the majority of school-age children, gross haematuria is secondary to renal haematoma formation after blunt trauma while falling astride bicycle handlebars. Urinary calculi themselves may lead to epithelial trauma with subsequent bleeding (Chapter 12).

Non-renal causes of haematuria

Any severe coagulopathy can present with haematuria. Indeed, microscopic haematuria is extremely common in patients with thrombocytopenia (e.g. with idiopathic thrombocytopenic purpura (ITP) or those receiving chemotherapy) and in those taking anticoagulants. Other drugs that may cause renal damage or cystitis may also precipitate haematuria (e.g. antibiotics, cytotoxics). Sickling within the kidneys can result in haematuria in children with both sickle cell disease and trait. **Renal vein thrombosis** is a complication seen in critically ill neonates and presents with renal mass(es) and haematuria. Some individuals develop haematuria after strenuous exercise, which resolves within a few days of rest. In all cases, tests of renal function and urinary tract imaging are normal.

7.7 Renal failure

Neonates have a diminished glomerular filtration rate

and ability to excrete ions such as hydrogen, potassium, sodium and phosphate and can concentrate urine to a maximum of 700 mosmol/l. Older children can concentrate urine beyond 1000 mosmol/l. Urine output below 1.0 and 0.5 ml/kg per hour for newborns and older children, respectively, constitutes **oliguria** and is indicative of renal failure. **Anuria** describes a total absence of urine output.

Acute renal failure

Most children who present in renal failure have a decreased renal perfusion pressure from prerenal causes. The majority have hypotension associated with dehydration, hypoxia, sepsis and diminished cardiac output (congenital heart disease or postcardiac surgery). Renal and postrenal causes of renal failure are listed in Box 21.

Patients with acute renal failure present with lethargy, pallor, vomiting and decreased urine output. Examination reveals anaemia, hypertension and fluid overload. The last manifests as dependent oedema, heart failure, pulmonary oedema, behavioural changes and even coma. Other signs related to the primary cause may be evident (e.g. diarrhoea, rashes, etc.). Investigative findings may vary widely depending on the cause, although anaemia, hyponatraemia, hyperkalaemia, hyperphosphataemia with hypocalcaemia, acidosis, uraemia and a raised serum creatinine are usual. With renal causes of renal failure, urine quality is poor with low osmolality (<400 mosmol/l) and high sodium ions (>30 mmol/l). Urgent abdominal X-rays and ultrasound scans are required to exclude an obstructive cause.

A stringent **fluid balance** must be kept in all cases of diminished renal function. Prerenal failure caused by hypovolaemia usually responds to careful fluid replacement using isotonic saline or colloid solutions (10–20 ml/kg over 0.5–1 hour). In under-filled oliguric (not anuric) patients, a bolus dose of 20 ml/kg colloid followed by a potent diuretic may encourage urine output. Frusemide (furosemide) may be repeated twice in increasing doses (2 and 10 mg/kg), whereas mannitol (up to 1 g/kg) should only be administered once. Dopamine at 5 µg/kg per minute may improve renal perfusion and urine output. No response implies incipient or established renal failure. In this situation, in order to maintain an accurate fluid balance, patients should be catheterised, weighed twice daily and, if possible, measurement of the central venous pressure established. Continuous ECG monitoring is also mandatory.

Fluid restriction should be limited to insensible losses (approximately 400 ml/m^2 daily), plus the daily urine output (if any) and any other losses (e.g. from gastrointestinal tract). Regular monitoring of serum electrolytes is paramount and fluid given as glucose solutions with the appropriate addition of electrolytes.

Hyperkalaemia is the most serious complication, resulting in arrhythmias and death if uncontrolled. No potassium-containing solutions should be given in any guise. A serum potassium ion level >6 mmol/l without ECG changes should be treated with a potassium chelating resin (orally or per rectum). Levels >7 mmol/l with peaked T waves or other ECG changes require urgent treatment with slow intravenous 10% calcium gluconate (0.5 ml/kg over 10 minutes) to counteract cardiac irritability. The elevated potassium can be lowered using 8.4% sodium bicarbonate (1 ml/kg over 30 minutes), β agonists (e.g. salbutamol) and a dextrose–insulin infusion. A poor response to these measures necessitates urgent dialysis.

Hyponatraemia usually responds to fluid restriction and extra NaCl given with sodium ion levels <120 mmol/l.

Acidosis with a pH <7.1 or a bicarbonate level <8 mmol/l is managed by partial correction to maintain the pH at above 7.2. Sodium bicarbonate is given intravenously in the acute setting and by the oral route as the situation stabilises.

Hypocalcaemia–hyperphosphataemia is controlled by phosphate-binding oral calcium carbonate.

Hypertension that is moderate is treated with salt and fluid restriction, frusemide and propranolol. Severe hypertension may respond to labetolol by infusion (or sodium nitroprusside).

Anaemia is corrected only in severe cases and by using small amounts of packed cells.

Renal dialysis. Failure to control the above complications, plus fluid overload, congestive heart failure and hypertensive seizures are indications for renal dialysis (Table 39). This can be performed by continuous or intermittent flushing of diasylate fluid across the peritoneum (**peritoneal dialysis**), or extracorporeal haemofiltration (**haemodialysis**).

BOX 21 Causes of acute renal failure		
Prerenal disease	**Renal disease**	**Postrenal disease**
Hypotension	Glomerulonephritis	Obstructive uropathy
Hypovolaemia	Acute tubular necrosis	Posterior urethral valves
Anoxia	Haemolytic uraemic syndrome	Reflux nephropathy
Sepsis	Renal vein thrombosis	Calculi, blood clot
Poor cardiac output	Drugs, toxins, uric acid	
	Congenital anomalies	

Table 39 Indications for acute renal dialysis

Complications	Manifestations
Electrolyte disturbance	Hyperkalaemia, hyperphosphataemia, acidosis
Fluid overload	Heart failure, pulmonary oedema
Hypertension	Uncontrolled, accelerated, with seizures

End-stage renal failure

Persistence of renal failure, often as a result of the causes listed in Box 21, results in **chronic renal failure** which, in due course, culminates in end-stage renal failure. Chronic renal failure is exacerbated by a high-protein diet, hypertension, persistent proteinuria and recurrent urinary infections. Management entails optimising nutritional intake utilising carbohydrate and fats, controlling electrolyte levels (especially potassium, hydrogen and phosphate ions) and provision of iron, folic acid and trace elements. Inadequate growth can be enhanced using growth hormone and chronic anaemia by means of erythropoeitin. Acidosis is corrected with bicarbonate to maintain levels above 20 mmol/l. Renal osteodystrophy is manifest by hyperphosphataemia, hypocalcaemia, raised alkaline phosphatase and parathyroid hormone, with ricket-like changes on X-ray examination. Treatment involves a low-phosphate diet, antacids such as calcium carbonate to bind phosphate in the gut, and vitamin D supplements. Hypertension and urinary infections must be treated aggressively. Renal replacement therapy via dialysis is instituted once the glomerular filtration rate falls below 20% of normal, usually with a serum creatinine level around 900 μmol/l.

Renal transplantation

Ultimately, all children on renal-replacement therapy will require a renal transplant. In the meantime, most patients are stabilised on **continuous ambulatory peritoneal dialysis** (CAPD) involving three to six daily exchanges via an abdominally sited Tenckhoff catheter. A minority require haemodialysis through a prosthetic arteriovenous fistula. Catheter/fistula failure and infection is an ever-present risk for these patients. Kidney transplantation is effected using a donor with matching human leucocyte antigens (HLA). These are encoded on the major histocompatibility complex (MHC) on chromosome 6. The best-fit is likely with an identical twin and, to a lesser extent, another living family member. Alternatively, a matched cadaveric donor organ is used. Up to 80% of living related and 65% of cadaveric grafts function adequately after 3 years. Despite the problems associated with immunosuppressive therapy (steroids, cyclosporin A), the improvement in quality of life of successful transplant recipients is tremendous. Transplant failure is primarily through rejection (50%), recurrence of primary renal disease (33%) and thrombotic phenomena (15%).

Renal dysfunction

Proximal renal tubular acidosis

In proximal renal tubular acidosis (RTA), bicarbonate is not sufficiently reabsorbed in the proximal tubules and the excess load spilling into the distal tubules cannot be totally reclaimed and is lost as sodium bicarbonate in the urine. Compensatory mechanisms including absorption of sodium (and chloride) in exchange for potassium ions results in hypokalaemia and hyperchloraemia. Loss of bicarbonate results in acidosis. Proximal RTA may be an isolated defect. However, in the **Fanconi syndrome** it is associated with generalised tubular dysfunction, resulting in RTA with glycosuria, phosphaturia and amino aciduria. Rickets is an added complication of this type of RTA.

Distal renal tubular acidosis

Defective hydrogen ion secretion in the distal tubules results in distal RTA, whereby the urine cannot be acidified below a pH of 5.8, even in the presence of marked systemic acidosis. Associated loss of sodium bicarbonate results in hypokalaemia and hyperchloraemia. Distal RTA, unlike proximal RTA, is also associated with hypercalciuria, leading to the formation of renal calculi and nephrocalcinosis.

The diagnosis is suspected when, in the presence of systemic acidosis with a serum bicarbonate level of less than 16 mmol/l, the urine pH remains above 5.5 or 5.8 for proximal and distal RTA, respectively. Treatment entails alkalinisation of the plasma with sodium bicarbonate (or citrate) and potassium supplementation.

Renal osteodystrophy

Loss of nephrons as well as significant glomerular and tubular dysfunction can result in renal osteodystrophy (renal rickets). Insufficient production of vitamin D at renal level, together with secondary hyperparathyroidism, results in malabsorption of calcium and phosphate from the gut. A compensatory increase in parathyroid hormone (PTH) ensures normocalcaemia but low or normal phosphate levels owing to increased excretion of phosphate in the urine. This leads to bone resorption, resulting in osteopenia, increased bone turnover and replacement with disorganised lamellae producing characteristic, ricket-like changes seen on X-ray film. Renal osteodystrophy contributes toward growth failure in children with chronic renal failure and is treated with calcium and vitamin D supplements, together with phosphate-lowering binding agents.

Renal diabetes insipidus

Failure to reabsorb water at renal level despite the presence of antidiuretic hormone (ADH) constitutes nephrogenic diabetes insipidus. This may be an

X-linked dominant condition where boys, and to a lesser extent girls, present with marked polydipsia and polyuria, sometimes with hypernatraemic dehydration. Hypernatraemia with serum hyperosmolality >295 mosmol/l in the presence of a dilute urine is suggestive of this diagnosis. Failure to concentrate the urine after intramuscular ADH and during a carefully monitored water deprivation test provides confirmatory evidence. Treatment includes regular fluid intake and, paradoxically, diuretics (e.g. chlorothiazide).

Self-assessment: questions

Multiple choice questions

1. The following statements describe urinary tract infection:
   a. It is the most common bacterial infection in childhood
   b. It is more common in those with ectopic ureters
   c. It carries a high risk of end-stage renal failure
   d. It is usually caused by *Proteus* species
   e. In school-age children, it is best treated with intravenous antibiotics

2. Asymptomatic bacteriuria:
   a. Is more common in girls
   b. Is always associated with significant urinary tract infection
   c. May be associated with vesicoureteric reflux (VUR)
   d. Is not associated with renal scarring
   e. Should be treated with antibiotics

3. The following features are observed in the nephrotic syndrome:
   a. Hypoalbuminuria
   b. Hyperlipidaemia
   c. Hypocalcaemia
   d. Increased intravascular volume
   e. Minimal change disease in the majority of idiopathic cases

4. The following are associated with a good prognosis for renal function:
   a. Nephrotic syndrome caused by glomerulosclerosis
   b. Nephrotic syndrome with minimal change disease
   c. Rapidly progressive glomerulonephritis
   d. SLE-related glomerulonephritis
   e. Poststreptococcal glomerulonephritis

5. The following are causes of haematuria in childhood:
   a. Urinary calculi
   b. Wilms tumour
   c. Haemolytic uraemic syndrome (HUS)
   d. Hyperbilirubinaemia
   e. Rifampicin therapy

6. The following are associated with acute renal failure:
   a. Hypertension
   b. Hypovolaemia
   c. Hypervolaemia
   d. Hypokalaemia
   e. Hypophosphataemia

7. The following statements describe the treatment of acute renal failure:
   a. Sodium supplements are an important addition to the diet
   b. Hyperkalaemia can be reduced using calcium gluconate
   c. Diuretics should not be used in oliguric patients
   d. Accelerated hypertension may be treated using labetolol
   e. Dialysis may be required for excessive fluid overload

8. The following are complications of chronic renal failure:
   a. Osteomalacia
   b. Hypertension
   c. Hypokalaemia
   d. Uraemia
   e. Alopecia areata

9. The treatment of chronic renal failure includes:
   a. A high-protein diet
   b. A low threshold for blood transfusion
   c. Potassium supplementation
   d. Growth hormone
   e. Phosphate-binding agents

10. In renal replacement therapy and transplantation:
    a. Most children are stabilised on haemodialysis not peritoneal dialysis
    b. Recurrent peritonitis is a serious complication with dialysis therapy
    c. Erythropoietin is only given after and not before transplantation
    d. Cyclosporin A therapy is commonly associated with hirsutism
    e. Cadaveric kidneys have an improved prognosis compared with live-related kidneys

Case histories

Case history 1

A 2-year-old girl presents with a fever and appropriate investigation confirms significant bacteriuria with *E. coli*. The fever settles within 24 hours of starting trimethoprim.

How would you plan follow-up for this child?

Case history 2

The numbers in parentheses at each question indicate the point weighting given for the answers.

As a senior house officer in casualty you see a 4-year-old girl who presents with a 2-day history of lower abdominal pain, fever and vomiting. Though undernourished for her age, clinically she appears well and there are no localising signs of infection though you cannot be sure that the left ear drum is not a bit congested. A full blood count shows a haemoglobin of 8 g/dl, a white cell count of 6×10^9 cells/l with a normal differential and a platelet count of 190×10^9 cells/l. A urine dipstick shows 2+ protein and 2+ blood. You send off a mid-stream urine (MSU) sample for culture, prescribe paracetamol and amoxycillin and ask the patient to come back the next day. The next day, you find that she has now stopped vomiting and her fever is less. The urine culture has been reported to show more than 10^5 colonies and the haematologist informs you that she has normochromic normocytic anaemia.

1. What is the most probable diagnosis? (2)
2. Why do you think she is anaemic? (4)
3. Is your choice of antibiotic appropriate? (4)
4. What advice would you give the parents regarding the immediate management? (10)

Microbiology informs you that the culture is growing *E. coli*.

5. Which part of the renal tract is most likely infected and why? (4)
6. How long should the therapy continue for? (4)
7. Name at least four other initial investigations that are needed and give the rationale (12)
8. Based on the results of these investigations what advice would you need to give to the parents on the long-term prognosis? (25)
9. Name three causes of haematuria other than the one illustrated here (6)
10. Name three possible complications of urinary tract infections (6)

Short notes

1. Outline the main problems and key points in the management of chronic renal failure.
2. Tabulate the tests that may be performed during the course of investigation of gross haematuria, indicating the reason for each test in a second column.

Self-assessment: answers

Multiple choice answers

1. a. **True**. It affects up to 1% of boys, 2% of girls.
    b. **True**. Ectopic ureters generally insert lower down the urinary tract (e.g. urethra or vagina) thereby allowing increased access to ascending organisms.
    c. **False**. There is a low risk at all ages although risk is greater in those under 3 years, especially if vesicoureteric reflux is also present.
    d. **False**. *E. coli* infection occurs in over 80%. *Proteus* sp. is associated with staghorn calculi, which are rare in childhood.
    e. **False**. Intravenous antibiotics are used in neonates.

2. a. **True**. It occurs in 1% of girls and 0.03% of boys.
    b. **False**. Hence, the dilemma of how to manage patients with asymptomatic bacteriuria.
    c. **True**. VUR occurs in 25%.
    d. **False**. Scarring occurs in 15%.
    e. **False**. Only treated with antibiotics if symptoms develop.

3. a. **False**. Hyperalbuminuria occurs with hypoalbuminaemia.
    b. **True**.
    c. **True**. This is secondary to hypoalbuminaemia.
    d. **False**. Decreased plasma oncotic pressure results in interstitial leakage, with decreased intravascular volume.
    e. **True**. The most common cause of nephrotic syndrome in childhood.

4. a. **False**. There is a high risk of end-stage renal failure.
    b. **True**. The majority of children with minimal change disease make a full recovery.
    c. **False**. It is associated with numerous glomerular crescents and renal failure.
    d. **False**. SLE-related disease often results in end-stage renal failure.
    e. **True**. Poststreptococcal glomerulonephritis is usually a transient disease.

5. a. **True**. Calculi may traumatise the urinary endothelium.
    b. **True**. Usually microscopic haematuria occurs.
    c. **True**. Usually associated with microscopic haematuria and proteinuria.
    d. **False**. Bilirubinuria occurs but no blood.
    e. **False**. Pink discoloration of urine occurs but no blood.

6. a. **True**. This is a major debilitating complication.
    b. **True**. It results in prerenal failure (e.g. following dehydration).

    c. **True**. Fluid overload occurs secondary to poor urine output.
    d. **False**. Hyperkalaemia is associated with acute renal failure.
    e. **False**. Hyperphosphataemia is associated with acute renal failure.

7. a. **False**. Sodium ion intake must be severely restricted.
    b. **False**. Calcium acts as a cardioprotective agent; it does not lower the potassium ion level.
    c. **False**. They may be very useful in establishing urine output, especially when given after a volume load.
    d. **True**. It provides both α and β blockade.
    e. **True**. Dialysis is appropriate with fluid overload, congestive heart failure, hypertension, acidosis, hyperkalaemia and central nervous system complications (e.g. seizures).

8. a. **True**. This is a feature of renal osteodystrophy.
    b. **True**. Hypertension is common in all types of renal failure.
    c. **False**. Hyperkalaemia can occur in chronic disease.
    d. **True**. This is a hallmark of renal failure.
    e. **False**. Acute hair loss may accompany severe (usually acute) illness but idiopathic alopecia areata does not occur.

9. a. **False**. A low-protein diet is used to reduce nitrogen load.
    b. **False**. Blood transfusion is avoided unless absolutely necessary.
    c. **False**. Potassium must be excluded.
    d. **True**. It is used to enhance growth potential.
    e. **True**. These are used to lower phosphate in renal osteodystrophy.

10. a. **False**. Most children cope well with peritoneal dialysis.
    b. **True**. It occurs with peritoneal dialysis.
    c. **False**. It is used both before and after transplantation.
    d. **True**. This is a common, cosmetically unwelcome, side-effect.
    e. **False**. The reverse is true.

Case history answers

Case history 1

This girl has a proven UTI and is in the 'at-risk' age group for further infections, possibly as a result of an underlying renal tract anomaly and reflux. Normal

Table 40 Tests performed in gross haematuria

Test performed	Reason for test
Blood tests	
Blood count*	Anaemia, thrombocytopenia
Blood film, sickle screen	Abnormal red cells/haemoglobin
Clotting profile	Clotting disorder
Electrolytes, urea, creatinine*	Renal dysfunction with glomerulonephritis, haemolytic uraemic syndrome
Calcium, uric acid, amino acids	Causes of urinary calculi
Antistreptolysin O titre (ASOT)/DNAase B	Poststreptococcal glomerulonephritis
C3 level*	Glomerulonephritis
Immunoglobulin levels	Glomerulonephritis
Antibody levels	For example antinuclear antibody (ANA) associated with systemic lupus erythromatosus (SLE) nephritis
Urine tests	
Urinalysis*	Amount of haematuria, also proteinuria
Urine culture*	To exclude UTI
Calcium and creatinine in 24 hour sample*	Hypercalciuria, renal concentrating ability
Microbiology	
Throat/skin cultures	Poststreptococcal glomerulonephritis
Mantoux, urine for acid-fast bacilli (AFB)	Tuberculosis
Imaging	
Plain abdominal X-ray	Renal calculi
Renal tract ultrasound*	Renal anomaly, malformation, tumour, renal vein thrombosis, haematoma
CT/MRI scan	Tumour, invasion of inferior vena cava
Invasive tests	
Cystoscopy	Renal calculi, bladder/urethral anomalies, tumours
Renal biopsy	Glomerulonephritis, SLE

*These tests are carried out on all patients.

renal function and absence of hypertension must be confirmed at the outset. The acute episode is treated with a 7–10 day course of trimethoprim (or an alternative once culture results are available), after which resolution of the UTI is confirmed on a repeat urine culture. Prophylactic single, night-time dose antibiotic is started and further investigations organised approximately 3 weeks later, once the urine is sterile. An anatomical abnormality of the renal tracts is assessed by ultrasound, renal scarring by DMSA scan, and vesicoureteric reflux by means of a micturating cystourethrogram (MCUG). If these are all normal, prophylactic antibiotics are not necessary and urine cultures are checked as a routine every 3–4 months. Prophylactic antibiotics are continued till the age of 4 years if there are risk factors for further UTIs (e.g. reflux, hydronephrosis or congenital abnormality) and if there is evidence of renal scarring. The latter requires monitoring with DMSA scans every 6–12 months. A repeat MCUG is required with non-resolution of hydronephrosis and reflux, prior to consideration for surgery. Annual blood pressure measurement and advice on the risks of hypertension in pregnancy must be organised.

Case history 2

1. The most likely diagnosis is a urinary tract infection. An acceptable alternative is cystitis.
2. Any child with an infection may have suppression of normal erythropoiesis. However, since this child has failed to thrive, a more chronic cause must be ruled out. Chronic renal insufficiency or failure could be a cause. Previous urinary tract infections may have been asymptomatic and resulted in reflux nephropathy and damage to the kidneys.
3. An antibiotic with action against Gram-negative bacilli is appropriate as they are the most common pathogens. Commonly co-trimoxazole, trimethoprim, nitrofurantoin or amoxycillin is used. The final choice should depend on the reported sensitivity of the organism. In this child, there appears to have been a therapeutic response and it is best to wait for the final culture and sensitivity report.
4. Urinary tract infections are a common childhood illness and are seen more often in girls. It is usually an ascending infection and responds quickly to a course of antibiotics. The course must be completed even though the symptoms may subside quickly; she can be managed as an outpatient and need not be hospitalised. Fever can be controlled with paracetamol and the child should be given small amounts of fluid frequently to ensure that she remains well hydrated. She will need to be followed up once she recovers and a repeat urine culture must be performed a week after stopping therapy to ensure that the urine remains sterile.
5. The bladder is the commonest site of infection. In this child, there is associated microscopic haematuria and lower abdominal pain, again a common presenting feature of cystitis. The absence of toxic signs and symptoms, colic and tenderness in the renal area argues against pyelonephritis.
6. The acute episode must be treated for 7–10 days.

135

Thereafter the child should be started on prophylactic antibiotics pending results of further investigations to rule out any underlying cause.

7. Four other investigations would be: serum creatinine to establish renal function; a plain abdominal X-ray to look for calculi and vertebral anomalies such as spina bifida; ultrasonography of the renal tract to rule out abnormalities of the renal tract and a $^{99\,m}$Tc-labelled DMSA scan to assess renal function.

8. The prognosis is based on the presence or absence of any underlying abnormality. Simple urinary tract infections, with normal imaging, may recur and if so acute exacerbations will need to be treated with a course of antibiotics. Cultures should be obtained at regular intervals and the child kept on a low single daily dose of either trimethoprim or nitrofurantoin for at least a year. The problem will resolve with age usually without any chronic sequelae. In those with renal scarring (shown by DMSA scan) or dilated renal tracts (ultrasound) further investigations including a MAG3 scan (to look for obstructive uropathy) and micturating cystourethrogram (for reflux) need to be performed. In some of these children, surgical reconstruction of the collecting tract may be required to prevent further damage to the kidney. In the majority with focal or reflux abnormalities, conservative management with long-term antibiotic prophylaxis is usually successful.

9. Causes can be divided into:

   - glomerular causes: IgA nephropathy, poststreptococcal glomerulonephritis, Henoch–Schönlein purpura
   - urinary calculi
   - systemic causes: sickle cell disease, idiopathic thrombocytopenic purpura
   - Drugs: cyclophosphamide.

10. Complications include pyelonephritis, renal scarring, hydronephrosis, perinephric abscess, chronic renal failure, anaemia and failure to thrive.

Short notes answers

1. The main complications associated with chronic renal failure include:

   - electrolyte imbalance: hyperkalaemia, hyponatraemia, hypocalcaemia, hyperphosphataemia
   - metabolic problems: acidosis with low bicarbonate, low pH, hyperuraemia
   - fluid imbalance: overload
   - anaemia: chronic disease, folate and iron deficiency
   - nutritional problems: catabolic state, rickets (renal osteodystrophy), growth failure
   - hypertension.

   The management is aimed at preventing further deterioration in renal function and controlling existing complications, initially by non-invasive means and, later, by renal replacement therapy (dialysis) prior to transplantation. A low-protein diet and aggressive treatment of UTIs and hypertension reduce the risk of exacerbating renal dysfunction. Electrolyte problems are controlled via a low-salt, low-potassium and low-phosphate diet and the use of phosphate-binding agents with vitamin D supplements. Bicarbonate supplements are required to maintain a serum bicarbonate level above 20 mmol/l. Anaemia is prevented with folic acid and iron, together with regular erythropoietin in those receiving renal replacement therapy. Growth is enhanced by optimising nutritional intake, mainly via a diet rich in carbohydrate and fat, if necessary via nasogastric tube feeding. Growth and an anabolic state may be augmented through the use of growth hormone. Failure of non-invasive therapeutic measures and inexorable progression of the underlying renal disease necessitates the introduction of regular dialysis, with a view to transplantation in the long term.

2. Tests performed during investigation of gross haematuria are given in Table 40.

The endocrine system

Key points

You should have an understanding of:

- The physiology of the various endocrine glands
- The symptoms and signs associated with various endocrinopathies
- The normal processes of growth and pubertal development, with particular emphasis on growth measurements (auxology)
- The management of short stature
- The acute and long-term management of diabetes mellitus
- The common endocrinological tests and their interpretation
- How to treat the common endocrinopathies.

8.1 Introduction

The endocrine system includes the pituitary, thyroid, adrenals, parathyroids, pancreas and gonads. These glands control the processes of growth and development in childhood and adolescence and are vital for the maintenance of normal homeostasis in the body and well-being of the individual.

8.2 Disorders of sexual differentiation

The gender of a newborn child is vital in determining the child's upbringing, although the sex of rearing does not always reflect the chromosomal sex: 1 in 4500 have **ambiguous genitalia** (Fig. 45) and, for those cases, it is essential to make an accurate diagnosis. Knowledge of the embryology of sexual differentiation is vital for understanding these conditions.

Physiology

The undifferentiated gonad develops into a male testis around the sixth week of gestation, under the influence of the sex-determining region on the Y chromosome (SRY). Testicular Leydig cells secrete testosterone in response to placental human chorionic gonadotrophin (hCG) and fetal luteinising hormone (LH), which in turn stimulates Wolffian ducts to develop. These form the epididymis, vas deferens and seminal vesicles. The external penis and scrotum develop as a result of the conversion of testosterone to dihydrotestosterone by the enzyme 5α-reductase. Testicular Sertoli cells produce anti-mullerian hormone (AMH), which, together with testosterone, directs the descent of the testes into the scrotum.

In the female ovary, primordial follicles develop and reach a peak at 20–25 weeks of gestation under the influence of fetal follicle-stimulating hormone (FSH). Wolffian ducts disappear and Mullerian ducts arise. The upper parts of these ducts develop into fallopian tubes, the middle into the uterus, and the lower parts into the upper third of the vagina. The clitoris is formed from the genital tubercle, the labia majora from the labioscrotal folds and the labia minora from the urethral folds. The urogenital sinus forms the lower two-thirds of the vagina.

Abnormal sexual development

Virilised females

Mullerian duct (female) differentiation proceeds normally in the absence of testes. However, the presence of androgens may result in a superimposition of masculine features onto the female phenotype. Clitoral hypertrophy is the most common problem, with labioscrotal fusion in extreme cases. Such virilisation usually follows congenital adrenal hyperplasia resulting from 21-hydroxylase deficiency (Box 22).

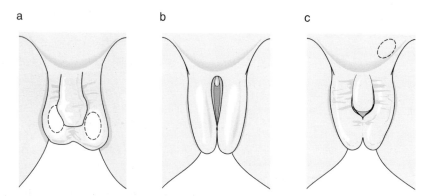

Fig. 45 External genitalia in the normal male (a), normal female (b) and in ambiguous genitalia (c), showing clitoromegaly (or underdeveloped penis), fused labia minora (or marked hypospadias), fused and rugose labia majora (or bifid scrotum). A partially descended gonad (if present) is usually a testis, implying XY karyotype.

Excess fetal androgens
Congenital adrenal hyperplasia: usually owing to
21-hydroxylase deficiency
Testis or ovotestis present: from partial gonadal
dysgenesis

Excess maternal androgens crossing placenta
Drugs: anabolic steroids, danazol, testosterone,
progestagens
Maternal disease: ovarian or adrenal tumours

Inadequately masculinised males

Incomplete masculinisation of the genital ducts and
external genitalia may result in a clinical appearance
ranging from the apparently normal female to a male
with hypospadias and cryptorchidism. Testes should be
looked for in all patients with intersex problems and, if
palpable, suggest a male karyotype. The causes of
incomplete masculinisation are shown in Box 23.

BOX 23
Causes of incomplete male masculinisation

Inadequate androgens
Gonadal dysgenesis: caused by the SRY gene
mutation
LH deficiency
Leydig cell agenesis or hypoplasia
Errors of testosterone synthesis: defect in adrenals,
testes or both

Impaired response to testosterone
Impaired conversion of testosterone to
dihydrotestosterone: 5α-reductase deficiency
Androgen insensitivity: androgen
receptor/postreceptor defect

Associated with dysmorphic syndromes
Smith–Lemli–Opitz
Aniridia–Wilms

Management, diagnosis and treatment
Parents will require expert counselling and registration
of the birth should be delayed until a decision has been
made regarding the sex of rearing. Attention should be
paid to a history of ingestion of drugs in pregnancy,
family history of primary amenorrhoea or infertility,
late puberty and unexplained neonatal deaths in relatives. Other congenital abnormalities, dysmorphic features and the presence of testes should be sought on
examination. Investigations include a pelvic ultrasound
scan to delineate the internal anatomy and a karyotype
to determine the genetic sex. In congenital adrenal
hyperplasia (CAH), 17α-hydroxyprogesterone and
adrenocorticotrophic hormone (ACTH) are usually
raised and the urinary steroid profile is abnormal. In
salt-losing CAH, serum electrolytes are abnormal, plasma renin activity is raised and aldosterone is reduced.

Testosterone and dihydrotestosterone levels are abnormal in androgen insensitivity and 5α-reductase
deficiency, whereas LH and FSH are low in
gonadotrophin deficiency. DNA analysis is helpful in
CAH, androgen insensitivity and 5α-reductase deficiency. Management is designed to achieve unambiguous
and functionally normal external genitalia and reproductive capacity. The penile size and its ability to
respond to testosterone are vital considerations.
Treatment may be medical (e.g. glucocorticoid and mineralocorticoid therapy in CAH, androgens in errors of
testosterone biosynthesis) or surgical (e.g. clitoral reduction, separation of labia and a limited vaginoplasty,
which should be performed early). In males with
hypospadias, reconstructive surgery is indicated to
ensure that the patients can urinate standing up before
going to school. Gonadectomy is indicated with dysge-
netic or non-functional gonads, especially in those with
Y-bearing cell lines, because of an increased risk of
malignant change in later life. Pubertal induction and
maintenance may be required.

8.3 Disorders of stature

Physiology

Growth is greatest in terms of height velocity in the second trimester of pregnancy, when the crown–heel
length increases at a rate of 52 cm/year. Influences on
fetal growth include ethnic origin, maternal height,
mid-pregnancy weight, nutrition, smoking and alcohol
intake, fetal sex, the presence of congenital abnormalities and growth factors. Postnatal growth is best
described by the infancy–childhood–pubertal model
(Fig. 46). The figure shows the height and velocity
curves of a normal child, highlighting the three phases
of growth in childhood and adolescence.

1. There is a rapidly decelerating growth phase in
   infancy, dependent on nutrition.
2. The steady, slowly decelerating growth phase in
   childhood is dependent on growth hormone (GH);
   growth rate may be enhanced by a mid-childhood
   growth spurt.
3. The rapidly accelerating and decelerating pubertal
   growth spurt is dependent upon the normal
   secretion of GH and sex steroids. This growth spurt
   occurs with breast development in girls (breast stage
   2–3), and a testicular volume of 10–12 ml in boys, as
   measured by a Prader orchidometer.

Assessment of growth

The assessment of growth is vital and involves several
parameters.
   Linear height should be measured using a stadiome-
ter and plotted onto a distance chart using the decimal

a

b

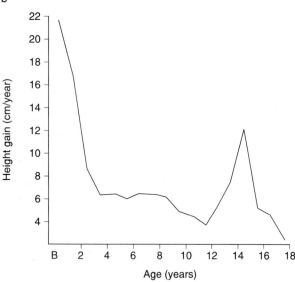

Fig. 46 The infancy–childhood–pubertal model of growth. (a) The height-distance chart and (b) the height-velocity chart of a normal child.

age. The parents' heights should also be plotted and the mid-parental centile calculated (add 12.5 cm to mother's height for a boy; subtract 12.5 cm from father's height for a girl). The distance chart simply compares the child's height to other children of the same age and a child may lie below the 3rd centile and still be normal.

Height velocity is often considered the 'gold standard' and is calculated by measuring the height at 3–4 monthly intervals and dividing the increment in height in centimetres by the time interval in years. A child's growth is normal if the height velocity lies close to the 50th centile on a height-velocity chart.

Bone age assesses skeletal maturity and is delayed in constitutional growth delay, hypothyroidism and systemic illness. It is advanced in precocious puberty, obesity and tall stature.

Pubertal staging employs standard references for breast, pubic hair, testicular and penile size development.

Short stature

Short stature is defined as a height below the third percentile for chronological age. Short stature may be disproportionate (e.g. achondroplasia, Turner syndrome) or symmetrical. The management of short stature is shown in Figure 47 and Table 41.

Achondroplasia

Children with achondroplasia, a common, autosomal dominant form of short-limbed dwarfism, may not have a positive family history as there is a high rate of spontaneous mutations. Patients have frontal bossing, hydrocephalus, a low nasal bridge, lumbar lordosis and the three middle fingers are trident-shaped. The use of growth hormone in this condition is currently under investigation.

Low-birth-weight infants

Low birth weight may be caused by problems during pregnancy such as hypertension and intrauterine infection. Children with the Russell–Silver syndrome have a low birth weight, feeding difficulties in the first year of life, clinodactyly and body asymmetry, especially pronounced in the face. Their growth velocity is generally normal; if so, no further investigation or treatment is indicated.

Turner syndrome

Girls with Turner syndrome have characteristic features (Section 9.3) including short stature and gonadal failure (Fig. 48). Although 20% of girls with Turner syndrome will start puberty spontaneously, most will require oestrogen at this stage. An anabolic steroid such as oxandrolone may promote growth prepubertally and GH can be used to maximise the blunted pubertal growth spurt. Psychological counselling is important, and the use of donor eggs to achieve pregnancy may be appropriate in later life.

Systemic causes of short stature

Short stature secondary to systemic diseases is often characterised by a delayed bone age and occurs in severe Crohn, coeliac, renal and cardiovascular disease, cystic fibrosis, asthma, rickets and metabolic disorders. The potential for catch-up growth is present if the underlying systemic disorder is treated successfully.

Psychosocial emotional deprivation

Infants suffering from severe neglect and non-accidental injury may develop endocrine abnormalities such as short stature and delayed skeletal and sexual maturation. The biochemical picture may indicate GH deficiency, with cortisol non-responsiveness. Following prolonged admission to hospital, an improvement in

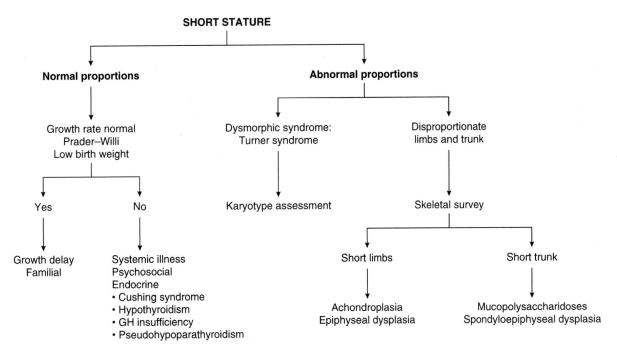

SHORT STATURE

Normal proportions

Growth rate normal
Prader–Willi
Low birth weight

Yes → Growth delay / Familial

No → Systemic illness
Psychosocial
Endocrine
• Cushing syndrome
• Hypothyroidism
• GH insufficiency
• Pseudohypoparathyroidism

Abnormal proportions

Dysmorphic syndrome:
Turner syndrome → Karyotype assessment

Disproportionate
limbs and trunk → Skeletal survey

Short limbs → Achondroplasia / Epiphyseal dysplasia

Short trunk → Mucopolysaccharidoses / Spondyloepiphyseal dysplasia

Fig. 47 Algorithm for the management of short stature.

Table 41 Investigations for short stature according to age

Age group	Investigations	Treatment
Infancy	Nutritional Karyotype Skeletal survey	Dietary management
Childhood	Growth hormone provocation test Thyroid function Adrenal function	Hormone replacement
Puberty	Hypothalamo– pituitary–gonadal function	Sex steroid treatment

height ensues, together with an increase in spontaneous and stimulated GH secretion. Treatment may involve placing the child in foster care, on a temporary or permanent basis.

Endocrine causes of short stature

The important hormones concerned with growth are thyroxine (T_4), GH and sex steroids. Deficiency of any of these hormones may result in short stature. Other endocrine disorders leading to short stature (e.g. hypothyroidism, Cushing syndrome) are discussed in the appropriate sections.

Growth hormone deficiency

Deficiency of GH may be isolated or may occur with other pituitary hormone deficiencies (Box 24). GH has a pulsatile secretion from the anterior pituitary gland that is controlled by growth hormone-releasing hormone (GHRH) and somatostatin which are themselves secreted by the hypothalamus. GH secretion is stimulated by

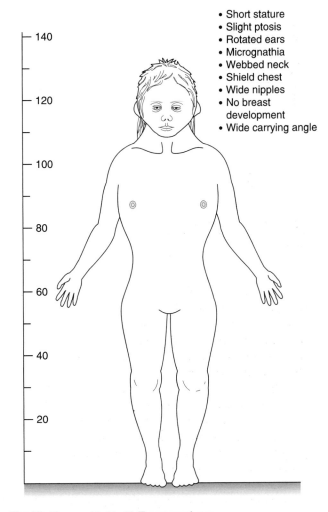

• Short stature
• Slight ptosis
• Rotated ears
• Micrognathia
• Webbed neck
• Shield chest
• Wide nipples
• No breast development
• Wide carrying angle

Fig. 48 12-year old girl with Turner syndrome.

sleep, exercise, hypoglycaemia, physical and emotional stress and a high protein intake. It is inhibited by REM sleep, psychogenic stress, malnutrition and CNS trauma. GH has indirect actions on the musculoskeletal system mediated via insulin-like growth factor I (IGF-I), leading to protein synthesis and cell proliferation. GH also has direct anti-insulin effects, resulting in lipolysis and breakdown of carbohydrate.

BOX 24
Causes of growth hormone deficiency

Congenital causes
GH gene deletion
Developmental abnormalities pituitary aplasia, pituitary hypoplasia, midline brain defects

Acquired causes
Hypothalamo–pituitary tumours: craniopharyngioma, Langerhans cell histiocytosis
Secondary to cranial irradiation
Secondary to head injury
Secondary to infection

Clinical features
GH deficiency is typified by a height equal to or less than 3 SDs (standard deviations) from the mean (Fig. 49), a slow height velocity, delayed bone age and delayed puberty. Normal body proportions are associated with crowded mid-face structures, high-pitched voice, increased skinfold thickness and small penis/scrotum.

Diagnosis
GH secretion can be assessed in several ways. GH

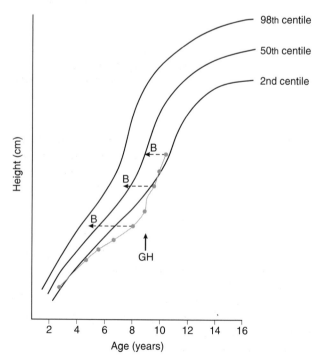

Fig. 49 Linear growth before and after treatment with GH in a patient with GH deficiency. After starting therapy, the height approaches and then crosses the 2nd percentile. The delay in bone age (B) is reduced and bone age becomes more appropriate for the chronological age.

profiles over 24-hour periods are mainly used as a research tool. Provocative tests induce GH secretion by means of a suitable stimulus such as sleep, exercise, insulin, arginine, L-dopa, glucagon, clonidine, propranolol and GHRH. The insulin-induced hypoglycaemia test is the most reliable but should only be performed in a tertiary centre under *strict medical supervision*. Glucagon is safer and more widely used. Normally a peak GH of 13.5–30 mU/l is achieved, although the absolute value depends on the assay used.

Treatment
The response to daily injections of recombinant human GH (hGH) is usually excellent, with an initial catch-up phase followed by a normal height velocity.

Constitutional delay of growth and puberty

Constitutional delay is more common in boys than girls and is often associated with a positive family history. It is the commonest cause of short stature, characterised by a delay in growth, puberty and bone age. The growth rate is normal, given the stage in puberty. The final height prognosis is good and treatment is unnecessary unless short stature leads to psychosocial distress. A short course of anabolic steroids (e.g. oxandrolone) or slow-release testosterone (sustanon), may accelerate the pubertal growth spurt in severe cases. The condition is difficult to differentiate from hypogonadotrophic hypogonadism.

Tall stature

Tall stature is defined as a height above the 97th percentile for chronological age. Tall children with normal body proportions and a normal appearance are unlikely to have any underlying pathological cause for tall stature. A height prediction can be made using the bone age and the height velocity. An algorithm for the assessment of children with tall stature is shown in Figure 50.

Tall stature in children with normal proportions

Tall stature associated with a normal height velocity
If a tall child has a normal appearance and normal growth velocity, constitutional tall stature is the most likely diagnosis. Obese children are often taller than average for their age and, if bone maturity is advanced, puberty may also occur earlier. Tall stature may represent a considerable handicap especially in girls and, if necessary, limitation of growth can be achieved using sex steroids.

Tall stature associated with increased growth velocity
Tall children with increased growth velocity and signs of puberty should be investigated for CAH and precocious puberty. In precocious puberty, accelerated linear

TALL STATURE

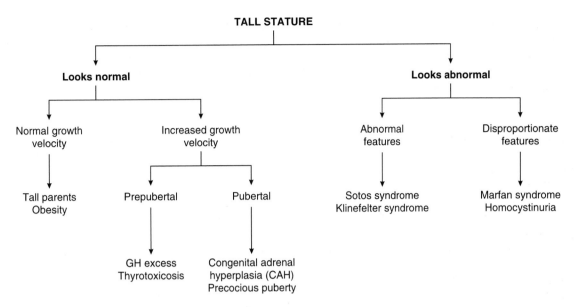

Fig. 50 Algorithm for the management of tall stature.

growth and bone maturation result in tall stature at presentation, but the final height is likely to be compromised because of early fusion of the epiphyses. If there are no signs of puberty, the following conditions should be considered.

Growth hormone excess. Excess GH secretion in childhood or adolescence causes gigantism. GH levels are elevated but the bone age is not advanced. The pituitary fossa may be enlarged because of a GH-secreting tumour. Patients present with rapid linear growth, overgrowth of soft tissues and hyperglycaemia. Treatment entails dopamine agonists (e.g. bromocriptine) to reduce the excess GH secretion and removal of an adenoma by trans-sphenoidal surgery and radiotherapy.

Thyrotoxicosis. An increase in growth rate and advanced bone age are seen in thyrotoxicosis. In addition, free thyroxine levels are high, thyroid-stimulating hormone (TSH) levels low and the TSH response to thyrotrophin-releasing hormone (TRH) is flat.

Tall stature in children with abnormal appearance

Sotos syndrome

Sotos syndrome is characterised by tall stature, a large elongated head, prominent forehead, large ears, elongated jaw, coarse facial features and subnormal intelligence.

Marfan syndrome

Patients with Marfan syndrome, an autosomal dominant condition, are tall with long limbs, narrow hands and slender fingers. Their arm span is greater than their height. Hyperextensible joints, kyphoscoliosis, rib cage deformities, upward lenticular dislocation, mitral and aortic valve lesions and aortic aneurysms are other features of this condition.

Homocystinuria

Homocystinuria is an autosomal recessive condition with features caused by the absence of cystathionine synthetase. Phenotypic features are similar to those of Marfan syndrome, except for downward dislocation of the lens. Mental retardation and venous and arterial thrombotic disease are also common.

Klinefelter syndrome

Klinefelter syndrome results from an XXY karyotype and results in tall stature, eunuchoid features, gynaecomastia, seminiferous tubule dysgenesis and testicular atrophy.

8.4 Disorders of puberty

Normal puberty

Puberty is the period during which sexual maturation occurs and reproductive capacity is attained. It is characterised by the adolescent growth spurt, appearance of secondary sexual characteristics and profound psychological changes.

In girls, puberty is heralded by an increase in height velocity followed by breast then pubic hair development and finally menarche. Peak height velocity coincides with stage 3 breast development and menarche with stage 4 so that only 5–8 cm of growth follows the first menstrual period. In boys, testicular enlargement is followed by penile growth, growth of pubic hair and increase in height velocity.

Profound changes in hormone levels occur with puberty. Pulsatile gonadotrophin (FSH and LH) secretion stimulates the release of testosterone and oestradiol to adult concentrations. In addition, in girls, gonadotrophin secretion is cyclical, resulting in increases in oestrogens in mid-cycle. Initially, the ovary does not secrete sufficient oestrogen to induce the LH surge required for ovulation and, during the first 2 years post-menarche, 50–90% of cycles are anovulatory, decreasing to <20% after 5 years. The initial appearance of multi-cystic ovaries is replaced by one with a dominant folli-cle. During this time, the uterus develops an adult configuration, with endometrium formation leading to menarche when the endometrium is 7–8 mm thick. At around 8 years of age, the adrenal gland matures and secretes adrenal androgens, leading to the development of pubic hair.

Delayed puberty

Delayed puberty may be a manifestation of severe systemic illness, central nervous system disease and gonadal disease (Box 25).

BOX 25
Causes of delayed puberty

Central disorders
Constitutional delay
Congenital abnormalities
Gonadotrophin deficiency
Panhypopituitarism
Severe systemic disease

Gonadal disorders
Turner syndrome
Noonan syndrome
Gonadal dysgenesis
Trauma and neoplasia

Constitutional delay of growth and puberty

This has been described earlier in this chapter.

Hypogonadotrophic hypogonadism

Children with hypogonadotrophic hypogonadism fail to achieve puberty without assistance. It may follow congenital or acquired malformations of the the hypo-thalamo–pituitary area (Box 26). Micropenis with small or cryptorchid testes are seen in boys, and the reproductive organs are prepubertal in size in girls. There is no FSH and LH response to luteinising hormone releasing hormone (LHRH).

Treatment includes pulsatile gonadotrophin-releasing hormone (GnRH) and testosterone or oestrogen replacement.

Prader–Willi syndrome

Prader–Willi syndrome results from deletion of paternally derived chromosome 15. Poor activity in utero is followed by hypotonia, obesity owing to an insatiable appetite, mental retardation and hypogonadotrophic hypogonadism. Patients have a characteristic facies

---

BOX 26
Causes of hypogonadotrophic hypogonadism

Congenital	Acquired
Malformations of hypothalamic area	Neoplasia
Intra-uterine infections	Encephalitis, meningitis
Perinatal hypoxia	Trauma
Kallman syndrome	

---

with almond-shaped eyes and often die prematurely through a Pickwickian syndrome with hypoventilation.

Anorexia nervosa

Anorexia nervosa usually arises in females and results in marked weight loss and secondary amenorrhoea. Gonadotophin secretion is reduced in these girls.

Precocious puberty

Though initially associated with tall stature, precocious puberty leads to early fusion of the epiphyses and short final height. The increased production of sex steroids results in early physical maturation and menstruation in mentally immature young children and behavioural problems are commonplace. Precocious puberty may be gonadotrophin dependent (central), or follow exogenous sex steroids (Box 27).

BOX 27
Causes of precocious puberty

Gonadotrophin-dependent causes
Idiopathic: common in girls, rare in boys
CNS disorders: space-occupying lesions (benign or malignant), congenital CNS anomalies, postinfection or trauma, hCG-producing neoplasms

Gonadotrophin-independent causes
Exogenous sex-steroids: tumours of the adrenal, ovary and testis, congenital adrenal hyperplasia
McCune–Albright syndrome
Testotoxicosis in boys

Gonadotrophin-dependent precocious puberty

Gonadotrophin-dependent precocious puberty is characterised by the normal pubertal sequence: breast development followed by pubic and axillary hair growth and menarche in girls; testicular development followed by penile enlargement, then pubic and axillary hair development in boys. The condition is more common in girls and is usually idiopathic. In boys, it often results from an intracranial lesion. Patients have a normal pubertal LH and FSH response after an LHRH test, and girls may have multicystic ovaries as a result of pulsatile gonadotrophin secretion. The bone age is usually advanced.

McCune–Albright syndrome

McCune–Albright syndrome is associated with gonado-trophin-independent precocious puberty, large unilateral irregular café-au-lait spots and polyostotic fibrous dysplasia. Excessive oestrogen in girls or excess testosterone in boys is seen together with no LH or FSH response to LHRH.

Premature thelarche

Isolated breast development (thelarche) is usually an isolated finding in children with a normal growth rate, appropriate skeletal maturity for chronological age and normal final height. Pelvic ultrasound is indicated to exclude an ovarian cyst.

Premature pubarche

Isolated pubic hair development may arise because of excess androgens (adrenarche), CAH, an adrenal neoplasm and Cushing syndrome.

Treatment of precocious puberty

LHRH analogues are only effective in centrally mediated, gonadotrophin-dependent precocious puberty. Cyproterone acetate can be effective in gonadotrophin-independent precocious puberty but can cause adrenal insufficiency.

Polycystic ovary syndrome

Polycystic ovaries may be idiopathic or follow treatment with GH, central precocious puberty or CAH. These girls are tall, obese and hirsute with acne, palpable ovaries, amenorrhoea, dysfunctional menstrual bleeding and infertility. Biochemical findings include hyperinsulinism, raised adrenal and ovarian androgens, testosterone, LH:FSH ratio, and lowered sex hormone-binding globulin.

Treatment entails cyclical oestrogen, progesterone and cyproterone acetate, with induction of ovulation using clomiphene/hCG.

8.5 Disorders of the thyroid gland

Physiology

The thyroid gland forms in the third week of gestation. Thyroid follicular cells synthesise, iodinate and store thyroglobulin and release the thyroid hormones thyroxine (T_4) and triiodothyronine (T_3) after organification of the trapped iodide. The gland stores thyroglobulin, T_3 and T_4 and is responsible for deiodination and recycling of the iodide.

TRH secreted by the hypothalamus leads to TSH secretion by the anterior pituitary, which in turn stimulates release of T_4 from the thyroid gland. Circulating T_4 levels are high in the neonate and when the thyroid gland is hyperactive in response to TSH and decrease during childhood and when the gland is underactive. TSH is inhibited by somatostatin, dopamine and T_3, thereby completing the negative feedback loop. The thyroid gland is the sole source of T_4 which is bound in plasma by thyroxine-binding globulin (TBG). It is monodeiodinated in peripheral tissues to form T_3, the more potent hormone, which is bound by both albumin and TBG. The latter binds to tissue receptors and stimulates mitochondrial activity, catecholamine release, lipid and amino acid turnover and growth factor production and action.

In the fetus, the pituitary–thyroid axis is independent of the mother's axis, as the placenta is impermeable to TSH and allows only small amounts of T_3 and T_4 to cross. TSH levels may be elevated in normal neonates and declines to normal levels within the first few days after birth.

Hypothyroidism

Congenital hypothyroidism

Congenital hypothyroidism occurs in 1 in 4000 live births and follows maldescent or dysgenesis of the gland, or dyshormonogenesis. Most affected neonates are initially asymptomatic, the majority being detected on routine screening. If untreated clinical features will eventually include coarse facies, large tongue, hoarse cry, hypotonia, lethargy, umbilical hernia, constipation, prolonged jaundice, feeding and respiratory problems (Fig. 51). Routine screening involves the measurement of TSH from blood collected on a Guthrie card between 5 and 7 days of age. If the initial TSH is elevated, free T_4 and TSH levels are measured. If free T_4 is low and TSH high, a radionuclide thyroid scan is performed to distinguish between thyroid dysgenesis and dyshormonogenesis. Deafness may be associated with dyshormonogenesis and congenital hypothyroidism (Pendred syndrome) and audiological assessment is also required.

Treatment. Replacement with T_4 is necessary for life, with monitoring of thyroid function, growth and skeletal maturation at regular intervals. Worsening neurodevelopmental delay is related to lower initial T_4 levels and increasing delay in starting hormone replacement, especially if left until after 6 weeks.

Secondary hypothyroidism

Hypothyroidism secondary to TRH or TSH deficiency is rare and usually associated with deficiency of other pituitary hormones and midline defects, e.g. cleft palate.

- Developmental delay
- Sparse hair
- Vacant expression
- Protuberant tongue

- Bradycardia
- Hypotonia
- Absent/slow reflexes

- Umbilical hernia
- Constipation

- Cool peripheries

- These signs may be associated with a goitre

HEART RATE 90

Fig. 51 Clinical features of hypothyroidism.

Transient hypothyroidism

Since T_4 concentrations increase with gestational age, all premature neonates have a degree of transient hypothyroidism. In addition, premature infants cannot convert T_4 to T_3 efficiently. Transient primary hypothyroidism should still be treated with T_4, and the dose reduced after a few months. In transient cases, the TSH level remains normal, whereas with permanent hypothyroidism, it continues to rise.

Acquired hypothyroidism

The most common cause of acquired hypothyroidism, worldwide, is iodine deficiency. Autoimmune disease (Hashimoto disease) is the usual cause in girls in childhood and adolescence, whereas local or total body irradiation is the usual cause in those treated for malignant disease. Disease secondary to TSH or TRH deficiency is rare. Poor height velocity, with consequent short stature, is associated with delayed skeletal age, gain in weight and subcutaneous fat, intolerance of cold, constipation and mental slowing. Examination may reveal a goitre, coarse facies, bradycardia, protuberant abdomen and slow relaxation of tendon reflexes. Isolated breast development or testicular enlargement follows excess FSH secretion. Signs of associated autoimmune disease may also be present, e.g. chronic mucocutaneous candidiasis, hypoparathyroidism, Addison disease, vitiligo, chronic active hepatitis, pernicious anaemia, myasthenia gravis and diabetes mellitus.

Treatment. Therapy with T_4 is indicated, initially in low dose to avoid dramatic behavioural changes. Cortisol deficiency must also be excluded since the commencement of T_4 may precipitate an Addisonian crisis if untreated hypoadrenalisim exists. Regular monitoring of growth and thyroid function is essential.

Hyperthyroidism

Hyperthyroidism is usually caused by autoimmune disease involving a multinodular goitre. The term Graves' disease is used when eye signs are present. Excess TSH production from the pituitary or T_4 from a single thyroid nodule is less common.

Thyrotoxicosis is seven times more common in girls than boys and generally occurs in the peripubertal period. A family history of other autoimmune disease is common. Patients may present with behavioural problems including hyperactivity, agitation, weight loss, tall stature, excessive sweating, intolerance of heat and palpitations. A goitre, occasionally with a bruit, tachycardia, tremor, lid lag, exophthalmos and ophthalmoplegia may be found on examination.

Levels of T_4 and free T_3 are raised while TSH is suppressed (often undetectable). TSH does not respond to TRH.

Treatment. Propranolol controls the acute symptoms and carbimazole or propylthiouracil suppresses the overactive gland. If medical treatment fails or side-effects are unacceptable, thyroidectomy or radioactive iodine is necessary.

8.6 Disorders of the adrenal gland

The adrenal cortex occupies 80% of the gland at term

BOX 28
Causes of adrenal insufficiency

	Primary adrenal insufficiency	Secondary adrenal insufficiency
All zones	Autoimmune adrenalitis	Pituitary hormone deficiencies
	Adrenal haemorrhage	Isolated ACTH deficiency
	Infections (including DIC)	Hypothalamo–pituitary tumours
	Iatrogenic, chemical or surgical	Glucocorticoid therapy
	Multiple endocrinopathy	Cranial radiotherapy
		Surgery
Zona glomerulosa	Hypoaldosteronism	
Zona fasciculata	Isolated glucocorticoid deficiency	
	Congenital adrenal hyperplasia	

and becomes active during the second trimester. The zona glomerulosa in the outer cortex produces aldosterone under the control of the renin–angiotensin system. Aldosterone modulates sodium and potassium exchange mainly in the renal distal tubule. The middle zona fasciculata comprises 75% of the adrenal cortex and secretes cortisol under the control of hypothalamic corticotrophin–releasing hormone (CRH) and especially pituitary ACTH. From 6 months of age, cortisol and ACTH levels vary in a circadian rhythm with higher levels in the morning than at night. The urinary steroid profile provides a useful assessment of the secretion of abnormal steroid metabolites.

The innermost zona reticularis matures in mid-childhood to release adrenal androgens, predominantly dehydroepiandrosterone sulphate.

Adrenal steroid deficiency

Adrenal insufficiency may involve all three zones or affect production of mineralocorticosteroids or glucocorticoids alone (Box 28). It may result from primary failure of the gland or be secondary to ACTH deficiency.

Primary adrenal insufficiency

Adrenal haemorrhage is the most common cause of adrenal insufficiency in the newborn whereas autoimmune adrenalitis is most common in the older child. Hypoglycaemia, salt loss and conjugated hyperbilirubinaemia predominate in infants, whereas anorexia, vomiting, fatigue, weight loss, hypotension and hyperpigmentation are seen in childhood. A family history of autoimmune disorders may be present.

Investigations show hyponatraemia with hyperkalaemia, raised ACTH, low cortisol throughout a 24-hour period, raised plasma renin with low aldosterone levels, and hypoglycaemia. There is failure of the adrenals to respond to exogenous ACTH (synacthen) by increasing cortisol levels. Positive antibodies to the adrenal glands arise in autoimmune adrenalitis. A CT scan of the adrenals may reveal large adrenal glands in CAH.

Secondary adrenal insufficiency

Secondary adrenal insufficiency should be excluded in those with hypopituitarism. GH, LH and FSH insufficiency are more common than isolated ACTH deficiency. However, ACTH deficiency combined with other pituitary hormone deficiencies is a late feature of hypopituitarism, especially when secondary to cranial irradiation. In congenital hypopituitarism, there may be associated midline defects, e.g. agenesis of the corpus callosum, cleft lip and palate.

Investigations reveal low cortisol and ACTH levels over a 24-hour period. MRI of the hypothalamo–pituitary area is essential to exclude local tumours, e.g. craniopharyngioma.

Treatment of adrenal insufficiency

In an Addisonian crisis, resuscitative measures are required to replete the plasma volume. Intravenous hydrocortisone should be administered, later replaced by oral hydrocortisone. Mineralocorticoid deficiency, indicated by increased renin levels, requires mineralocorticoid replacement in the form of 9α-fludrocortisone. Regular assessment of growth, ACTH, cortisol and plasma renin profiles is mandatory in all those on adrenal replacement treatment.

Adrenal steroid excess

Cushing syndrome

Cushing syndrome describes the clinical features of adrenal steroid excess. This is usually iatrogenic through exogenous steroids but may follow excess corticosteroids from pituitary tumours (Cushing's disease) and, less commonly, adrenal and other neoplasms (Box 29).

A moon-like plethoric facies with acne, interscapular fat pad (buffalo hump), truncal obesity, striae, hirsutism, growth arrest, easy bruising, hypertension, proximal myopathy, cataracts, hypogonadism and glucose intolerance characterise this syndrome (Fig. 52). Loss of the normal diurnal variation in plasma cortisol, with an elevated midnight level, is associated with ele-

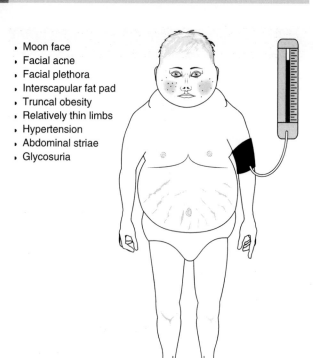

- Moon face
- Facial acne
- Facial plethora
- Interscapular fat pad
- Truncal obesity
- Relatively thin limbs
- Hypertension
- Abdominal striae
- Glycosuria

Fig. 52 Manifestations of Cushing syndrome.

vated urinary cortisol. There is failure of suppression of cortisol secretion by exogenous low-dose dexamethasone in all cases, although levels may suppress with high-dose dexamethasone in pituitary-dependent Cushing's disease but not in adrenal-dependent Cushing syndrome. ACTH levels are raised in Cushing's disease but suppressed in Cushing syndrome. CT or MRI scanning of the pituitary and adrenal glands is required to exclude hormone-secreting adenomas or carcinomas.

Management. Surgery is required, via an abdominal approach (adrenal tumours) or transphenoidal resection (pituitary tumours). Following total hypophysectomy, replacement therapy in the form of hydrocortisone, T_4, gonadotrophins or sex steroids, and GH is indicated.

Adrenal tumours

Patients with adrenal tumours develop Cushing syndrome and virilising features, e.g. accelerated growth velocity, advanced bone age, pubic hair, acne, hirsutism and clitoromegaly.

Investigation confirms elevated adrenal androgens and urinary steroids.

Management. Surgical resection is followed by regular monitoring of the growth rate and 24-hour urinary steroid profile.

Congenital adrenal hyperplasia

CAH describes a group of autosomal recessive conditions where an enzyme block in cortisol synthesis results in excessive CRH–ACTH drive to the adrenal gland, promoting the incorporation of cholesterol into the adrenal

---

BOX 29
Causes of adrenal steroid excess

Primary adrenal disorders
Glucocorticoids
    Nodular adrenal hyperplasia
    Adrenal neoplasm
Mineralocorticoids
    CAH (11β, 17α-hydroxylase)
    Neoplasm (Conn syndrome)
    Dexamethasone-suppressible
    hyperaldosteronism
Androgens
    CAH (11β, 21-hydroxylase)
    Adrenal neoplasm
    Premature adrenarche

Secondary adrenal disorders
CRH- and ACTH-secreting tumours
Renin-secreting tumours

Iatrogenic
Excess steroids

---

cortex, leading to adrenal hyperplasia. The incidence of CAH is 1 in 4000. The mutation can be identified in many patients, allowing for antenatal diagnosis. The enzyme defect prevents the production of particular adrenal steroids with accumulation of others higher up the biochemical pathway. Clinical features depend upon which steroids are deficient and which are present in excess.

The commonest defect is 21-hydroxylase deficiency. Female patients have ambiguous genitalia, whereas males may have a large penis with pigmented scrotum, and all may develop hypertension. In later childhood, males develop precocious puberty with excessive growth and bone maturation, and virilisation occurs in females. Salt-losing crises occur in early life in two-thirds of patients. Low levels of cortisol and elevated ACTH are associated with hyponatraemia, hyperkalaemia and excess urinary sodium in salt losers. Identification of urinary steroid metabolites will delineate the enzymic block, e.g. elevated 17-hydroxyprogesterone with 21-hydroxylase deficiency. A karyotype and pelvic ultrasound scan are essential to ascertain the gender and internal genitalia in those who present with ambiguous genitalia (Fig. 45).

Management. Treatment entails hydrocortisone and mineralocorticoid replacement. Follow-up includes measurement of the growth rate and estimation of plasma renin activity. The prognosis for fertility is guarded and girls develop polycystic ovarian disease. If well-controlled, the prognosis for final height is good.

8.7 Disorders of calcium homeostasis

Physiology

Three hormones, vitamin D, parathyroid hormone

BOX 30
Causes of rickets

Calcium deficiency	Vitamin D deficiency	Phosphate deficiency
Dietary	Dietary	Decreased intake
Malabsorption	Malabsorption	Renal tubular acidosis
	Lack of sunlight	Renal tubular loss
	Hepatic disease	Fanconi syndrome
	Anticonvulsants	X-linked hypophosphataemia
	Renal disease	Nephrotoxic agents
	1α-Hydroxylase deficiency	
	Vitamin D receptor defect	

(parathormone, PTH) and calcitonin, are vital in the maintenance of normal calcium homeostasis. Vitamin D is synthesised in the skin, converted to 25-hydroxyvitamin D in the liver and to 1,25-dihydroxyvitamin D in the kidney (Fig. 5, p. 14). The latter induces the synthesis of mRNA and, in turn, protein messengers that stimulate transport of calcium and phosphate across the intestine into the blood and assist PTH-stimulated osteoclastic bone resorption. 1,25-Dihydroxyvitamin D has an inhibitory feedback effect on 1α-hydroxylation and PTH secretion.

The secretion of PTH by four parathyroid glands is regulated by plasma calcium concentration. Secretion is maximal with a calcium concentration of 2 mmol/l, but is not totally suppressed even with very high calcium levels. PTH promotes calcium reabsorption in the distal renal tubules and inhibits phosphate and bicarbonate reabsorption in the proximal tubule. It also stimulates 1α-hydroxylation of 25-hydroxyvitamin D and induces osteoclasts to resorb calcium from bone.

In response to a fall in calcium concentration, PTH release leads to reduced renal calcium excretion and, in conjunction with 1,25-dihydroxyvitamin D, to mobilisation of calcium from bone. In addition, enteral calcium and phosphate absorption is promoted. The phosphate concentration remains stable because of the phosphaturic effect of PTH. With hypercalcaemia, PTH secretion is inhibited, leading to increased calcium excretion, decreased bone resorption and suppression of calcium binding in the gut. Phosphate loss increases vitamin D synthesis independently of PTH, while phosphate retention inhibits it. The primary role of calcitonin, produced by thyroid C-cells, is the inhibition of bone resorption by PTH and vitamin D.

Hypocalcaemia

Neonatal hypocalcaemia

Hypocalcaemia is a common, usually transient problem in the first few days of life. Hypocalcaemia between 4 and 28 days can be caused by transient or congenital hypoparathyroidism, a high phosphate intake, hypomagnesaemia, calcium malabsorption or maternal vitamin D deficiency. Neonates present with irritability, jitteriness and apnoea.

Treatment. Initial correction using intravenous calcium gluconate is followed by maintenance oral calcium lactate.

The older child with hypocalcaemia

Intractable fits, paraesthesiae, muscle cramps, weakness and laryngospasm together with carpopedal spasm, positive Chvostek and Trousseau signs may all be manifestations of hypocalcaemia. Chronic hypocalcaemia leads to mental retardation, cataracts and dental enamel hypoplasia. Clinical features of rickets may be present (see below).

The plasma phosphate concentration may provide the clue to the underlying diagnosis. If high with a low PTH, the cause of the hypocalcaemia is likely to be hypoparathyroidism. Low plasma phosphate suggests hypophosphataemic rickets, while a normal phosphate concentration indicates calciopenic rickets.

Rickets

Rickets follows calcium, phosphate and vitamin D deficiency (Box 30). In the first year of life, the child presents with craniotabes, widened cranial sutures, frontal bossing, swollen epiphyses (especially wrists), bulging costochondral joints (rachitic rosary) and a Harrison's sulcus. Later, patients present with growth failure, genu varum and valgum, bone pain, proximal myopathy and/or retarded motor development. The clinical features can be attributed to hypocalcaemia, secondary hyperparathyroidism and hypophosphataemia, resulting in defective bone mineralisation with excessive bone resorption.

Investigation. Low calcium and phosphate levels are observed with an elevated alkaline phosphatase. The 1,25-dihydroxyvitamin D level may also be low and serum PTH high. Radiological features include expansion of the growth plate with fraying, cupping and widening of metaphyses, pseudofractures and signs of secondary hyperparathyroidism, e.g. subperiosteal erosions. Other abnormalities may be found, depending upon the underlying cause, e.g. acidosis, aminoaciduria, chronic renal failure.

Treatment. Calcium, phosphate and vitamin D supplements help correct the bony abnormalities. Treatment of end-organ (receptor) resistance to vitamin D can be very difficult, requiring large doses of calcium. Hypophosphataemic rickets is treated with very high doses of phosphate, and compliance may be a major problem.

Hypoparathyroidism

Hypoparathyroidism may result from agenesis or hypoplasia of the parathyroid glands and presents with hypocalcaemia in the neonatal period. This abnormality may be a feature of DiGeorge syndrome, when it is associated with thymic abnormalities, T cell defects, cardiac and facial abnormalities. In older children, hypoparathyroidism usually results from an autoimmune process and may be part of the polyglandular autoimmune syndrome with chronic mucocutaneous candidiasis, Addison's disease, thyroid disease and malabsorption. Hypoparathyroidism may follow inadvertent removal of the parathyroids during thyroidectomy. End-organ receptor resistance to PTH causes **pseudohypoparathyroidism**, with short stature, round facies, mental retardation, ectopic calcification and short fourth and fifth metacarpals and metatarsals.

Diagnosis. A high plasma phosphate, low plasma calcium and low PTH level are diagnostic of hypoparathyroidism. In pseudohypoparathyroidism, the PTH level is elevated. Treatment entails calcium and vitamin D supplements to achieve normocalcaemia.

Hypercalcaemia

Hypercalcaemia occurs with vitamin D intoxication, familial hypocalciuric hypercalcaemia and hyperparathyroidism. The last is an uncommon condition caused by a primary parathyroid adenoma, sometimes as part of the multiple endocrine neoplasia syndromes (MEN). Infantile hypercalcaemia may be an isolated abnormality that runs a benign and self-limiting course or is a feature of Williams syndrome, associated with supravalvular aortic stenosis, peripheral pulmonary artery stenosis, mental retardation and dysmorphic features (elfin-like facies).

Anorexia, nausea, vomiting, constipation and polyuria are symptoms of hypercalcaemia. Urinary stones develop if hypercalciuria is present. With all causes of hypercalcaemia, with the exception of hyperparathyroidism and familial hypocalciuric hypercalcaemia, the PTH level is suppressed. In hyperparathyroidism elevated plasma calcium level is associated with hypophosphataemia and inappropriately elevated PTH.

Management. In infantile hypercalcaemia, adequate hydration and a low-calcium diet should be maintained. If calcium levels remain high, then glucocorticoids should be commenced. In the emergency setting with very high calcium levels, a calcitonin infusion can be effective. Surgery remains the definitive treatment for primary hyperparathyroidism.

8.8 Disorders of glucose homeostasis

Physiology

The blood glucose reflects the balance between glucose intake, its mobilisation from glycogen stores in the liver (glycogenolysis), its formation from protein (glyconeogenesis) and fat (lipolysis) and the consumption of glucose by body tissues. Glucose mobilisation is controlled by hormones including cortisol, GH, glucagon and catecholamines, while its utilisation is controlled by insulin. In the fed state, an increase in blood glucose and amino acid levels leads to the secretion of insulin from beta cells in the islets of Langerhans in the pancreas. Insulin inhibits gluconeogenesis and glycogenolysis and stimulates deposition of glucose as glycogen in the liver, uptake of glucose and amino acids by muscle and by adipocytes to form triglycerides. In the fasting state, blood glucose levels fall and insulin secretion is switched off. Counter-regulatory hormones such as GH, cortisol and catecholamines inhibit glucose uptake and stimulate glycogenolysis, gluconeogenesis, the release of amino acids by muscle, and lipolysis and the release of free fatty acids from adipose tissue. Subsequent β-oxidation of free fatty acids results in the production of ketone bodies, an alternative fuel for the brain.

Insulin-dependent diabetes mellitus (IDDM)

Insulin-dependent diabetics are insulin deficient and cannot utilise carbohydrate as fuel. Blood glucose levels are elevated and the ability of the proximal renal tubules to reabsorb the glucose is exceeded; as a result, glycosuria followed by an osmotic diuresis results. The incidence of IDDM varies markedly from 5.3 to 35.3 new cases/100 000 in different countries, with 16.5/100 000 in the UK.

Genetically susceptible individuals with the HLA antigens B8, B15, DR3 and DR4 develop islet cell antibodies that destroy the beta cells of the pancreas. The autoimmune process is probably triggered off by environmental factors, including viruses such as coxsackievirus. IDDM may be a feature of other conditions, e.g. cystic fibrosis and chronic pancreatitis. Non-insulin-dependent diabetes mellitus occurs in obesity, Prader–Willi syndrome, acanthosis nigricans and polycystic ovarian disease.

Clinical features

IDDM usually presents insidiously at any age, with glycosuria, polyuria, dehydration, thirst and polydipsia. Inefficient energy utilisation results in weight loss despite polyphagia, and lassitude. Diabetic ketoacidosis is the mode of presentation in 25% of diabetics. Clinical signs include those of severe dehydration, sometimes coma, with dry mucous membranes, decreased skin turgor, muscle and subcutaneous tissue wasting, odour of ketones on the breath and Kussmaul (deep sighing) respiration.

Initially, shortly after diagnosis, some endogenous insulin secretion is still present and the requirement for exogenous insulin is low. This 'honeymoon phase' is characterised by improved insulin sensitivity but is invariably followed by further destruction of islet cells and an increase in the insulin requirement.

Investigation

The presence of hyperglycaemia, glycosuria and ketoacidosis confirm the diagnosis. Other useful investigations include blood gas analysis, urea and electrolytes and a glycosylated haemoglobin level.

Ketoacidosis

Ketoacidosis is a medical emergency that must be managed in a controlled fashion if severe complications are to be avoided. The following steps should be observed:

- careful assessment of the degree of dehydration, with slow rehydration over 24–48 hours, using isotonic fluids
- adequate replacement of electrolyte losses, especially potassium, with regular measurements of electrolytes and pH
- gradual reduction of hyperglycaemia and suppression of ketone production using an insulin infusion
- careful monitoring of the cerebral state and prompt measures to counteract cerebral oedema.

Long-term management of IDDM

Time should be spent discussing the condition, its treatment and possible complications with the entire family prior to discharge. During the inpatient stay, an adequate insulin regimen tailored to the individual patient must be devised, ensuring that the control of blood glucose in hospital is not 'perfect', thereby allowing for the inevitable increase in energy requirements once discharged. An approximate insulin requirement of 0.5–1.0 unit/kg is usually needed, administered in a twice or three times daily dose, with one-third given as soluble, rapid acting insulin and two-thirds as a long-acting preparation. A balanced, complex carbohydrate-rich, low-fat diet is recommended. Careful manipulation of the diet and insulin regimen allows for strenuous exercise, provided exercise-associated hypoglycaemia is avoided. Family education, with emphasis on self blood-glucose monitoring and urinalysis for ketones, particularly during intercurrent illnesses, is essential. Patients should be referred to a diabetic health visitor and reviewed regularly in the diabetic clinic, where measurement of glycosylated haemoglobin at 3-monthly levels gives a good index of dietary control.

Complications
Acute complications

- cerebral oedema is usually the result of over-rapid correction of hyperglycaemia during ketoacidosis
- hypoglycaemia follows insulin overdosage or inadequate carbohydrate intake
- patients with IDDM, especially if poorly controlled, have an increased susceptibility to infection.

Chronic complications. Good diabetic control in childhood reduces the risk of late microangiopathic complications in adults. Chronic complications are rare in children and include:

- impaired growth
- limited joint mobility
- early cataract formation
- hypertension
- hyperlipidaemia
- nephropathy
- retinopathy
- neuropathy.

Changes in insulin requirements
During puberty, insulin requirements increase probably because of the increased secretion of growth and sex hormones. The requirements decrease after puberty and in adulthood they are lower than in adolescence. Any intercurrent illness may disrupt diabetic control by increasing insulin requirements as a result of the increased secretion of catecholamines. Control is also impaired as a result of the dawn and Somogyi phenomena. Nocturnal increase in GH secretion increases circulating glucose concentrations in the early hours of the morning, without preceding hypoglycaemia, and results in the **dawn phenomenon**. The **Somogyi effect** is defined as posthypoglycaemic hyperglycaemia and is thought to be caused by the increase in counter-regulatory hormones during hypoglycaemia, which leads to insulin resistance.

Hypoglycaemia

Hypoglycaemia, is usually defined as a blood glucose level of less than 2.6 mmol/l. Its causes are listed in Box 31.

Clinical features

Hypoglycaemia in the neonatal period presents with feeding problems, irritability, jitteriness, apnoea, hypotonia, convulsions and coma. Older children develop lassitude, headaches, abdominal pain, hunger, irritability, pallor, sweating, confusion, behavioural abnormalities, convulsions and coma.

Investigations

The normal infusion rate of glucose required to main-

BOX 31
Causes of hypoglycaemia

Inadequate glucose production	**Excessive glucose utilisation (hyperinsulinism)**
Inadequate glycogen stores	Infant of diabetic mother
Glycogen storage disease	Beckwith–Wiedemann syndrome
Galactosaemia, fructose intolerance	Nesidioblastosis
Fat oxidation defects	Insulinoma
GH, ACTH, glucocorticoid deficiency	Excessive insulin administration
Liver disease	Oral hypoglycaemic agents
Alcohol, salicylate poisoning	

---

tain euglycaemia is 5–8 mg/min per kg body weight in neonates and infants. A blood sample taken during hypoglycaemia should be analysed for glucose, insulin, cortisol, growth hormone, lactate, free fatty acids, ketone bodies and C-peptide. A urine sample taken simultaneously should be analysed for organic acids.

Hypoglycaemia associated with low ketone and free fatty acid levels is typical of hyperinsulinaemic states. In factitious hyperinsulinism, insulin levels are elevated, but C-peptide levels are reduced. In endogenous hyperinsulinism insulin and C-peptide are produced in equimolar amounts.

Treatment

Hypoglycaemia is a medical emergency and must be treated promptly with the administration of glucose (given intravenously in the unconscious patient) after taking the appropriate blood and urine samples. Intravenous glucose should not exceed 10–20% as higher concentrations can cause cerebral oedema. Glucagon can be used as an emergency short-term measure but can lead to hyperinsulinism, with subsequent rebound hypoglycaemia. The mainstay of long-term treatment is diazoxide, which switches off insulin secretion and stimulates glycogenolysis. When medical therapy fails or its side-effects are unacceptable, a 95% pancreatectomy is indicated. Prompt control of hypoglycaemia is crucial as the neurological outlook of these patients is related to the duration of hypoglycaemia.

8.9 Disorders of antidiuretic hormone secretion

Physiology

Water balance is maintained by the action of the hypothalamic thirst centre: osmoreceptors and neurones secrete antidiuretic hormone (ADH or vasopressin) which limits urinary output. ADH is synthesised in the supraoptic nuclei and migrates to the posterior pituitary for storage and release. Its release into the circulation is inhibited at a plasma osmolality of approximately 275 mosmol/l, thereby allowing maximal urinary dilu-

tion. Conversely, an osmolality of 295 mosmol/l stimulates sufficient ADH release to permit maximal urinary concentration.

Diabetes insipidus

Without normal ADH activity, water is lost through the renal tubules; if the thirst mechanism is intact this will lead to polydipsia. Hence, thirst, polydipsia and polyuria are the cardinal features of diabetes insipidus (DI). This may result from central ADH deficiency (central DI) or renal causes (nephrogenic DI).

Cranial diabetes insipidus
Cranial DI is caused by ADH deficiency and may follow congenital abnormalities of the hypothalamo–pituitary axis (e.g. septo-optic dysplasia), surgical or accidental trauma, inflammation (e.g. postmeningitis, autoimmune disease) and local infiltrative or invasive lesions (e.g. histiocytosis, sarcoid, craniopharyngioma, optic nerve glioma). Genetic causes of cranial DI include autosomal dominant and X-linked hereditary conditions, and the DIDMOAD syndrome (DI, diabetes mellitus, optic atrophy and deafness).

Nephrogenic diabetes insipidus
Nephrogenic DI is an X-linked disease resulting in resistance of the renal tubules to ADH. It may also be associated with sickle cell disease and renal abnormalities, e.g. hypokalaemia, hypercalcaemia, polycystic kidneys and chronic renal failure.

Clinical features

Loss of more than 80% of ADH secretory capacity is required before symptoms of thirst, polydipsia and polyuria develop. If fluids are restricted, severe dehydration with hypernatraemia ensues. In children with associated ACTH deficiency, DI will only become evident once glucocorticoid treatment is started, since the ability to excrete a water load is dependent on adequate glucocorticoid secretion.

Investigations

If hypernatraemia with a high plasma osmolality is present simultaneously with a low urine osmolality a water deprivation test is not necessary. Indeed, this test can be extremely dangerous and should only be performed under careful supervision. However, in children with compulsive water drinking, the kidneys may develop a chronic inability to concentrate urine, and a water deprivation test may be the only method of differentiating this condition from DI. A dose of DDAVP (D-amino-D-arginine vasopressin) will restore the concentrating ability of the kidneys in cranial DI, thereby distinguishing this from nephrogenic DI.

Treatment

DDAVP given parenterally, orally or intranasally is used to treat cranial DI. The dose is titrated against symptoms, urine output and biochemical results. Access to water should not be restricted in those with normal thirst sensation. In patients who lack thirst sensation, a strict regimen of fluid intake and DDAVP replacement should be instigated, with careful monitoring of the sodium level, paired plasma and urine osmolalities.

In nephrogenic DI, treatment consists of free access to fluids and therapy with indomethacin or, paradoxically, diuretics such as hydrochlorothiazide and amiloride.

Syndrome of inappropriate ADH secretion

The syndrome of inappropriate ADH secretion (SIADH) arises with abnormalities of the respiratory and nervous systems, malignancy and drugs (Box 32).

BOX 32
Causes of SIADH (inappropriate ADH secretion)

Nervous system abnormalities
Tumours
Haemorrhage
Trauma
Infection, e.g. meningitis, encephalitis
Guillain–Barré syndrome
Ventriculo–atrial shunt blockage

Respiratory disease
Pneumonia
Tuberculosis
Hyaline membrane disease

Malignancies
Thymoma
Lymphoma

Drugs
Narcotics and analgesics
Cytotoxics

Clinical features of SIADH include headaches, apathy, nausea, vomiting, abnormal neurological signs and impaired consciousness, occasionally convulsions and coma.

Investigations reveal hypo-osmolality, hyponatraemia, inappropriately high urinary osmolality and sodium loss with inappropriately elevated ADH levels.

Treatment entails restriction of fluid intake and replacement of sodium losses. In severe cases, ADH secretion may be inhibited using demeclocycline.

Self-assessment: questions

Multiple choice questions

1. Development of a normal male phenotype is dependent on:
   a. The SRY region of the Y chromosome
   b. Gonadotrophin secretion by the anterior pituitary gland
   c. Normal secretion of adrenal androgens
   d. Normal testicular function
   e. Normal prolactin secretion

2. The following should be performed in a child with ambiguous genitalia:
   a. Abdominal ultrasound scan
   b. Karyotype analysis
   c. Urinary steroid profile
   d. hCG test
   e. Thyroid function

3. The following are causes of short stature:
   a. Constitutional delay of growth and puberty
   b. Thyrotoxicosis
   c. Cushing syndrome
   d. Rickets
   e. Soto syndrome

4. The following are manifestations of Turner syndrome:
   a. Delayed puberty
   b. Webbing of the neck
   c. Abdominal striae
   d. Renal abnormalities
   e. Lenticular dislocation

5. In normal puberty:
   a. Breast development is the first stage in girls
   b. Pubic hair development heralds the onset of puberty in boys
   c. The growth spurt is only dependent on the normal secretion of growth hormone
   d. Menarche is an early event in girls
   e. Pulsatile gonadotrophin secretion is mandatory for normal puberty

6. The following are causes of delayed puberty:
   a. Anorexia nervosa
   b. Cranial irradiation
   c. Poorly controlled insulin-dependent diabetes mellitus
   d. Neurofibromatosis
   e. Marfan syndrome

7. The McCune–Albright syndrome is associated with:
   a. Precocious puberty
   b. Hypothyroidism
   c. Insulin-dependent diabetes mellitus

   d. Cushing syndrome
   e. Growth hormone insufficiency

8. Congenital hypothyroidism:
   a. Because of dyshormonogenesis is an autosomal recessive condition
   b. Can be associated with development delay
   c. Is detected in the UK by screening for free thyroxine levels
   d. Is usually the result of an autoimmune process
   e. Resulting from secondary causes can be missed on screening

9. Thyrotoxicosis:
   a. Frequently presents with difficulties in behaviour and schooling
   b. Is associated with delayed relaxation of reflexes
   c. Is invariably associated with exophthalmos
   d. May be associated with vitiligo
   e. May be associated with an absent TSH response to TRH

10. The following are features of Addison disease:
    a. Hypotension
    b. Retinal haemorrhages
    c. Virilisation
    d. Hyponatraemia
    e. Hyperpigmentation

11. In Cushing syndrome, the following may be helpful in the diagnosis:
    a. Plasma renin activity
    b. Loss of diurnal variation in cortisol secretion
    c. Synacthen test
    d. Urinary free cortisol
    e. Dexamethasone suppression test

12. The following are clinical features of rickets:
    a. Proximal myopathy
    b. Bone pain
    c. Ectopic calcification
    d. Genu varum
    e. Craniotabes

13. The following may be associated with infantile hypercalcaemia:
    a. Mental retardation
    b. Elfin-like facies
    c. Supravalvular aortic stenosis
    d. Ectopic calcification
    e. Chronic diarrhoea

14. The following can be used in the treatment of hypercalcaemia in children:
    a. High-dose phosphate
    b. Increased fluid intake
    c. EDTA

d. Calcitonin
e. Glucocorticoids

15. With regard to cranial diabetes insipidus:
    a. It can present with convulsions
    b. Neuroradiological imaging is vital in all cases
    c. A water deprivation test is essential for diagnosis
    d. Water restriction is the treatment of choice
    e. It is a feature of Langerhans cell histiocytosis

16. Causes of nephrogenic diabetes insipidus include:
    a. An X-linked recessive condition
    b. Meningitis
    c. Heavy metal poisoning
    d. Hypokalaemia
    e. Intracranial neoplasia

Case histories

Case history 1

A 6-month-old baby girl presents with bilateral inguinal swellings. A karyotype is performed and shows 46XY.

How would you manage this child?

Case history 2

A prepubertal 8-year-old boy presents with tall stature and headaches. The bone age is 6 years and growth velocity 12 cm/year, equivalent to the 97th centile on the height velocity chart.

How would you investigate this child?

Case history 3

A 4-year-old boy presents with tall stature. Examination reveals bilateral papilloedema and penile and testicular enlargement. The bone age is 10 years, and the growth velocity lies on the 97th centile.

Give two further essential investigations and the most likely diagnosis.

Case history 4

A 6-year-old girl presents with short stature and isolated breast development. Examination confirms a height well below the third centile, weight on the 25th centile and breast stage III with no pubic or axillary hair development. Bone age was delayed at 2 years of age. Follow-up revealed a height velocity that lay on the 3rd centile.

What is the most likely diagnosis?

Case history 5

A 2-year-old girl presents with tall stature and a rapid rate of growth. Examination revealed marked clitoromegaly, and the bone age was advanced, at 7 years.

Name two diagnostic investigations and give the most likely diagnosis.

Case history 6

A 9-year-old boy presents with a history of recurrent croup, epilepsy, alopecia and mental retardation. His corrected plasma calcium level was 1.3 mmol/l (normal 2.25–2.6 mmol/l), phosphate 2.4 mmol/l (normal 1.4–1.8 mmol/l) and magnesium 0.5 mmol/l (normal 0.8–1.4 mmol/l).

Name one further diagnostic investigation and the most likely diagnosis.

Short notes

Write short notes on the following:

1. The management of short stature
2. The management of persistent hypoglycaemia in a week-old baby
3. The immediate management of diabetic ketoacidosis in a comatose 10-year-old child.

Self-assessment: answers

Multiple choice answers

1. a. **True**. This regulates testicular development.
   b. **True**. Vital for the stimulation of the testis.
   c. **False**. They have no role in the development of the male phenotype.
   d. **True**. Testosterone is produced by the testis.
   e. **False**. It has no role in the development of the male phenotype.

2. a. **True**. This will enable assessment of adrenal size/masses, internal genitalia and gonads.
   b. **True**. This is essential.
   c. **True**. In order to diagnose congenital adrenal hyperplasia.
   d. **True**. This assesses functioning testicular tissue, if testes are present.
   e. **False**. Thyroid disease is not associated with ambiguous genitalia.

3. a. **True**. Although these children have a late growth spurt.
   b. **False**. This causes tall stature.
   c. **True**. Excess steroids result in impaired growth, the height often falling below the 3rd percentile.
   d. **True**. Poor skeletal maturation and stunting.
   e. **False**. This is linked with tall stature.

4. a. **True**. Atretic ovaries occur, with failure of sexual maturation.
   b. **True**. This is a typical feature of Turner syndrome.
   c. **False**. This is a feature of obesity and Cushing syndrome.
   d. **True**. Abnormalities include horseshoe kidneys.
   e. **False**. This is a feature of Marfan syndrome or homocystinuria.

5. a. **True**. It is followed by pubic hair, female habitus and finally menses.
   b. **False**. Puberty in the male is heralded by testicular enlargement.
   c. **False**. It also requires sex steroids.
   d. **False**. This is a late event in girls.
   e. **True**. This is the driving force behind pubertal development.

6. a. **True**. Undernutrition results in generalised growth and pubertal delay, including amenorrhoea.
   b. **True**. This results in inhibition of pituitary gonadotrophins.
   c. **True**. Metabolic derangement will impair normal developmental processes.
   d. **False**. This usually leads to precocious puberty.

e. **False**. It is usually associated with normal pubertal timing.

7. a. **True**. It is the most common endocrinopathy.
   b. **False**. Although thyrotoxicosis is associated with this condition.
   c. **True**. This is a rare association.
   d. **True**. It is caused by corticosteroid-secreting adrenal nodules or adenomas.
   e. **False**. Although pituitary gigantism is an association.

8. a. **True**. As with most hereditary enzyme deficiencies.
   b. **True**. This is a characteristic feature.
   c. **False**. Screening is based on a raised TSH level.
   d. **False**. It is caused by thyroid agenesis or dyshormonogenesis.
   e. **True**. Congenital hypothyroidism secondary to pituitary failure is associated with a low TSH, which may be missed on many screening programmes that are initially designed to identify *high* TSH levels (and only then go on to check the free thyroxine levels).

9. a. **True**. Aggressive, unruly behaviour and poor concentration with poor school performance can be the presenting picture.
   b. **False**. This is a feature of hypothyroidism.
   c. **False**. Exophthalmos is a feature of Graves' disease but is not *invariably* associated with thyrotoxicosis.
   d. **True**. This is an unusual association.
   e. **True**. Suppression of the hypothalamic–pituitary axis by excess circulating thyroxine occurs.

10. a. **True**. Collapse with hypotension is typical of Addison disease.
    b. **False**. These are a feature of hypertension and, therefore, are seen in Cushing syndrome.
    c. **False**. Virilisation is caused by excessive adrenal androgen secretion.
    d. **True**. In the absence of mineralocorticoids there is a subsequent loss of sodium in the urine.
    e. **True**. This is a consequence of lack of cortisol and excess corticotrophin.

11. a. **False**. Plasma renin activity is of little use in diagnosing Cushing syndrome.
    b. **True**. Flattening or loss of the diurnal rhythm in cortisol is a major indicator toward the diagnosis of Cushing syndrome.
    c. **False**. Synacthen test is diagnostic in Addison disease.
    d. **True**. This would be elevated in Cushing syndrome.

e. **True**. This test is useful to determine whether the excess corticosteroid secretion can be suppressed (i.e. cases that are ACTH dependent) or not (e.g. ACTH-independent steroid secretion by tumours).

12. a. **True**. It may prevent or delay walking in severely affected patients.
   b. **True**. Pain usually occurs in the long bones.
   c. **False**. Ectopic calcification is a feature of pseudohypoparathyroidism.
   d. **True**. The distal limb is bowed inward below the knee.
   e. **True**. Softening of the skull is a feature seen in young infants.

13. a. **True**. This is part of Williams syndrome.
   b. **True**. Williams syndrome.
   c. **True**. Williams syndrome.
   d. **False**.
   e. **False**.

14. a. **False**. High-dose phosphate is toxic and contraindicated.
   b. **True**. This will help to enhance urinary clearance.
   c. **False**. EDTA is toxic and contraindicated.
   d. **True**. Calcitonin lowers serum calcium levels.
   e. **True**. Steroids also lower serum calcium.

15. a. **True**. Convulsions are caused by dehydration and electrolyte disturbance.
   b. **True**. Imaging is necessary to exclude hypothalamic–pituitary tumours.
   c. **False**. This test can be very dangerous and is not essential for diagnosis; paired plasma:urine osmolalities may be sufficient.
   d. **False**. This can lead to devastating consequences and death in cranial DI.
   e. **True**. Together with multiple bony osteolytic lesions.

16. a. **True**. This is the usual mode of inheritance.
   b. **False**. This causes cranial DI.
   c. **True**. This is a rare renal complication of poisoning with toxic heavy metals.
   d. **True**.
   e. **False**. This causes cranial DI.

Case history answers

Case history 1

The diagnosis in this child is that of complete androgen insensitivity. The bilateral inguinal swellings contain testes. Management is as follows.

History. Family history of infertility in phenotypic female members. The condition is inherited as X-linked recessive condition.

Investigations. hCG test to assess gonadal function and exclude Leydig cell hypoplasia, in which there is no response to hCG.

Treatment. Sex of rearing should be female, and the gonads removed because of the risk of malignant change in the late teenage years.

Case history 2

In a tall, prepubertal child with a rapid growth rate, the differential diagnosis lies between pituitary gigantism and thyrotoxicosis. A GH profile may reveal high basal GH and increased secretion after provocation. The normal secretory pattern of GH peaks and troughs (when GH secretion may be undetectable) is absent. An MRI scan may show a pituitary adenoma. In thyrotoxicosis, there are high free T_4 and T_3 levels with undetectable TSH and a flat TSH response to TRH.

Case history 3

Precocious puberty in boys is never idiopathic. In this instance, the presence of papilloedema suggests an underlying brain tumour. The investigations indicated are an LHRH test, which will show an elevation of LH and FSH in response to LHRH, and a CT or MRI scan of the brain.

Case history 4

Early breast development in a child with short stature, a delayed bone age and a poor height velocity is caused by primary hypothyroidism. All other causes of breast development are associated with a normal or rapid growth rate. The breast development is caused by elevated FSH concentrations, which are increased probably because of an excessive TRH drive.

Case history 5

Virilisation with tall stature and an advanced bone age in a girl is suggestive of excessive secretion of adrenal androgens as a result of congenital adrenal hyperplasia or a virilising adrenal tumour. The diagnostic investigations include a plasma 17-hydroxyprogesterone level, a urinary steroid profile and a CT/MRI scan of the adrenal glands.

Case history 6

The hypocalcaemia, hypomagnesaemia and hyperphosphataemia are indicative of hypoparathyroidism; a serum parathyroid hormone level is, therefore, the diagnostic investigation of choice.

Short notes answers

1. The management can be divided into several areas:

   History. The following should be assessed: symptoms of raised intracranial pressure, systemic illness, birth weight, feeding difficulties in infancy, family history of short stature, thyroid disease.

   Examination. Important points are dysmorphic features, features of Russell–Silver syndrome, signs of systemic illness, wasting, abdominal distension, raised intracranial pressure, hypothyroidism or Cushing syndrome.

   Auxology. Compare the child's height with target mid-parental centile; calculate height velocity.

   Investigations. Exclude systemic illness, investigate for endocrine causes of short stature, e.g. insulin tolerance test, insulin-like growth factor I (IGF-I), IGF-I binding protein 3.

   Treatment. Treat according to diagnosis.

2. The management can be considered in various sections:

   History. Take details of birth weight, maternal diabetes mellitus, family history of neonatal hypoglycaemia and neonatal deaths.

   Examination. Look for polycythaemia, dysmorphic features, Beckwith–Wiedemann syndrome (macrosomia, macoglossia, transverse crease in ears, exomphalos, hepatomegaly).

   Investigations. Measure glucose requirement to maintain normoglycaemia. During spontaneous or induced hypoglycaemia, sample blood for glucose, insulin, growth hormone, cortisol, free fatty acids, ketone bodies, C-peptide, lactate.

   Treatment. This depends upon underlying cause. Maintain euglycaemia with 10–20% glucose infusion; use glucagon and/or somatostatin if unresponsive. Diazoxide with hydrochlorothiazide is useful in hyperinsulinism; 95% pancreatectomy is required if the child is unresponsive to drugs. In glycogen storage disease, use frequent feeds including corn starch.

3. Management includes:

   History. Take details of weight loss, anorexia, polyuria, polydipsia, fatigue, family history of insulin-dependent diabetes mellitus and other autoimmune conditions.

   Examination. Look for dehydration, Kussmaul respiration, altered level of consciousness, ketone odour on breath, signs of precipitating infection.

   Investigations. Measure blood glucose, analyse urine for glycosuria and ketonuria, measure arterial blood gas, urea and electrolytes, glycosylated haemoglobin, do blood cultures, and cultures of mid-stream urine (MSU).

   Treatment. Rehydrate slowly over 48 hours using normal saline initially and sliding scale insulin infusion to reduce the blood glucose slowly. Substitute fluid with dextrose/saline when blood glucose is <10 mmol/l; replace potassium. Carefully monitor electrolytes, pH and blood glucose at regular intervals over the first 24 hours; use antibiotics if sepsis suspected.

Hereditary and metabolic diseases

Key points

You need to have an understanding of:

- The basis of inheritance of disease
- The basis of molecular detection in genetic disorders
- The features of the common chromosomal disorders of childhood
- How to examine a child for dysmorphological features
- The different manifestations of the common inherited metabolic disorders of childhood
- The principles of genetic counselling.

9.1 Introduction

Molecular basis of genetic disorders

Each human cell contains two copies of the entire human genetic programme or **genome**. This is packaged into 46 chromosomes (23 pairs), amounting to approximately 6 billion base pairs of DNA. **Genes**, the functional units of the DNA, comprise approximately 10% of the human genome and there are approximately 100 000 of them encoded for by human DNA. Their size varies from several hundred to more than 2 million base pairs. In any one cell, subsets of these genes are actually active and genes will be expressed at varying levels from cell to cell. Genes **transcribe** messenger RNA (mRNA). To do this, the double-stranded DNA separates and a complementary strand is synthesised. The cellular machinery takes out (splices out) the non-coding sequences or **introns** and the sequences that are retained represent the coding sequences or **exons**. The mRNA is transported to the ribosomal cytoplasm where it is **translated** into protein. Proteins can then be further modified. Some functional proteins are the products of more than one gene and these genes do not necessarily lie on the same chromosome. For example, the various components of the human heavy chain immunoglobulin protein are all located on the large arm of chromosome 14. However haemoglobin is composed of α chains coded for by genes on chromosome 16 and β chains coded for by a gene on chromosome 11.

While the majority of genes are present in the nucleus, the mitochondrion has its own genome and genes. Peculiarly, the sperm does not carry mitochondria into the oocyte, so all mitochondrial DNA is of maternal origin.

Genetic variation

Mutations

Human genetics deals with variations between humans. A change in the linear sequence of bases along the DNA is a **mutation**. Mutations can affect the functioning of a gene or may have no apparent impact on the organism. The latter type are called **polymorphisms** and will include changes in the intronic sequences. The effect of mutation varies with the number of base pairs affected and with the role of the genes involved.

Mutations in the coding sequence. These may result in a change in a single amino acid (**missense mutation**) or may truncate a protein (**nonsense mutation**). They may also destroy stop or start codons. Small deletions (or insertions) can cause a **frameshift** affecting all subsequent translation.

Mutations in introns. These may destroy or create splicing sites.

Mutations in other areas. Mutations in promoter sites can prevent or alter transcription rates; mutations within mRNA untranslated end regions can destroy ribosome recognition sites and alter mRNA stability.

Gross changes

A number of larger changes to the genetic material can also have functional consequences.

Chromosome segregation. Whole chromosome mis-segregation at meiosis can lead to monosomy or trisomy and cause a range of conditions.

Translocations. Gross rearrangements can alter the 'dosage' of genes or may result in loss of gene function or control of gene expression.

Deletions. Small deletions of all or part of a gene may destroy its function leading to a 50% reduction in gene dose (a carrier state if 50% is adequate).

Repeats. Tandemly repeated nucleotide triplets are found normally in non-coding sequences but are capable of increasing in number to form unstable repeats.

Analysis of genetic material

Restriction analysis

Restriction endonucleases recognise typical DNA sequences at which they will cut DNA. A change in the nucleic acid sequence can alter the enzyme cutting sites and change the lengths of DNA produced when genomic DNA is digested with a restriction endonuclease. These are called **restriction fragment length polymorphisms (RFLP)** (Fig. 53). The figure shows a stretch of DNA that contains three enzymatic sites in the wild-type (A) and the loss of the second enzymatic site in the mutant (B). The squiggle represents a radioactively labelled probe that recognises DNA at the site of the second restriction site. Restriction digestion will result in two similar size fragments in the wild type but only one larger fragment in the mutant. When these are electrophoresed on a gel, the smaller fragments will migrate faster. The separated fragments are then **denatured** (DNA is made single stranded), blotted onto a nylon membrane (**Southern blot**) and **hybridised** with the radioactively labelled probe. On autoradiography, in this instance, the wild type is detected as two smaller

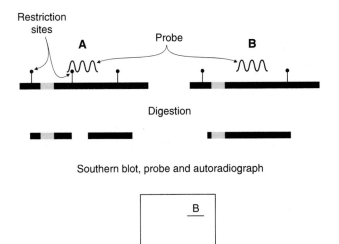

Fig. 53 Restriction fragment length polymorphism. See text for details.

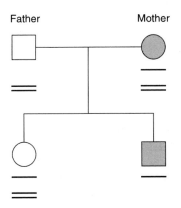

Fig. 54 Pedigree showing segregation of a sex-linked recessive disorder by restriction analysis.

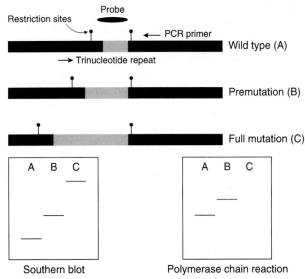

Fig. 55 Molecular analysis of increased tandem repeats. See text for details.

blot with labelled DNA from the region of the gene reveals a single band in a normal male subject (wild type, A in Fig. 55). An asymptomatic male carrier will have a band of higher molecular weight (B), and a subject with a full mutation will have a very large, diffuse band because of the instability of the full-mutation allele (C). The normal and asymptomatic carrier alleles can also be detected by the **polymerase chain reaction** (PCR). This is a method that allows a small targeted DNA sequence to be amplified to assist in its analysis. The full-mutation allele cannot be amplified by PCR because it is too large (Fig. 55).

PCR-based techniques are used for direct analysis of mutations and can be used as shown in the example for the detection of a triplet-repeat mutation or for mutations within the coding sequence of a gene.

These powerful molecular techniques are being used to diagnose disease in affected individuals and as prenatal testing for those with a familial history. Prenatal screening for β thalassaemia using **chorionic villi biopsy** or **amniocentesis**, and termination of affected fetuses, has almost wiped out the disease within a generation in Cyprus. The administration of steroids to a mother carrying a fetus with congenital adrenal hyperplasia will prevent virilisation in a female fetus. The same principle applies to an increasing number of conditions such as Duchenne muscular dystrophy, haemolytic anaemias and inherited malignancies such as retinoblastoma.

9.2 Mendelian patterns of inheritance

Not all **dysmorphic** syndromes are inherited.

Deformation. A deformation is an alteration in the shape or structure of a part that has differentiated normally. This is often the result of an abnormal physical

bands and the mutant as a single larger band. The use of this procedure in clinical practice is illustrated in Figure 54. The mother clearly has one mutant and one normal **allele** (gene), while the father is normal. In this case, the daughter has inherited the mother's **genotype**, but the son only has the mother's mutant gene. This is an example of an X-linked recessive disorder such as Duchenne muscular dystrophy or haemophilia A.

Another form of mutation is the expansion of tandemly repeated nucleotide triplets. The prototype for disease caused in this way is the fragile X syndrome and other examples are Huntington disease and myotonic dystrophy. Figure 55 illustrates the molecular diagnosis of such conditions. In the fragile X syndrome, a CGG repeat occurs near the 5′ end of the gene. The number of repeats ranges from 5 to 50 in the general population, from approximately 50 to 200 in asymptomatic carriers and exceeds 200 in those with the fragile X syndrome. To detect the abnormality, DNA is treated with a restriction enzyme that cuts at recognition sites flanking the CGG repeat. Hybridisation on a Southern condition in utero. An example of this occurs with oligo-hydramnios. The fetus is squeezed and unable to turn; as a result a breech presentation with deformation of the feet (talipes) may occur.

Disruption. The term disruption is used for the destruction of a part that has previously developed normally. This may result from either physical severance (e.g. amputation of a digit by an amniotic band) or the interruption of the blood supply to a developing organ (e.g. gastroschisis, porencephaly).

Malformation. By comparison, a malformation is a primary structural defect arising from a localised error in morphogenesis. Single malformations such as pyloric stenosis and cardiac septal defects tend to be multifactorial in origin.

Multiple malformations. These can occur as part of a syndrome, where the same malformations are seen consistently and may be caused by a single gene change, chromosomal defects or teratogenesis.

Association. This term is used for non-specific malformations involving groups of organs. An example is the VATER association, where non-specific vertebral malformations are found to coexist with anal atresia, tracheo-oesophageal fistula and non-specific radial defects.

Sequence. These conditions must be distinguished from a sequence, which refers to a series of events occurring after one initiating defect. In the Pierre–Robin sequence, there is hypoplasia of the mandible. As a result the tongue is pushed posteriorly and interferes with the development of the soft palate. Consequently the child has micrognathia, cleft of the soft palate and glossoptosis.

Autosomal dominant inheritance

Examples of autosomal dominant conditions include achondroplasia, Marfan syndrome and neurofibromatosis. An affected individual carries the abnormal gene on one pair of autosomes (chromosomes 1–22). The heterozygote, carrying one copy of the abnormal gene manifests the condition, i.e. a single copy of the mutant gene is sufficient for expression of the disease phenotype. The affected person passes to each offspring either the normal or the abnormal allele. Each offspring has a 1 in 2 (50%) chance of inheriting the abnormal gene (Fig. 56). A family history is, therefore, highly predictive of these disorders. Occasionally an autosomal dominant condition may occur as the result of a new mutation, in which case there will be a negative family history. The gene may also be varyingly expressed. For example in a family with tuberous sclerosis, the parent may only have skin abnormalities while the child has, in addition, neurological defects. Sometimes the effect of inheriting the abnormal gene (genotype) is not expressed in the phenotype, and this is referred to as **non-penetrance.** An example of this is otosclerosis where only 40% of the gene carriers become deaf.

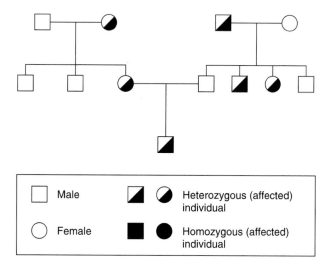

☐	Male	◪ ◐	Heterozygous (affected) individual
○	Female	■ ●	Homozygous (affected) individual

Fig. 56 Example of autosomal dominant inheritance.

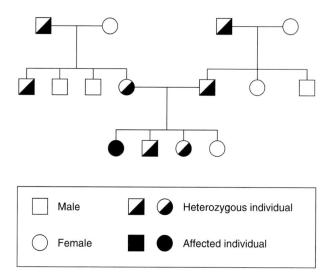

☐	Male	◪ ◐	Heterozygous individual
○	Female	■ ●	Affected individual

Fig. 57 Example of autosomal recessive inheritance.

Autosomal recessive inheritance

Numerous disorders result from autosomal recessive inheritance and include cystic fibrosis, congenital adrenal hyperplasia, phenylketonuria and galactosaemia. Unlike autosomal dominant inheritance, the heterozygous (single abnormal allele) individual is healthy. The affected individual is one who is homozygous (both alleles are abnormal). In most instances, both parents are heterozygotes or carriers (though one or both may also be homozygous). The risk of each child of two carrier parents being affected is 25% (Fig. 57). Although the abnormal gene may be transmitted from one generation to the next, there is usually no positive history outside the sibship. This is because other members of the family will usually have non-carrier partners. In communities where **consanguinity** (marrying one's close relative) is practised, there is an increased incidence of autosomally recessive diseases and here the family history may be positive. Mostly, autosomal dominant conditions involve non-lethal structural defects while autosomal recessive conditions often involve

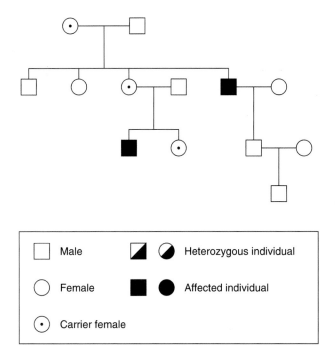

Male	Heterozygous individual
Female	Affected individual
Carrier female	

Fig. 58 Example of X-linked recessive inheritance.

metabolic disorders resulting from enzyme deficiencies and are more often life threatening. Some conditions, such as β thalassemia, do not strictly fit the description of being autosomally recessive. In this case, heterozygotes produce abnormal haemoglobin and can be symptomatic, though severe disease is only seen in homozygotes. Such conditions have also been called **autosomal co-dominant**.

Sex-linked inheritance

X-linked disorders are usually inherited in a recessive fashion. The abnormal gene is carried on the X chromosome. In the carrier female, the normal allele on her other X chromosome 'protects' her from disease. In the male, however, the abnormal allele on his X chromosome is not balanced by a normal allele and he manifests the disease. Daughters of affected males will be carriers but sons will not be affected (Fig. 58). The family history is often negative, as many cases are a result of new mutations. Examples of X-linked recessive disorders include colour blindness, Duchenne and Becker muscular dystrophies, glucose 6-phosphate dehydrogenase deficiency, haemophilia A and B and Hunter syndrome.

X-linked dominant disorders

X-linked dominant inherited disorders such as vitamin D resistant rickets are rare. No serious genetic defects apart from some rare intersex conditions and a gene for azoospermia are linked with the Y chromosome. After all, half the population lives very happily without a Y chromosome!

Mitochondrial or cytoplasmic inheritance

There are rare metabolic disorders such as the mitochondrial myopathies and Leber optic neuropathy that are inherited as part of the mitochondrial DNA. Inheritance is not strictly Mendelian; while the defect can only be maternal in origin, it is not related to the X chromosome.

Imprinting

Normally one allele each is inherited from either parent and usually only one gene is active in a random fashion. In some cases, genes only express the copy derived from a parent of a given sex and this process is called imprinting. In some cases, this is because both chromosomes of a pair are inherited from one parent (**uniparental disomy**). The classical examples of this are the Prader–Willi (learning difficulties, hypotonia, obesity) and Angelman (severe learning difficulties, ataxia, characteristic facies, epilepsy) syndromes, which are associated with deletion and uniparental disomy of chromosome 15. In Prader–Willi syndrome, it is the paternally derived and in Angelman the maternally derived genetic information on chromosome 15 which is missing.

Multifactorial inheritance

Multifactorial inheritance describes a pattern of inheritance observed for several relatively common conditions that appear to result from the interactions of a genetic predisposition with environmental factors. The conditions vary from those seen in childhood such as cleft lip / palate, congenital dislocation of the hip, neural tube defects, congenital heart disease and pyloric stenosis to those seen in later life such as asthma, depression, diabetes mellitus, hypertension and epilepsy. The concept of multifactorial inheritance is not entirely satisfactorily understood but a few characteristic features are present.

- There is a similar rate of recurrence in first-degree relatives and the risk declines sharply as the relationship with the affected person becomes more distant. For example, the risk of a neural tube defect in first-degree relatives is 4–5%; it is 1–2% in second-degree relatives and is similar to the general population in third-degree relatives.
- The risk of recurrence is related to the incidence of the disease.
- The risk is higher if more than one first-degree relative has the defect. For example, if parents have two children with a neural tube defect the risk that the third child will be affected rises to 10–12%.
- The risk of recurrence may be greater when the disorder is more severe. An infant with long segment Hirschsprung disease has a greater chance of having an affected sibling than the infant who has short segment Hirschsprung disease.
- Some disorders have sexual predilection; pyloric

stenosis is more common in males while congenital dislocation of the hip is more common in females.

• The frequency of concordance in identical twins is 21–63%.

9.3 Chromosomal disorders

Chromosomal abnormalities are either numerical or structural, occur in 0.4% of live births and are an important cause of mental defects and congenital anomalies.

Down syndrome (trisomy 21)

Down syndrome is the most common autosomal trisomy and the commonest genetic cause of severe learning difficulties. The incidence is 1 in 650 liveborn infants. Table 42 lists the characteristic clinical manifestations of children with Down syndrome. As shown in Table 43, the risk of Down syndrome is related to maternal age.

The presence of Down syndrome is often suspected by the failure to grow in utero. In women with a fetus with Down syndrome, the maternal serum oestriol and α-fetoprotein are lowered and the human chorionic gonadotrophin raised. If any of these are abnormal and/or there are fetal anomalies on ultrasonography, an amniocentesis is performed and the fetal karyotype is confirmed.

Table 42 Clinical features of Down syndrome

	Features
Head	Brachycephaly, low set hairline, flattened occiput
Face	Round face, epicanthic folds, Brushfield spots in the iris, protruding tongue, small low set ears.
Limbs	Single palmar (simian) crease, fifth finger clinodactyly, short stubby digits, abnormal dermatoglyphics, wide gap between first and second toes
Other	Generalised hypotonia, small stature, congenital heart defect (atrioventricular canal defects), anal and duodenal atresia
Later problems	Severe learning difficulties (IQ usually around 50), growth failure, recurrent respiratory infections, auditory and visual handicaps, hypothyroidism, Alzheimer disease, increased risk of leukaemia

Table 43 The risk of Down syndrome and maternal age

Maternal age (years)	Risk of Down syndrome
All ages	1:650
30	1:900
35	1:380
37	1:240
40	1:110
44	1:37

The commonest mechanism (~94%) by which an extra chromosome 21 is acquired is by **non-disjunction**. This results from an error at meiosis, when one pair of chromosome 21 fails to separate so that one gamete has two chromosomes 21 and one has none (Fig. 59.) In 80% of children, the extra 21 chromosome is maternal in origin. If females with trisomy 21 conceive, there is a 50% chance that they will have a baby with trisomy 21. Males with Down syndrome are generally infertile.

In about 5% of individuals there is a translocation involving chromosome 21 (Fig. 60). Half of the translocations arise de novo and half are inherited from a carrier parent. The majority of translocations are examples of fusion at the centromeres (Robertsonian) of chromosomes 13, 14 and 15 with 21. As shown in Figure 60, parents who are carriers produce three types of live offspring, a normal phenotype and karyotype, a phenotypically normal translocation carrier and a translocation trisomy 21. In practice, however, the risk of Down syndrome is 2–5% for a carrier male and 10–15% for a carrier female. Rarely, the parent carries a balanced 21q21q Robertsonian translocation and the risk of Down syndrome in the live born offspring is then 100%. About 1% of Down syndrome babies have **mosaicism**. This is

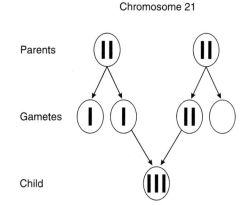

Fig. 59 Non-disjunction in Down syndrome.

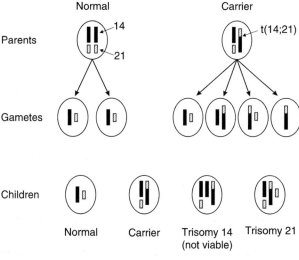

Fig. 60 Down syndrome with an inherited t(14;21) translocation.

the result of non-disjunction after the zygote has been formed and occurs during mitosis. Variable proportions of cells in the body are of the normal karyotype while others have trisomy 21. The phenotype is, therefore, often milder in mosaic Down syndrome.

Other trisomies

Trisomy 18

Trisomy 18 (Edward syndrome) affects approximately 1 in 3000 neonates. Intrauterine growth retardation is a common feature and 90% of the babies have congenital heart disease. Most die within the first year of life. The clinical features include mental retardation, prominent occiput, low set dysplastic ears, small mouth and jaw, clenched hands with second and third fingers overlapping the third and fourth fingers, and rocker bottom feet.

Trisomy 13

Trisomy 13 (Patau syndrome) is rare and is characterised by a structural defect of the brain (holoprosencephaly), polydactyly, scalp defects, microphthalmia and cardiac and renal anomalies. Survival beyond a few weeks is unusual.

Klinefelter syndrome

Klinefelter syndrome occurs in approximately 1:1000 live-born males. These children have a 47XXY karyotype. Children are usually phenotypically normal though they may have mildly impaired verbal IQ. Adults are taller than average with long limbs; 30% have gynaecomastia and all are infertile.

Turner syndrome

The incidence of Turner syndrome is 1:5000 of live-born females but it can be detected in 3–5% of abortus material as most cases result in miscarriage. The affected individuals have a delayed maturation of the lymphatic system, which manifests as a cystic hygroma and puffy hands and feet in the neonate and later on with residual neck webbing. Short stature is the commonest presenting feature and is often associated with a low posterior hairline, increased carrying angle, widely spaced nipples (shield-shaped chest) and congenital heart disease (15% have a coarctation of the aorta). Facial abnormalities (e.g. micrognathia, rotated ears, ptosis and high arched palate), multiple pigmented naevi, dysplastic nails, renal anomalies (horse shoe kidney), autoimmune conditions, deafness and osteoporosis are other associations. Presentation in adult life is with primary amenorrhoea and infertility resulting from ovarian dysgenesis, though 20% will start puberty spontaneously. In 50% there is only one sex chromosome (45XO), which is of maternal origin. In the others

there is either deletion of the short arm of one X chromosome or an isochromosome with two long arms and no short arm. Intellectual development is normal and the children benefit from growth hormone therapy during childhood, with oestrogen-replacement therapy at puberty. Boys and girls with **Noonan** syndrome display the Turner phenotype but the disorder is autosomally dominantly inherited and the classic cardiac malformation is that of peripheral pulmonary artery stenosis.

9.4 Inborn errors of metabolism

An inborn error of metabolism is any of a wide group of inherited conditions caused by a genetically determined deficiency in a particular enzyme. Many hundreds of enzyme defects have been identified and they are all rare. An inborn error of metabolism may be suggested from a positive family history or previous unexplained deaths in the family. In the neonatal period, these disorders must be considered whenever infants become severely ill without an adequate explanation. Other presenting features include poor feeding with recurrent vomiting; lethargy, convulsions and coma; jaundice with hepatomegaly; and unusually smelly body or urine. There may be severe metabolic acidosis, ketosis or raised plasma ammonia. Inborn errors of metabolism should also be considered in children with learning difficulties, coarse facies and abnormal hair, skeleton and pigmentation.

Disorders of amino acid metabolism

Phenylketonuria (PKU)

This rare disorder is caused by deficiency of the enzyme phenylalanine hydroxylase or the synthesis or recycling of the biopterin cofactor for this enzyme. Untreated, it presents with infantile spasms and developmental delay in late infancy. There is a characteristic musty odour and many of the children are fair haired and blue eyed with eczematous skin. Raised phenylalanine is detected once milk feeding has been established for 5–7 days and most children are detected in the neonatal stage by the national screening programme in the UK. Treatment is with the restriction of dietary phenylalanine while ensuring that there is sufficient protein for optimal physical and neurological growth. The plasma phenylalanine level needs to be monitored regularly. The majority (75%) on this regimen will be able to attend normal school, though there is a higher incidence of behavioural and learning difficulties. While dietary restrictions should be in place lifelong, this is often difficult to achieve in practice. Maternal PKU is devastating to the fetus (microcephaly, severe handicap) unless dietary restrictions have been strictly followed

Table 44 Disorders of amino acid metabolism

Disorder	Enzyme deficiency	Characteristics
Phenylketonuria	Phenylalanine hydroxylase	Infantile spasms, developmental delay, microcephaly, severe mental deficiency, convulsions
Tyrosinaemia	Fumarylacetoacetate hydrolase	Failure to thrive and acute hepatic failure in infancy, cirrhosis, renal tubular dysfunction, neuropathy in childhood
Homocystinuria	Cystathionine synthetase	Failure to thrive, developmental delay, marfanoid features, ectopia lentis, thromboembolic episodes
Albinism	Defects in the production and distribution of melanin	Oculocutaneous albinism, Chédiak–Higashi syndrome (neutrophil dysfunction), Hermansky–Pudlak (platelet dysfunction), piebaldism

Table 45 Glycogen storage disorders

Type	Enzyme deficiency	Symptoms
I	Glucose 6-phosphatase	Growth failure, asymptomatic hypoglycaemia and enlarged kidneys; the prognosis is good and most children can be managed with dietary regimens such as frequent night-time feeding
II (Pompe disease)	Lysosomal enzyme	Lysosomal enzyme deficiency; excess glycogen is deposited in both liver and muscle, especially in cardiac muscle; most patients present in early infancy with marked hypotonia, poor feeding, severe cardiomegaly and congestive cardiac failure; the prognosis is poor
III	Debranching enzyme	Milder form of type I
V	Muscle phosphorylase	Muscle cramps
VI	Liver phosphorylase	Milder form of type I
VII	Phosphofructokinase	Muscle cramps
XI		Rickets and renal tubular problems

prior to conception. Other disorders of amino acid metabolism are listed in Table 44.

The organic acidaemias

The organic acidaemias disrupt the catabolic pathways of several essential amino acids (the branched-chain amino acids leucine, isoleucine and valine and the odd-chain amino acids, e.g. threonine) resulting in **maple syrup urine disease** (MSUD), **methylmalonic** and **propionic acidaemia** among others. MSUD most often presents in the neonatal period with severe metabolic acidosis, hypoglycaemia and seizures. There is increased excretion of the branched-chain amino acids. The urine has the characteristic maple syrup smell. A delay in diagnosis leads to learning difficulties and neurological dysfunction and there remains a high risk of death during any acute illness. The management of organic acidaemias centres on the restriction of dietary protein. During acute decompensation, catabolism is limited by a high-carbohydrate, low-protein intake. Acidosis is corrected and the hyperammonaemia is treated by peritoneal dialysis or haemoperfusion. Some disorders respond to large dosages of vitamin cofactors but the outcome is often poor.

Urea cycle defects

Enzyme defects have been identified for all stages of the urea cycle. They tend to cause neonatal encephalopathy owing to high blood ammonia levels but the onset can be delayed; if so the patients present with coma and infection.

Liver enzyme deficiencies

Galactosaemia

Galactosaemia results from a deficiency in the enzyme galactose 1-phosphate uridyl transferase. The infant is unable to convert galactose to glucose and, therefore, will become hypoglycaemic while on a pure milk diet. The affected neonate feeds poorly, vomits and develops jaundice and hepatomegaly and, ultimately, liver cell failure. Management is with a lactose and a galactose-free diet. In those untreated, chronic liver disease and cataracts are the ultimate end result.

Glycogen storage disorders

The glycogen storage diseases are mostly recessively inherited disorders that have specific enzyme defects which prevent mobilisation of glucose to glycogen. Most enzymes are liver based although some defects affect other tissues as well and a few affect only muscle. There are eleven main enzyme defects (types I–XI), which all lead to an abnormal storage of glycogen in different tissues (Table 45).

Hereditary fructose intolerance

Fructose intolerance arises from deficiency of aldolase B. Again prompt recognition and action can be life saving. Ingestion of fructose results in the toxic accumulation of fructose 1-phosphate in the liver and other tissues. Once fructose-containing foods are started, the child presents with abdominal pain, nausea, vomiting and symptoms of hypoglycaemia. In the long term, hepatomegaly, growth reduction and liver failure occur. Therapy involves eliminating all fructose-containing items from the diet.

Defects in the conjugation of bilirubin

Hepatic glucuronyl transferase activity is deficient in the **Crigler–Najjar syndrome** and produces congenital, non-haemolytic, non-obstructive, unconjugated hyperbilirubinaemia. It is a rare cause of kernicterus. Low levels of unconjugated hyperbilirubinaemia are also seen in the benign **Gilbert syndrome**. Inherited conjugated hyperbilirubinaemia, a mild benign disorder, is seen in the **Dubin–Johnson** and **Rotor** syndromes.

Deficiency in α_1-antitrypsin

Deficiency of the protease inhibitor (Pi) α_1-antitrypsin is associated with emphysema in adults and liver disease in infancy and childhood. There are more than 25 phenotypes of the Pi, coded for by a gene on chromosome 14. Liver disease is associated with the phenotype PiZZ. It is a cause of neonatal hepatitis and ultimately will progress to cirrhosis and portal hypertension. Replacement therapy using fractionated plasma α_1-antitrypsin and milk from transgenic sheep has been used in adults with emphysema, but its use in children with hepatitis is still experimental. The current therapeutic goal is to transplant the liver as the cirrhosis decompensates. This is also a disease that is a potential target for gene therapy.

Lipid storage disorders

The lipid storage disorders are rare and have a predominantly fatal neurodegenerative presentation.

Tay–Sachs disease is a **gangliosidosis**. The enzyme hexosaminidase D is deficient and there is an increased deposition of GM2 ganglioside in the grey matter. The affected infant presents with developmental regression, exaggerated startle response and visual inattention. Findings include severe hypotonia, enlarging head and a cherry-red spot on the macula.

Gaucher's disease is caused by glucocerebroside deposition in the reticuloendothelial system and has an early-onset neuropathic and a late-onset non-neuropath-

ic presentation. The former presents with feeding problems, stridor and spasticity. There is progressive enlargement of the liver and spleen and Gaucher cells can be identified in the bone marrow. The late-onset variety presents with hepatosplenomegaly and bone disease.

Niemann–Pick disease causes an abnormal storage of sphingomyelin in the reticuloendothelial system. Of the four varieties, two resemble Tay–Sachs disease and are neuropathic and the others present with a hepatitic picture with hepatosplenomegaly.

Mucopolysaccharidoses

The mucopolysaccharidoses (MPS) are a group of inherited disorders caused by incomplete degradation and storage of acid mucopolysaccharides (glycosaminoglycans). Mucopolysaccharides are the major components of the intracellular substance of connective tissue. The clinical manifestations result from its accumulation in various organs. The clinical features are listed in Table 46. There are various characteristic syndromes, but the most severe is **Hurler syndrome** which results from deficiency of α-L-iduronidase. The features of some of them are given in Table 47. Treatment is supportive according to the child's needs. Enzyme replacement by bone marrow transplantation has been performed for Hurler syndrome, which is also a target for gene therapy.

Lipid metabolism

Hyperlipidaemia

Hyperlipidaemia is one of the main risk factors for coronary heart disease. Identification and treatment of

Table 46 Clinical features of mucopolysaccharidoses

	Features
Eyes	Corneal clouding, retinal degeneration, glaucoma
Skin	Thickened skin, coarse facies
Heart	Valvular lesions, cardiac failure
CNS	Developmental regression
Skeletal	Thickened skull, conductive deafness, broad ribs, claw hand, thoracic kyphosis, lumbar lordosis, carpal tunnel syndrome
Other	Umbilical and inguinal hernias, hepatosplenomegaly

Table 47 Types of mucopolysaccharidose

Type	Inheritance	Cornea	Heart	Brain	Skeletal	Visceral
MPS IH (Hurler)	AR	+++	++	+++	++	+++
MPS IS (Scheie)	AR	+++	++	–	–	+/–
MPS II (Hunter)	XR	–	+	++	+	+++
MPS III (Sanfilippo)	AR	+/–	–	+	+	+/–
MPS IV (Morquio)	AR	+	+	–	+	+/–
MPS VI (Maroteaux–Lamy)	AR	+++	++	–	++	+
MPS VII	AR	+/–	–	++	++	++

AR, autosomal recessive; XR, sex-linked recessive.

Table 48 Immunodeficiency disorders of childhood

Defect	Disorder	Characteristics
B cell	X-linked agammaglobulinaemia (Bruton's disease)	X-linked; caused by abnormal Bruton tyrosine kinase on Xq22, which leads to panhypogammaglobulinaemia Presents with **bacterial** sinopulmonary infections
	Selective IgA deficiency	Autosomal inheritance, gene on 6p21 leads to selective deficiency of IgA **Bacterial** infections of the renal, pulmonary and gastrointestinal systems
T cell	Thymic hypoplasia (DiGeorge syndrome)	22q11 deletion, dysmorphogenesis of the 3rd and 4th pharyngeal pouches; aplasia of parathyroids and hypocalcaemia; aortic arch, palatal and mandibular malformations Predominantly **fungal**, **viral** and ***Pneumocystis carinii*** infections
	Hyper-IgM syndrome	X-linked, owing to abnormal CD40 on Xq26 in defective T cells; leads to defective signalling of B cells Boys present with frequent **bacterial** otitis media, tonsillitis and pneumonia
B and T cell	Severe combined immunodeficiency (SCID)	Genetically diverse; some are X-linked (Xq13); absent T and B cell function from birth Pulmonary, gastrointestinal, cutaneous and systemic infections
	Nezelof syndrome	
	Wiskott–Aldrich syndrome	X-linked
	Adenosine deaminase (ADA) deficiency	Adenosine deaminase gene on 22q13
	Ataxia-telangiectasia	Autosomal recessive
Complement	Primary	Manifests as recurrent infections of capsulated bacterial organisms such as *Neisseria* and *Pneumococcus* or as autoimmune diseases such as systemic lupus erythematosus or glomerulonephritis
	Secondary	Nephrotic syndrome, sickle cell disease, cirrhosis, splenectomy
Phagocytic cells	Chronic granulomatous disease (CGD)	X-linked (50–60%): defective expression of the cytochrome *b* 91 kDa subunit (gene on Xp21) Autosomal recessive: defective expression of 47 kDa and 67 kDa cytosolic factor Chronic recurrent pyogenic infections with unusual organisms and granuloma formation in skin and viscera

hyperlipidaemia in childhood may delay the onset of cardiovascular disease in later life. Children should be screened for hyperlipidaemia if there is a family history of coronary heart disease, peripheral vascular disease, cerebrovascular disease or sudden death before 55 years of age.

Familial hypercholesterolaemia

Familial hypercholesterolaemia is an autosomal dominant disorder of lipoprotein metabolism resulting from a defect in the low-density lipoprotein (LDL) receptor. About 1:500 are heterozygous and affected. The serum LDL cholesterol concentration is markedly raised (>3.3 mmol/l). The condition is associated with premature coronary heart disease, which occurs in 50% of patients by 50 years of age in males and 60 years of age in females. Skin and tendon xanthomata may be present but are uncommon in childhood. Homozygous disease is very rare and much more severe, causing xanthomata in childhood and clinical cardiovascular disease in the second decade.

Familial combined hypercholesterolaemia

Familial combined hypercholesterolaemia is an autosomal dominant condition associated with an increased risk of premature coronary heart disease in adult life. Management involves attention to accompanying risk factors such as obesity, hypertension, diabetes mellitus and smoking.

Management in lipid disorders

Diet remains the main component of lipid-lowering strategies. Anion-exchange resins such as cholestyramine are effective in lowering LDL cholesterol but compliance is a problem. Hydroxymethylglutaryl (HMG) CoA reductase (the rate-limiting enzyme in cholesterol synthesis) inhibitors pravastatin and simvastatin have been shown to be effective in preliminary trials.

9.5 Immunodeficiency disorders

Immunodeficiencies may be primary when there is an intrinsic, often inherited, defect in the immune system or, more commonly, they may be secondary to another phenomenon such as malnutrition, malignant disease, immunosuppressive therapy or infections such as HIV. Many of the primary immunodeficiency disorders are inherited as autosomal recessive or X-linked disorders. There may be a family history of unexplained death, particularly in boys, and parental consanguinity. Children will usually present with a history of recurrent, persistent or unusual infections (Table 48) or with protein-losing enteropathy and failure to thrive. The management involves aggressive treatment of infections, antibiotic prophylaxis (e.g. co-trimoxazole for *Pneumocystis carinii* and penicillin for pneumococcal infections), replacement immunoglobulin for defects in antibody function, replacement of missing factors such as adenosine deaminase and bone marrow transplanta-tion for severe immunodeficiency. With the discovery that most of these disorders have a genetic defect they have become prime targets for gene therapy.

Self-assessment: questions

Multiple choice questions

1. Methods used to look for DNA that has been rearranged include:
   a. In situ hybridisation
   b. Southern blotting
   c. Polymerase chain reaction
   d. Northern blotting
   e. Fingerprinting

2. With regard to diseases of autosomal recessive inheritance:
   a. A child of two heterozygotes has a 25% chance of being homozygous for the condition
   b. The frequency of the carrier state will be many times higher than those with disease
   c. It is the commonest form of inherited disease
   d. Most homozygotes will have affected children
   e. It is the result of a single gene mutation

3. The following diseases and their Mendelian inheritance are correctly matched:
   a. Glucose 6-phosphate dehydrogenase deficiency and X-linked recessive
   b. Cystic fibrosis and autosomal recessive
   c. Hereditary spherocytosis and autosomal dominant
   d. Vitamin D-resistant rickets and X-linked dominant
   e. Beta-thalassaemia and autosomal codominance

4. The following describe chromosomal anomalies:
   a. 90% of karyotypically abnormal conceptions do not survive pregnancy
   b. They occur in 50% of cases of primary amenorrhoea
   c. They are associated with 20% of cases with mental retardation
   d. They account for 10% of male sterility
   e. They are seen in approximately 10% of human conceptions

5. Syndactyly is seen in:
   a. Apert syndrome
   b. Carpenter syndrome
   c. Laurence–Moon–Biedl syndrome
   d. Fanconi anaemia
   e. Trisomy 13

6. Chromosomal breakage can be seen in children with:
   a. Congenital telangiectatic erythema and dwarfism
   b. Constitutional aplastic anaemia
   c. Louis–Bar syndrome
   d. Xeroderma pigmentosum
   e. Chickenpox

7. Maternal serum α-fetoprotein may be altered when the fetus has:
   a. Trisomy 21
   b. Anencephaly
   c. Myelomeningocoele
   d. Died
   e. Congenital nephrotic syndrome

8. Teratogenic drugs include:
   a. Diethylstilboestrol
   b. Thalidomide
   c. Warfarin
   d. Lysergic acid diethylamide
   e. Cocaine

9. Metabolic acidosis is feature of:
   a. Phenylketonuria
   b. Maple syrup urine disease
   c. Insulin-dependent diabetes mellitus (IDDM)
   d. Isovaleric acidaemia
   e. Galactosaemia

10. A cherry-red spot can be seen in the macula in:
    a. Tay–Sachs disease
    b. Laurence–Moon–Biedl syndrome
    c. I-cell disease
    d. Niemann–Pick disease
    e. Central retinal artery occlusion

11. Hepatosplenomegaly is seen in:
    a. Tay–Sachs disease
    b. Niemann–Pick disease
    c. I-cell disease
    d. Laurence–Moon–Biedl syndrome
    e. Hurler syndrome

12. Ectopia lentis is seen in:
    a. Marfan syndrome
    b. Homocystinuria
    c. Sulphite oxidase deficiency
    d. Ehlers–Danlos syndrome
    e. Congenital rubella syndrome

13. Hepatic failure may be seen in the following:
    a. Wilson's disease
    b. Gaucher's disease
    c. Tyrosinaemia
    d. Galactosaemia
    e. Von Gierke disease

14. Hypoglycaemia can occur in:
    a. Glucose 6-phosphate dehydrogenase deficiency
    b. Galactosaemia
    c. Tyrosinosis

    d. Maple syrup urine disease
    e. Salicylate poisoning

15. Secondary hyperlipidaemia is often seen in:
    a. Nephrotic syndrome
    b. Von Gierke disease
    c. Diabetes mellitus
    d. Hypothyroidism
    e. Use of oral contraceptives

16. Cardiomyopathy is seen in:
    a. Pompe disease
    b. Primary carnitine deficiency
    c. Kwashiorkor
    d. Hunter syndrome
    e. Friedreich ataxia

17. Mental retardation is a feature of the following mucopolysaccharidoses:
    a. Hunter
    b. Hurler
    c. Scheie
    d. Maroteaux–Lamy
    e. Morquio

18. An altered colour of fresh urine can be expected in:
    a. Porphyria
    b. Indicanuria
    c. Antituberculous therapy
    d. Alkaptonuria
    e. Congenital biliary atresia

Case history

A young Asian couple come to ask you for advice. They have been married for 3 years and have an 18-month-old son who was investigated for anaemia and has just been diagnosed to have β thalassaemia. They have been planning to have another child but are now worried that the second child can also be affected.

Outline the steps you would take to help them with their dilemma.

Short notes

Write short notes on:

1. The investigations required in a child with a suspected immunodeficiency
2. Gene therapy.

Self-assessment: answers

Multiple choice answers

1. a. **True**. For example fluorescent in situ hybridisation is often used to detect known chromosomal rearrangements.
    b. **True**. The method used to detect a change in or differences between DNA samples.
    c. **True**. This is a highly specific technique that allows even point mutations to be detected.
    d. **False**. A method for RNA analysis.
    e. **True**. This is a restriction fragment length polymorphism (RFLP) technique and an example of its use is in the establishment of paternity/maternity.

2. a. **True**. As there is a 1:4 chance that the offspring will inherit both affected alleles.
    b. **True**. As those who have only one affected allele are phenotypically normal.
    c. **False**. Multifactorial inheritance is the most common.
    d. **False**. Not unless the other partner is heterozygous, but all children will be carriers.
    e. **True**.

3. a. **True**. It is, therefore, more likely to cause haemolytic anaemia in boys.
    b. **True**. This is the commonest inherited condition in the Caucasian population.
    c. **True**. Therefore there is no carrier state!
    d. **True**. It is a rare condition.
    e. **True**. This is because even those with one abnormal allele may show a phenotypic change; the number of alleles involved influences the severity of the clinical condition.

4. a. **True**. These are considered to be 'blighted' ova.
    b. **True**. Usually 45XO involved.
    c. **True**. This includes Down and Turner syndromes.
    d. **True**. This includes Klinefelter syndrome.
    e. **True**.

5. a. **True**. Syndactyly is fusion of the digits and is most often seen as an isolated anomaly; Apert is an example of an autosomal dominant condition characterised by craniosynostosis and syndactyly.
    b. **True**. Acrocephaly with polysyndactyly occurs in this autosomal recessive syndrome.
    c. **True**. It occurs with obesity, mental retardation, retinal dystrophy, hypogonadism and polysyndactyly.
    d. **True**. Though they usually have radial hypoplasia with hyperpigmentation and marrow failure.
    e. **True**. Polydactyly is more common.

6. a. **True**. This is Bloom syndrome (short stature, malar hypoplasia, telangiectatic erythema of the face).
    b. **True**. This is Fanconi anaemia (radial hypoplasia, hyperpigmentation, pancytopenia).
    c. **True**. This is ataxia telangiectasia (ataxia, telangiectasia, lymphopenia, immune deficit).
    d. **True**. Increased sensitivity to sunlight occurs, atrophic and pigmentary skin changes, actinic skin tumours.
    e. **True**.

7. a. **True**. Lowered.
    b. **True**. Raised.
    c. **True**. Raised.
    d. **True**. Raised.
    e. **True**. Raised.

8. a. **True**. It causes carcinoma and adenosis of the vagina.
    b. **True**. It causes phocomelia.
    c. **True**. It causes abnormal facies.
    d. **False**.
    e. **True**. It causes prematurity and addiction.

9. a. **False**. PKU involves mental retardation, hypopigmentation, skin rashes, seizures.
    b. **True**. Neonatal onset of hypertonicity, convulsions, hypoglycaemia.
    c. **True**. It occurs in diabetic ketoacidosis.
    d. **True**. Neonatal onset of vomiting, lethargy and convulsions.
    e. **True**. Neonatal onset of liver cell failure, hypoglycaemia and convulsions.

10. a. **True**. It is caused by deposition of GM2 ganglioside.
    b. **False**. Retinitis pigmentosa occurs.
    c. **True**. This is a mucolipidosis; the clinical picture resembles both the lipidoses and mucopolysaccharidoses.
    d. **True**. It is caused by deposition of sphingomyelin and cholesterol.
    e. **True**.

11. a. **False**. Though it is seen in other gangliosidoses.
    b. **True**. Other findings include neurological and mental deterioration.
    c. **True**. Sufferers also have coarse facial features, congenital dislocation of hips, gum hypertrophy and psychomotor retardation.

d. **False**. This syndrome includes retinal pigmentation, polydactyly and obesity.

e. **True**. Patients also have coarse facial features, clouding of the cornea and progressive neurological and mental deterioration.

12. a. **True**. Supratemporal displacement of the lens occurs together with arachnodactyly, joint hyperextensibility and aortic dilatation. Inheritance is autosomal dominant and the gene responsible is thought to be the fibrillin-1 gene (*FBN1*) at 15q21.

    b. **True**. Inferonasal displacement occurs.

    c. **True**. This is a defect of cysteine metabolism.

    d. **True**. It also causes hyperextensibility of joints and skin, poor wound healing. It has autosomal dominant inheritance with a wide variety of expression.

    e. **False**. Cataract formation occurs.

13. a. **True**. It is caused by copper deposition.

    b. **True**. This is rare in Gaucher disease and results from deposition of glucocerebroside.

    c. **True**. Intermediate metabolites of tyrosine are thought to be hepatotoxic.

    d. **True**. Galactose 1-phosphate, which is not metabolised, is hepatotoxic.

    e. **False**. Deposition of glycogen leads to hepatomegaly but not liver cell failure.

14. a. **False**. Glucose 6-phosphate deficiency (type I, glycogen disorder) is associated with hypoglycaemia.

    b. **True**. The inability to metabolise galactose leads to hypoglycaemia in babies who are dependent on milk.

    c. **True**. It occurs in addition to hepatic failure.

    d. **True**. However, correcting the hypoglycaemia alone does not improve the clinical condition.

    e. **True**. Usually occurs in the later stages along with dehydration, hypokalaemia and metabolic acidosis (which overrides the respiratory alkalosis).

15. a. **True**. Hypoproteinaemia also occurs.

    b. **True**. It may present as xanthomas.

    c. **True**. Hyperinsulinaemic states lead to lipogenesis.

    d. **True**.

    e. **True**. Ingestion of oestrogen-containing pills increases the production of very-low-density lipoproteins.

16. a. **True**. This is a lysosomal storage disorder.

    b. **True**. This is a lipid myopathy.

    c. **False**. Fatty infiltration of the liver occurs.

    d. **False**. Hurler syndrome includes cardiomyopathy (Hunter syndrome does not).

    e. **True**. Ataxia, degeneration of the posterior columns and late-onset cardiomyopathy occur.

17. a. **True**.

    b. **True**.

    c. **False**.

    d. **False**.

    e. **False**.

18. a. **True**. Burgundy red urine caused by uroporphyrin; this is most common in congenital erythropoietic porphyria.

    b. **True**. This is blue diaper syndrome.

    c. **True**. Rifampicin alters urine colour (it turns pink).

    d. **False**. Urine turns black only on standing.

    e. **True**. Colour change is caused by the presence of conjugated bilirubin in the urine.

Case history answer

The main aim in genetic counselling is to provide parents with greater autonomy over decision-making and a choice in reproductive decisions. The first step in this direction is to confirm the diagnosis. In this case, the diagnosis of β thalassaemia at such an early age suggests that the child has thalassaemia major and will be transfusion dependent and have a shortened lifespan. This is an autosomal recessive or codominant condition and it is likely that both the parents are carriers. The history needs to determine to at least three generations whether there is a family history of anaemia requiring transfusion, and early deaths. The parents need to be screened to determine whether they are anaemic (as carriers can be in this condition) and if they have abnormal haemoglobins other than the thalassaemic β globin (such as HbE).

Once the carrier status is known, the next step is to explain to the parents what it means to have this disorder. Details of this disease are discussed in detail in Chapter 11. However, they include the fact that the child is producing an abnormal haemoglobin and has an increased breakdown of the red blood cells for which there is no current medical treatment available other than blood transfusion. The risks of frequent blood transfusions include iron overload and infections such as hepatitis. The child will require to be on a regular transfusion–chelation programme to allow normal growth, but in the end this will not be enough to provide a normal lifespan.

Explain the risk for the second child. Assuming that both parents are carriers, the risk estimation for the second child to be affected is 25%. Drawing the pedigree chart and explaining how the disease is transmitted is an essential part of counselling. Information should be presented in an unbiased way; for example, the impact of saying that the risk of recurrence is 1 in 4 is different from saying that the risk of no recurrence is 3 in 4. Both should be presented.

The final goal is to discuss the options. These include not having any more children, ignoring the risk, artificial insemination or ovum donation or antenatal diagnosis and termination of pregnancy of an affected fetus.

The counselling should be non-directive but should assist in the decision-making process. The counsellor should be aware of the psychological issues such as denial, grief and anger that are evoked by genetic illness and of the ethnic, social, religious and educational backgrounds of the family. A compassionate and patient approach is required and counselling should be carried out over several sessions with an adequate follow-up. The latter is essential particularly where there has been a termination of pregnancy. In the UK, most regional health authorities have at least one clinical genetics centre where genetic counselling is carried out as a special service. As antenatal diagnosis becomes established for more genetic disorders, it will be important to develop a more coordinated approach to the community, which includes education of the community and medical profession about genetic issues, the setting up of comprehensive screening programmes and the training of non-medical genetic counsellors.

Short notes answers

1. The investigations are outlined in Table 49.
2. Gene therapy is a novel form of drug delivery that enlists the synthetic machinery of the patient's cells to produce a therapeutic agent. The targets of gene therapy are either intracellular or extracellular. In the latter case, the cell releases the product of the new gene, which can act locally on neighbouring cells or enter the circulation for delivery to distant cells. A gene delivered to the cell itself can replace a defective or missing gene or provide a product that kills or inhibits the growth of cells. Most gene therapy to date has involved the use of viruses as carriers of the gene of interest. The carrier virus may be a retrovirus that lacks virtually all viral genes except those required for infecting mammalian cells. As vectors, retroviruses have two major limitations. First, they can harbour genes of only limited size, approximately 7 kb; although most therapeutic

genes of interest can be accommodated, some are too large. Second, retroviruses infect only dividing cells, whereas most tissues in adults consist primarily of non-dividing cells. For this reason, retroviruses are generally used for ex vivo gene delivery, i.e., the injection of cells that were genetically engineered by infection outside the body, rather than by in vivo infection with the retrovirus itself. Adenoviruses are the second most commonly used viral vector for gene delivery. These viruses have the same size constraints as retroviruses but they have certain advantages. Adenoviruses readily infect non-dividing cells and can be produced in large numbers, making infection of tissues in an adult more efficient. Moreover, these viruses remain extrachromosomal, thereby reducing the chance of disrupting the cellular genome. A limitation of adenoviruses is that if delivered in vivo they infect all tissues including the germline, and thus could affect subsequent generations. Another problem is that they are not as defective as retroviruses and could more readily yield infectious virus in the body. A third problem is that the current generation of adenoviral vectors is immunogenic, which reduces the length of time available for the expression of the gene and makes repeated administration of the vector impossible. There are also non-viral methods of gene delivery. Liposomes, or lipid vesicles, which combine readily with cell membranes, are being used to deliver genes, sometimes as aerosols. Liposomes are also being tested in conjunction with viruses to enhance localised delivery of genes. Direct injection of naked DNA plasmids is possible, but for unknown reasons this method appears to function primarily in heart and skeletal muscle. A disadvantage of this method is that relatively few cells take up the DNA (1–3%), and, therefore, only small amounts of the encoded protein are produced. As a result, the primary and most important current use of DNA plasmids as gene vectors is in vaccine development, since the small amount of protein

Table 49 Investigations in suspected immunodeficiency

Test	Measurements
Full blood count	Determine the white cell and differential count. Is there neutropenia or lymphopenia? Is there thrombocytopenia?
Lymphocyte subsets	Determines the number of T cells (and CD4/CD8 ratio), B cells, monocytes and natural killer cells
Immunoglobulins	Level of IgM, IgA, IgE and IgG (with subclasses) to determine whether there is deficiency of all or a single immunoglobulin class and to assess B cell function
Antibody screen	Another test of B cell function; antibodies to type A and B blood groups or childhood vaccines are the commonest used
Candida skin test	Intradermal candida antigen test; a positive reaction will rule out virtually all primary T cell deficiencies
T cell proliferation with mitogens	Functional test of cell-mediated immunity
Complement assay	Total haemolytic complement is a functional test for the complement system and, when suspected, individual complement components can also be looked for
Neutrophil function	Nitroblue tetrazolium (NBT): defective in chronic granulomatous disease (CGD) Chemotaxis: decreased in leucocyte adhesion defects Oxygen release: decreased in CGD, increased in neutrophil granule defects
Imaging	X-ray of the superior mediastinum to detect an absent thymus (DiGeorge syndrome), visceral ultrasonography (multiple pyogenic granulomas in CGD)

produced by the few cells that take up the plasmid can elicit a protective immune response. Yeast- or bacterial gene regulatory systems have been adapted for use in mammalian cells. These inducible systems appear advantageous because they affect the expression introduced but not resident genes. There is no toxicity and the gene-inducing agent can be administered orally. For example, it is possible to regulate the expression of a gene of interest, such as one encoding a hormone, by means of a hybrid of microbial and mammalian proteins and microbial DNA regulatory elements that respond to either the antibiotic tetracycline or the progesterone antagonist mifepristone (RU 486). In principle, these new

regulatory systems allow genes to be turned on and off, and the level of the therapeutic protein can be varied over time. The complex goal of regulating genes through the use of endogenous biological signals, such as glucose levels in the case of diabetes, is also being pursued but will take time to reach. A number of clinical trials of gene therapy have been completed or are under way. These include inherited disorders such as α_1-antitrypsin deficiency, chronic granulomatous disease (CGD), cystic fibrosis, Hunter syndrome, Fanconi anaemia, severe combined immune deficiency (SCID) and familial hypercholesterolaemia as well various malignancies.

Infectious diseases

Key points

You should have an understanding of:

- The way common infections of childhood present and their predisposing factors
- The varying host response to different infections
- The investigation of a child with suspected infections and interpretation of the results
- The management of common infections and their complications
- Passive and active immunisation.

10.1 Introduction

This chapter will deal with only the common systemic infections seen in children. Localised infections of organs such as the gastrointestinal tract, the urinary system and respiratory system are covered in their respective chapters.

10.2 Symptoms and assessment

Fever

The commonest symptom of an infection is fever. Usually, either an identifiable microbiological agent can be found or the fever subsides after a short time. Body temperature follows a circadian rhythm, being lowest in the morning and highest around 4–6 p.m. An alteration of this normal homeostatic mechanism can be brought about by numerous clinical causes other than an infection, for example, drugs, inflammatory disorders, tissue injury, malignancies and metabolic disorders. Regardless of the aetiology, the final pathway of most common causes of fever is the production of endogenous pyrogens that directly alter the hypothalamic temperature set-point by increasing local production of prostaglandin E_2 (PGE_2). As a result, heat is both generated (increased cell metabolism, muscle activity and involuntary shivering) and conserved (vasoconstriction). The neonate, lacking muscle mass, is able to generate heat by the oxidation of brown fat (**non-shivering thermogenesis**). The diurnal variation of temperature is usually preserved in patients with febrile illnesses.

Fever patterns may be:

- remittent: daily elevated temperature returning to a baseline but above normal
- intermittent: daily fever returning to normal
- hectic: intermittent or remittent with temperature excursion of more than 1.4°C
- sustained.

Other than in specific infections like malaria, the pattern of fever is of little diagnostic importance.

Fever can be controlled with paracetamol, aspirin and other non-steroid anti-inflammatory agents (NSAIDs) (e.g. ibuprofen). These are all inhibitors of hypothalamic cyclooxygenase and, therefore, inhibit PGE_2 synthesis. These drugs are equally effective but because of the association of aspirin with Reye syndrome in childhood, paracetamol (10–15 mg/kg every 4 hours) is the drug of choice.

The child with pyrexia of unknown origin

In most children with prolonged fever, the development of additional clinical manifestations over a relatively short period makes the infectious nature of the illness apparent. Therefore, pyrexia of unknown origin (PUO) is defined as persistence of documented fever in a child for more than 1-week duration with no apparent diagnosis 1 week after investigation has begun. There is an extensive list of causes of PUO in children but in general most are caused by infections, connective tissue disorders, atypical presentations of common disease, or malignancies.

History
The evaluation of a child with PUO should start with the history. The younger child is more likely to have genitourinary tract, respiratory or localised infection (e.g. osteomyelitis) or juvenile chronic arthritis. The adolescent is more likely to have tuberculosis, inflammatory bowel disease or an autoimmune process. Leading questions may provide vital clues:

- Has the child been to the zoo recently? – zoonosis
- Is there pica? – *Toxocara* and *Toxoplasma* spp. infection
- Are their dietary habits unusual? – brucellosis, tuberculosis, salmonellosis
- Have they travelled recently? – malaria
- Is the child on any medications (including eye drops)? – drug fever
- What is the genetic background? – nephrogenic diabetes, Riley–Day syndrome, anhidrotic ectodermal dysplasia.

Symptoms and signs
Symptoms and signs may provide a clue to the diagnosis (Table 50). Physical examination should include tapping over the sinuses and teeth and palpating the muscles and bones. For example, point tenderness over a bone may suggest occult osteomyelitis or malignant infiltration, and tenderness over the trapezius provides a clue to a subdiaphragmatic abscess.

Investigations
Laboratory investigations should include:

- a full blood count and examination of the blood film for parasites
- urine and blood cultures (repeated serially)
- chest X-ray
- tuberculin skin testing.

Table 50 Symptoms and signs in pyrexia of unknown origin (PUO) of diagnostic importance

Symptom/sign	Possible cause
Absence of sweating	Nephrogenic diabetes insipidus, anhidrotic ectodermal dysplasia, atropine poisoning
Absent tears, absent corneal reflex	Riley–Day syndrome
Red weeping eyes	Connective tissue disorder
Palpebral conjunctivitis	Viral infections
Bulbar conjunctivitis	Kawasaki syndrome, leptospirosis
Petechial conjunctival haemorrhages	Endocarditis
Oral candidiasis	Immune deficiency
Repetitive chill and temperature spikes	Systemic onset juvenile chronic arthritis, septicaemia
Fever blisters	Pneumococcal, streptococcal infection
Congested pharynx	Viral infection, Kawasaki syndrome, leptospirosis
Absolute neutrophil count >10 × 10^9 cells/l	Bacterial infection

Dictated by the condition, other roentgenographic and ultrasonographic examination may be necessary as well as examination and culture of a bone marrow aspirate. Bone marrow cultures are often more sensitive for occult *Salmonella*, mycobacterium and fungal infections. Serologic evidence may aid diagnosis in some viral and bacterial infections as well as in juvenile chronic arthritis (JCA). Radioactive scans are helpful in localising osteomyelitis and abdominal abscesses and echocardiography in identifying endocarditis. On occasion, total body imaging with computed tomography (CT) or magnetic resonance imaging (MRI) and ultimately biopsy via laparoscopy or endoscopy may be required.

Sepsis and shock

In children, beyond the neonatal period, *Streptococcus pneumoniae*, *Haemophilus influenzae* type b, *Neisseria meningitidis*, *Salmonella* spp. and *Staphylococcus aureus* are the most common microorganisms causing bacteraemia. One potential consequence of bacteraemia is septic shock, a state characterised by inadequate tissue perfusion and frequently associated with endotoxaemia. Although this is more often seen with infections with Gram-negative organisms (*Pseudomonas aeruginosa* being a frequent culprit) it is also seen with Gram-positive (*Streptococcus pneumoniae*), viral and fungal pathogens. A **systemic inflammatory response syndrome** (SIRS) is thought to occur as a result of tissue damage following host response to endotoxin from Gram-negative bacteria and the lipoteichoic acid–peptidoglycan complex from Gram-positive bacteria. SIRS is recognised to be a cytokine-mediated process involving tumour necrosis factor (TNF), interleukin (IL) 1, 6 and 8, platelet-activating factors and interferon-γ. Alone or in combination, bacterial products and proinflammatory cytokines trigger physiological responses to stop microbial invasion. These responses include:

- activation of the complement system
- activation of coagulation factor XII
- adrenocorticotrophic hormone (ACTH) and β-endorphin release
- stimulation of the kallikrein–kinin system
- stimulation of neutrophils.

Table 51 Signs and symptoms of septic shock

	Signs/symptoms
Primary effects	Fever, shaking chills, hyperventilation, tachycardia, hypothermia, cutaneous lesions (petechiae, ecchymoses, ecthyma gangrenosum, diffuse erythema, cellulitis), mental obtundation
Secondary effects	Hypotension, cyanosis, symmetric peripheral gangrene (purpura fulminans), oliguria or anuria, jaundice, congestive cardiac failure, tissue hypoxia and lactic acidosis

These result in diffuse capillary leakage, reduced vascular tone and an imbalance between tissue perfusion and the increased metabolic requirements of the tissues.

The primary signs and symptoms of septic shock are listed in Table 51. As shown in Figure 61, ultimately irreversible organ failure may occur.

Children with septic shock need to be treated in an intensive-care unit where central venous and continuous intra-arterial monitoring are possible. Broad-spectrum synergistic bactericidal anti-microbials should be started while awaiting the results of cultures. Shock should be managed by infusing i.v. fluids, 20 ml/kg body weight of colloid, which can be repeated. If the blood pressure remains low, inotropic drugs such as dopamine and dobutamine may be used. Where there is bradycardia or a poorly contracting myocardium, adrenaline or isoprenaline may help. Sodium bicarbonate is only infused in severe acidosis (pH <7.1), and glucose and calcium supplements may be required. Oxygen and ventilation may be required. The routine use of corticosteroids has not been shown to be of benefit except in the treatment of adrenal haemorrhage (Waterhouse–Friderichsen syndrome). A poorer prognosis is seen in those who are initially refractory to resuscitative measures and those with multiorgan failure.

The immunocompromised child

A child with a defective immune system, whether caused by disease or therapy, is at risk of infection with the usual pathogens and with organisms that would not normally be able to cause infection and disease.

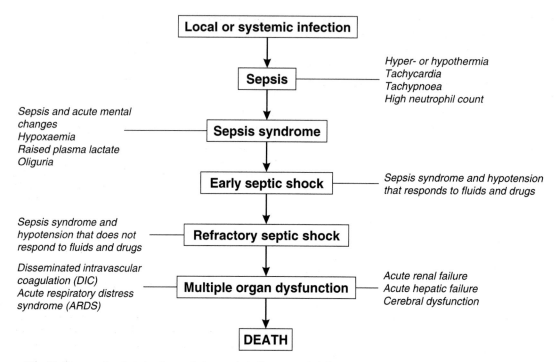

Fig. 61 Progression from bacteraemia to sepsis to the systemic inflammatory response syndrome (SIRS) and its complications.

Table 52 Common opportunistic infections associated with defective anatomic barriers

Defects in anatomic barriers	Common opportunistic organism
Dermal sinus tracts	*Staphylococcus epidermidis*, diphtheroids
Cerebrospinal fluid shunts	*Staphylococcus epidermidis* and *S. aureus*
Intravenous catheters	*Staphylococcus, Pseudomonas* and *Candida* spp.
Urinary catheters	*Pseudomonas, Serrati* and *Candida* spp.
Burns	*Pseudomonas, Serrati, Candida* and *Staphylococcus* spp.
General surgery	*Staphylococcus, Pseudomonas* spp.
Cardiac surgery	*Staphylococcus epidermidis*, diphtheroids and *Candida* sp.
Congenital cardiac defects	*Streptococcus viridans, Corynebacterium* and *Pseudomonas* spp.

Table 53 Opportunistic infections in immunodeficiency

Predisposing cause	Common organisms isolated
Chronic granulomatous disease	*Staphylococcus* spp., Gram-negative enteric organisms
Job syndrome (Hyper-IgE)	*Staphylococcus aureus*
Complement deficiencies	*Streptococcus pneumoniae, Streptococcus pyogenes, Neisseria meningitidis*
Splenic insufficiency	*Streptococcus pneumoniae, Salmonella* spp.
Sickle cell disease and other haemoglobinopathies	*Streptococcus pneumoniae, Salmonella* spp., *Haemophilus influenzae* type b
Humoral immunodeficiency	Bacterial pathogens, *Pseudomonas* spp.
Cellular immunodeficiency	*Mycobacterium, Listeria, Candida* spp., cytomegalovirus (CMV), varicella zoster (VZV), *Pneumocystis carinii*
Cystic fibrosis	*Staphylococcus, Pseudomonas* spp.
Diabetes mellitus	*Staphylococcus* spp., *Escherichia coli*
Nephrotic syndrome	*Streptococcus pneumoniae, Salmonella* spp.

Opportunistic infections are generally caused by organisms indigenous to the host or commonly found in the environment. The skin and mucous membranes represent important barriers to infections and any breaches in these protective layers can predispose to infections by opportunistic organisms (Table 52).

Table 53 shows some of the diseases in which a defect in immunity predisposes to certain kinds of infection.

Children with cancer or those undergoing transplantation are at a particularly high risk for three different reasons.

Indwelling catheters. Most of these children have an indwelling central venous catheter, which breaches the mechanical skin barrier. This increases the incidence of Gram-positive infections especially with skin-dwelling commensals such as *Staphylococcus aureus* and *S. epidermidis*.

Drug therapy. Many cytotoxics are highly immuno-suppressive and can predispose to fungal, viral and pro-tozoal (*Pneumocystis carinii*) infection.

Neutropenia. Most children receiving chemotherapy will go through periods when they are severely neu-tropenic. During these periods they are highly suscepti-ble to both Gram-negative and Gram-positive infections.

Prevention of infection

Prevention of infection in the immunocompromised child varies with the type and severity of the individual defect. Often simple measures like improving personal hygiene and the use of non-touch techniques when inserting internal devices and attending to their routine maintenance are far more effective than the use of anti-microbial agents. The use of prophylactic co-trimoxa-zole has been extremely successful in decreasing the incidence of *Pneumocystis carinii* infections in children being treated for acute lymphoblastic leukaemia. Similarly, prophylactic antibiotics used in children with valvular or septal heart defects prevent endocarditis. Routine prophylactic antibiotics have not proved to be useful, and indeed may be detrimental, in children with immunodeficiency, immunosuppression and severe neutropenia. Therapy with broad-spectrum antibiotics is started empirically in these children when an infec-tion is suspected. Often a combination of a third-genera-tion cephalosporin and an aminoglycoside is given until symptoms subside or an organism is isolated, when more specific therapy can be instituted.

10.3 Immunisation

Two hundred years ago, Edward Jenner was able to demonstrate that vaccination with material from cow-pox provided protection against smallpox. At that time smallpox caused 20% of all deaths in Glasgow and 90% of those who died were below the age of 5 years. In 1980, smallpox was eradicated worldwide. We are now poised to eradicate poliomyelitis and measles will hope-fully follow.

Many countries have an immunisation programme targeting children and intended to reduce the incidence of infectious diseases (Table 54).

Immunity can be induced either actively (long term) or provided by passive transfer (short term) against a variety of bacterial and viral agents.

Active immunity

Active immunity is induced by using inactivated or attenuated live organisms or their products. Live atten-uated vaccines include those for poliomyelitis (OPV), measles, mumps, rubella and Bacillus–Calmette–Guérin (BCG) vaccine. Pertussis, whole cell typhoid and inacti-vated poliomyelitis (IPV) vaccines contain inactivated organisms. Others such as influenza and pneumococcal

Table 54 The UK immunisation schedule (1997)

Age	Immunisation
2 months	DTP, OPV, Hib
3 months	DTP, OPV, Hib
4 months	DTP, OPV, Hib
12–15 months	MMR
3–5 years	Booster DT, OPV, MMR second dose
10–15 years	BCG (can be given in infancy)
13–18 years	Booster dT and polio

DTP, diphtheria/tetanus/pertussis; OPV, oral polio vaccine; Hib, *Haemophilus influenzae* type b; MMR, measles/mumps/rubella; BCG, Bacillus–Calmette–Guérin (tuberculosis); dT, low-dose diphtheria and tetanus toxoids used to immunise adults.

vaccine contain immunising components of the organ-isms. Tetanus and diphtheria vaccines contain toxoid, which is toxin inactivated by treatment with formalde-hyde. A first injection of inactivated vaccine or toxoid in a subject without prior exposure to the antigen pro-duces a slow antibody or antitoxin response of predom-inantly IgM antibody, called the **primary response**. Depending on the potency of the product and time interval, further injections will lead to an accelerated response in which the antibody or antitoxin titre (IgG) rises to a higher level, called the **secondary response**. Following a full course, the antibody or antitoxin level remains high for months or years. Even if the level of detectable antibody falls, the immune mechanism has been sensitised and a further dose of vaccine reinforces immunity. Some inactivated vaccines contain adjuvants (substances that enhance the antibody response). Examples are aluminium phosphate and aluminium hydroxide, which are contained in adsorbed diphthe-ria/tetanus/pertussis vaccines and adsorbed diphthe-ria/tetanus vaccine.

Passive immunity

Passive immunity results from the injection of human immunoglobulin. The protection afforded is immediate but lasts only a few weeks. There are two types of immunoglobulin available. Human normal immunoglobulin (HNIG) derived from pooled plasma donors contains antibody to infectious agents currently prevalent in the general population. It is used, for exam-ple, to protect an immunosuppressed child against measles or individuals against hepatitis A. Specific immunoglobulins for tetanus, hepatitis B, rabies and varicella-zoster are obtained from the pooled blood of convalescent patients or those recently immunised with the relevant vaccine. Each specific immunoglobulin, therefore, contains antibody at a higher titre than that present in normal immunoglobulin.

Special risk groups

Some conditions increase the risk of complications from infectious diseases and children and adults with such conditions should be immunised as a matter of priority. These conditions include asthma, chronic lung disease, congenital heart diseases, Down syndrome, HIV infection, small-for-dates babies and those born prematurely. These children should be immunised according to the recommended schedule from 2 months of birth irrespective of the extent of prematurity.

Those children who, for a variety of reasons, have not been immunised or for whom the immunisation history is unknown should be immunised fully. For children under 10 years of age, this should be the full primary immunisation schedule. *Haemophilus influenzae* type b (Hib) is only given up to the age of 4 years: three doses for those under 1 year and one dose for those aged 1–4 years. Children over the age of 10 years should receive dT (low-dose diphtheria and tetanus toxoids).

Children with no spleen or functional hyposplenism are at an increased risk from the bacterial infections most commonly caused by encapsulated organisms. Such infection occurs most often in the first 2 years after splenectomy. The following vaccines are recommended in addition to the routine schedule: pneumococcal vaccine in those over 2 years of age; Hib vaccine irrespective of age; and influenza, meningococcal A and C vaccines. When possible, immunisation should be completed 2 weeks before splenectomy.

Children on haemodialysis or those who have a hepatitis B virus (HBV) carrier in the family should be immunised against HBV. In addition, HBV vaccination is now being adopted as part of the routine schedule by many countries. The age of vaccination with HBV will depend on the 'risk level' of the individual country; it is given in the first few years of life in those countries with an incidence of HBV carriage in over 3% of the population.

Indications and contraindications

The following are *not* contraindications to immunisation:

- family history of any adverse reaction following immunisation
- previous history of pertussis, measles, rubella or mumps infection
- prematurity: immunisation should not be postponed
- stable neurological conditions such as cerebral palsy and Down syndrome
- contact with infectious disease
- asthma, hay fever, snuffles, diarrhoea, upper respiratory infections, otitis media
- treatment with antibiotics or locally acting steroids (topical or inhaled)
- child's mother is pregnant or child is breast fed
- history of jaundice at birth
- under a certain weight
- over the age recommended in the immunisation schedule.

HIV-positive children with or without symptoms should receive MMR (measles, mumps, rubella), DTP (diphtheria, tetanus, pertussis), HBV and Hib. Injectable polio vaccine (IPV) may be used instead of oral vaccine

(OPV) for symptomatic patients. BCG should not be given as dissemination of the bacillus can occur in these children.

Immunisation should not be carried out in individuals who have a definite history of severe local or general reaction to a preceding dose. A general reaction includes fever of at least 39.5°C within 48 hours of vaccine, anaphylaxis, bronchospasm, laryngeal oedema, shock, prolonged unresponsiveness, prolonged inconsolable or high-pitched screaming for more than 4 hours, convulsions or encephalopathy occurring within 72 hours.

Children who are immunosuppressed through treatment for cancer or have undergone a bone marrow transplant should not be immunised until at least 6 months have elapsed after stopping treatment. Children who have received prednisolone 2 mg/kg daily for at least 1 week or 1 mg/kg daily for 1 month should not have live vaccines until at least 3 months after stopping the steroids.

Adverse effects of vaccines

Every now and then concern is raised about the so-called toxicities of vaccines. The truth is that they are among the safest 'drugs' known, but like all drugs have some possible side-effects.

DTP. Adverse effects include acute encephalopathy, shock and unusual shock-like state, and protracted inconsolable crying. There is little evidence to suggest that the whole cell pertussis vaccine causes permanent brain damage or death. However, acellular pertussis vaccines being developed seem to have fewer side-effects and their immunogenicity is currently being assessed. A combination Hib–DTP and Hib–DTP–IPV vaccine is now available.

OPV/IPV. OPV has been implicated in vaccine-induced paralysis. Since IPV is a killed vaccine, it does not have this disadvantage. IPV, however, has to be given as an injection and does not produce herd immunity, unlike OPV. IPV is available as a quadruple vaccine along with DTP.

MMR. While thrombocytopenia and anaphylaxis have been reported, this is one of the safest of the commonly used vaccines. Lately, there have been anecdotal reports linking the combined vaccine with infantile autism and inflammatory bowel disease. However, a scientific committee has examined the evidence and has stated that there is no evidence to suggest that MMR is implicated in the aetiology of these disorders.

10.4 Bacterial infections

Staphylococcal infections

Staphylococcus aureus is ubiquitous. Most neonates are colonised within the first week of life and 20–30% of adults carry *S. aureus* in the anterior nares. It is the commonest cause of pyogenic skin infections and may cause furuncles, osteomyelitis, septic arthritis, lower respiratory infections, septicaemia, pericarditis, endocarditis and deep-seated abscesses. The organism releases exotoxins that can cause tissue necrosis. Exfoliative toxins can result in bullous impetigo or the scalded skin syndrome (Ritter disease). Enterotoxins A and B are associated with diarrhoea and vomiting and may cause food poisoning. TSS-1 is associated with toxic shock syndrome (TSS), which is related to menstruation and focal staphylococcal infections. Enterotoxins A and B can also cause non-menstrual TSS.

Management

Staphylococcal infection is transmitted primarily by direct contact. Strict attention to hand-washing techniques is the most effective measure for preventing the spread of staphylococci from one individual to another. Antibiotic therapy alone is rarely effective in individuals with undrained abscesses or foreign bodies. Loculated collections need to be drained and foreign bodies such as cannulae and lines removed. Therapy should always be initiated with a penicillinase-resistant antibiotic, as over 90% of all staphylococci isolated are resistant to penicillin. In serious infections, parenteral therapy is employed along with an aminoglycoside. Sodium fusidate can also be used adjunctively in localised infections. The glycopeptide antibiotics vancomycin and teicoplanin are used where the organism is resistant to semi-synthetic penicillins (methicillin-resistant *S. aureus* (MRSA)). The coagulase-negative staphylococci *S. epidermidis* and *S. haemolyticus* are nosocomial pathogens and can cause infections in immunosuppressed patients or those with indwelling foreign devices such as catheters, shunts and valves. In most of these cases, glycopeptide antibiotics are required to eradicate the organism.

Streptococcal infections

Streptococci are Gram-positive cocci classified on their ability to haemolyse red blood cells. Complete, partial and non-haemolytic strains are classified as β, α and γ haemolytic strains. They are further classified according to the carbohydrate components of the cell wall into the A through H, and K through V type (Lancefield groups). The β haemolytic group A and B are major pathogens in children, affecting the skin, soft tissues, blood and respiratory tract (Table 55).

Clinically, it is difficult to distinguish streptococcal pharyngitis from that caused by other bacterial and viral pathogens. A mixture of staphylococcal and streptococcal infection often cause pyoderma. Similarly streptococcal septicaemia, meningitis, arthritis, etc. are diagnosed only on recovery of the organism from culture. While direct culture of infected tissue is the best way to confirm the diagnosis of streptococcal infection, serological tests may also be of value. The anti-streptolysin O (ASO) titre is more than 166 Todd units in 80% of children with untreated streptococcal pharyngitis within the first 3–6 weeks. In those with skin infections, ASO is not a good test but anti-deoxyribonuclease B (Anti-DNAase B) provides the best serological test and is detectable 6–8 weeks after the start of the infection. Rheumatic fever is a late complication of streptococcal pharyngitis; a raised ASO (>330 Todd units) is one of the criteria used to establish a diagnosis. Poststreptococcal glomerulonephritis occurs after streptococcal skin infections; elevated anti-DNAase B titres (>170 units) help to confirm the diagnosis.

Management

Therapy is directed at preventing suppurative and non-suppurative complications of the infection. In most cases, the organism is exquisitely sensitive to penicillin. At least 10 days of therapy is required with oral penicillin or a single dose of long-acting intramuscular penicillin. In those allergic to pencillin, cefadroxil, erythromycin or clindamycin may be used. Those with severe infections require high doses of intravenous penicillin given every 3–4 hours (400 000 U/kg over 24 hours). Prophylactic use of penicillin is effective in preventing further attacks in those with a history of rheumatic fever. Many of the non-typable streptococci

Table 55 Common streptococcal infections of childhood

Lancefield group	Species	Haemolysis	Site of colonisation	Common human diseases
A	*S. pyogenes*	β	Pharynx, skin, rectum	Pharyngitis, tonsillitis, erysipelas, impetigo, septicaemia, wound infections, cellulitis, meningitis, toxic shock-like syndrome, rheumatic fever, glomerulonephritis
B	*S. galactiae*	β	Pharynx, vagina	Puerperal sepsis, chorioamnionitis, neonatal sepsis, pneumonia, meningitis, osteomyelitis, endocarditis
C–H, K–O	Various	β, α	Mouth, pharynx, skin, vagina	Puerperal sepsis, endocarditis, wound infections, nosocomial or opportunistic brain abscess
Non-typable	*S. viridans*	α	Pharynx	Endocarditis
Non-typable	*S. mutans*	α	Pharynx	Endocarditis
Non-typable	*Enterococcus* (*faecalis, faecium*)	α, β, γ	Colon contents	Endocarditis, urinary tract, biliary tract and intestinal infections, peritonitis, bacteraemia

are only sensitive to the glycopeptide antibiotics (vancomycin, teicoplanin), though clinically significant strains of enterococci resistant to glycopeptide antibiotics are emerging.

Pneumococcal infections

Streptococcus pneumoniae is a Gram-positive, lancet-shaped, encapsulated diplococcus. It is a normal inhabitant of the upper respiratory tract but can also be an invasive pathogen. It is the most common cause of community-acquired bacterial pneumonia and otitis media and the second most common cause of meningitis. Its frequency and severity are increased in those with functional or anatomic asplenia (splenectomy, sickle cell disease, after total body irradiation) and humoral and complement deficiencies. The signs and symptoms are related to the site of infection. The severity of disease is related to the virulence and number of organisms causing the infection. Pneumococcal septicaemia may have a fulminant onset with a high mortality unless promptly treated. In such children a high white cell count (>30 × 10^9 cells/l) may be helpful in suspecting pneumococcal septicaemia.

Management

While penicillin remains the drug of choice, resistance to third-generation cephalosporins and treatment failures are being reported. A pneumococcal vaccine containing purified polysaccharide from 23 pneumococcal serotypes responsible for more than 85% of infections is available, though the clinical efficacy of the vaccine is controversial. Immunisation is currently recommended for those aged 2 years or older with functional or anatomic asplenia; chronic renal disease or nephrotic syndrome; cerebrospinal fluid leaks; chronic heart, lung or liver disease; diabetes mellitus; and those with immunodeficiencies or who are immunosuppressed, including those with HIV infection. Since the vaccine does not protect against all strains, these children will also require oral penicillin prophylaxis.

Haemophilus influenzae infections

H. influenzae is a normal commensal of the respiratory tract in 60–90% of healthy children. Disease is caused mainly by serotype b and invasive disease occurs primarily in those under the age of 2 years. Before the advent of an effective vaccine, *H. influenzae* was the leading cause of bacterial meningitis in children. Another potential life-threatening complication was epiglottitis, which presents with acute upper airway obstruction. This too has become a rare disease with the advent of the vaccine. The organism is also an important pathogen in soft tissue infections. It is responsible for 10% of cellulitis in young children and can present as orbital or preseptal cellulitis. Osteomyelitis, septic arthritis, pneumonia and peri-

carditis are other examples of invasive disease. Non-b serotypes are associated with acute otitis media, sinusitis and conjunctivitis.

Management

Currently the third-generation cephalosporins and the fluoroquinolones are the antibiotics of preference. Children with invasive *H. influenzae* infections carry the organism in their upper airway. They and all close contacts need chemoprophylaxis with rifampicin if there are unvaccinated children in this group younger than 48 months. The goal of chemoprophylaxis is to prevent a susceptible child from acquiring *H. influenzae* type b from contacts by eliminating the colonisation in all close contacts.

Meningococcal infections

At least 13 serotypes of meningococci have been identified, but groups A, B, C, W, and Y account for most meningococcal disease. Heterogeneous groups of meningococcal serotypes cause endemic disease while epidemics are caused by a single serotype. Individuals with primary or acquired complement deficiency have an increased risk of developing meningococcal disease. The spectrum of disease can vary widely from occult bacteraemia to septic shock and death. Acute meningococcaemia can present with pharyngitis, fever, myalgias, weakness and headache. With widespread haematogenous dissemination, the disease progresses rapidly to septic shock, characterised by hypotension, disseminated intravascular coagulation, acidosis, adrenal haemorrhage (Waterhouse–Friderichsen syndrome), renal failure, myocardial failure and coma. More often meningococcal disease manifests as acute meningitis. Less common manifestations include pneumonia, myocarditis, purulent pericarditis and septic arthritis. Uncommon manifestations include endocarditis, purulent pericarditis, pneumonia, osteomyelitis and septic arthritis. Chronic meningococcaemia is a rare disease manifested by fever, rash, arthralgias and headache.

Management

Penicillin is still the drug of choice, with ceftriaxone and cefotaxime as alternatives in those who are penicillin sensitive. Despite the use of appropriate antibiotics, the mortality rate for disseminated meningococcal disease remains around 10% and the majority of patients will require intensive management. Poor prognostic features include hypothermia, hypotension, purpura fulminans, seizures or shock at presentation, leukopenia and thrombocytopenia. Close contacts of patients are at risk and prophylaxis with rifampicin is indicated as soon as possible for household and other contacts as well for as the patient.

Pertussis

Bordetella pertussis is the sole cause of epidemic pertussis and the usual cause of sporadic disease, the other pathogens being *B. parapertussis* and *B. bronchiseptica*. In the unvaccinated population, pertussis is endemic, with superimposed epidemic cycles every 3–4 years after accumulation of a sizeable susceptible cohort. It is a highly contagious disease, with attack rates as high as 100% in susceptible individuals. However, with widespread use of pertussis vaccine there has been a dramatic decline in cases. The dramatic increase in the number of cases when immunisation was halted attests to the protective efficacy of the vaccine. Pertussis is a lengthy disease (it was known in ancient China as the 100-day cough), divided into **catarrhal**, **paroxysmal** and **convalescent** phases. After a non-distinctive period of low-grade fever, sneezing, rhinorrhoea and lacrimation, the paroxysmal stage sets in. Coughing begins first as a dry intermittent hacking cough and then progresses to the full-blown paroxysms. The rapid bursts of coughing preclude an adequate inspiration and often the child's face becomes suffused and cyanosed. The cycle is broken by a forced inspiratory gasp, often against a closed glottis producing the characteristic whoop. The last is often absent in those younger than 3 months of age. The episode may end with the expulsion of a thick plug of inspissated tracheal secretions and post-tussive emesis is common. Not 'all that whoops' is pertussis, however. A paroxysmal cough can also result from lower respiratory tract infections with adenovirus, chlamydia, mycoplasma and respiratory syncytial virus. Diagnosis can be difficult as isolation and identification of the organism is not always possible. Complications of pertussis infection include pneumonia (25%), seizures (4%), encephalopathy (1%), apnoea, physical sequelae of forceful coughing, and death (1%).

Management

Goals of therapy are to limit the paroxysms, provide supportive care and to maximise nutrition, rest and recovery without sequelae. Erythromycin is almost always prescribed for potential clinical benefit and to limit the spread of the organism.

Tuberculosis

Mycobacteria tuberculosis is spread from person to person by droplet infection and, rarely, by ingestion. Once inhaled, some bacilli remain at the site of entry and the rest are carried to the regional lymph nodes. The bacilli multiply at both sites and the **primary focus** along with the regional lymph nodes is described as the **primary complex**. As the organism multiplies, it can be disseminated via the bloodstream and lymphatic system. In about 4–8 weeks, the body defence mechanisms react and the primary complex heals and disappears or occasionally calcifies. Sometimes disease progresses either at

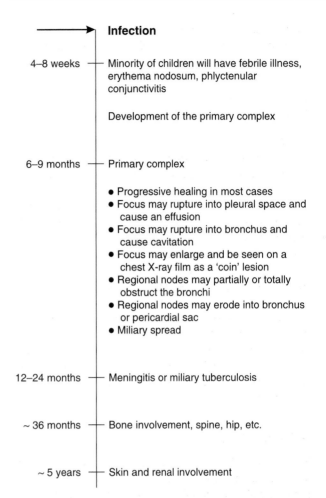

Fig. 62 Evolution of untreated primary tuberculosis in children.

Fig. 63 Radiological appearance of miliary mottling due to tuberculosis.

the site of the primary complex or at a more distant site such as the brain or spine. The greatest risk of dissemination occurs in the first year of infection. Particularly at risk are infants and the immunosuppressed as a result of malnutrition, infection with pertussis or measles or

Fig. 64 CT brain scan showing intracerebral tuberculoma.

because of immunosuppressive therapy. Figure 62 illustrates the natural history of untreated tuberculous infection in children along with some of the complications. The most serious complication is miliary or disseminated tuberculosis (Fig. 63), which involves the liver, spleen and often the brain; choroidal tubercules can even be seen on fundoscopy. Central nervous system disease is characterised by an insidious onset of basal meningitis, which often results in acute hydrocephalus and cranial nerve palsies. Tuberculomas (Fig. 64) present as space-occupying lesions and are typically seen as ring lesions on a CT scan. A diagnosis of tuberculosis is considered on the clinical features. In progressive pulmonary disease or pleural effusion a positive Mantoux tuberculin test (an induration of more than 10 mm 48 hours after an intradermal injection of 10 TU with Tween 80) is helpful. However, the Mantoux is often unhelpful when other organs are involved. Children do not cough up sputum but tend to swallow it, and culture and acid-fast staining of fasting gastric juice is more productive.

Management

The current recommended treatment for pulmonary infection is isoniazid and rifampicin for 6 months, adding pyrazinamide for the first 2 months. For miliary or meningitic disease, three drugs should be used for

---

BOX 33
Differential diagnosis of fever with a rash

Rubeola (measles)
Rubella
Echovirus
Coxsackievirus
Adenovirus
Infectious mononucleosis (Epstein–Barr virus)
Toxoplasmosis
Kawasaki disease
Serum sickness
Drug fever

---

the first 3 months and then isoniazid and rifampicin continued for 12–18 months. TB is a notifiable disease. It is essential to trace contacts of newly diagnosed patients and perform a tuberculin test and chest roentgenogram. BCG vaccination appears to be protective against miliary spread.

10.5 Viral infections

There are a number of illnesses that present with a rash, many of which are viral (Box 33).

Measles

In the unvaccinated population, measles is a common and highly contagious disease. It is characterised by an incubation period of about 10–12 days after which there is a prodromal illness with fever, conjunctivitis, coryza and cough. General lymphadenopathy may be found as well as tiny grey-white dots surrounded by erythema on the buccal mucosa and soft and hard palate (Koplik spots). After 3–4 days, the fever increases and a maculopapular erythematous rash spreads downwards from the head and neck to cover the whole body. The rash begins to fade by the third day and by the fifth day after the rash first appeared the affected child is no longer infective. The chief complications of measles are otitis media, pneumonia and encephalitis. A rare late complication occurring 4–10 years after an attack of measles is subacute sclerosing panencephalitis (SSPE). This is characterised by slow progressive dementia and deterioration. In developing countries, measles tends to occur in infants and younger children, with a high morbidity and mortality. Measles mortality rate directly correlates with the state of nutrition. An attack of measles in malnourished children results in a period of anergy, apathy and often diarrhoea. This may result in severe and often intractable states of malnourishment such as marasmus and kwashiorkor.

Management

Passive immunisation with measles-specific immunoglobulin is effective for the prevention and attenuation of infection in infants and immunocompromised children. In the USA and the UK, where measles immunisation is practically universal (>95%), the disease has been practically eradicated. The World Health Organization has included this in its Expanded Programme of Immunisation (EPI) and with sufficient coverage measles, like smallpox, can also be eradicated.

Rubella

Rubella is a mild illness and often passes unrecognised. The incubation period is 14 to 21 days and there may be no prodrome prior to the appearance of a pink maculopapular rash that generally lasts for 3 days.

Generalised lymphadenopathy, especially involving the suboccipital nodes, is a common finding. Virus is generally shed 5–7 days before the appearance of and after the disappearance of the rash. Complications are rare and include thrombocytopenia, encephalitis and arthritis. The importance of this infection lies in the devastating effect on the developing fetus during the first trimester (Chapter 2). The state of immunity to rubella should be determined in all pregnant women. If a pregnant woman, whose immune status is unknown, is exposed to a person with rubella infection, she should have an antibody test performed as an emergency measure. If she has been infected during the first 3 months of gestation and is not willing to undergo a therapeutic abortion, human immunoglobulin may provide some protection.

Mumps

With the advent of the MMR vaccine, mumps is now a rare disease. Painful enlargement of one or more parotid and occasionally submandibular glands usually follows a long incubation period (16–21 days). The swelling settles in 7–10 days. Aseptic meningitis is a common complication (60%), is often asymptomatic and usually follows a benign course. Rare complications include sensorineural deafness, and in older children epididymoorchitis and pancreatitis.

Chickenpox (varicella)

Primary infection with the varicella-zoster virus causes chickenpox. The reactivation of dormant viral infection in the dorsal root ganglia manifests as zoster. In chickenpox, the rash appears first on the trunk after an incubation period of 14–16 days and little prodrome. The spots appear in crops, progressing rapidly from macule to papule to vesicle and spread centripetally; they may appear in the mouth and mucous membranes. The pustules start drying by 48–72 hours after they first appear and the child is no longer infective once all the lesions have scabbed. The commonest complication of chickenpox is secondary bacterial infections with either *Staphylococcus aureus* or *Streptococcus pyogenes*. Meningoencephalitis and acute cerebellitis are well-recognised neurological complications. Pneumonia can be either primary or secondary to varicella infection and rarely the rash can be haemorrhagic, both conditions being associated with considerable morbidity. Progressive disease sometimes with hepatitis is seen in the immunocompromised.

Herpes zoster

Herpes zoster presents usually as a self-limiting vesicular rash in a dermatomal distribution with prodromal symptoms of localised pain, hyperaesthesia and pruritus. It can follow an indolent or recurrent course in the immunosuppressed.

Management

For those at risk, an attenuated live virus vaccine is available along with zoster immunoglobulin. Acyclovir, either orally or parenterally, is the drug of choice in those who have progressive disease or are immunocompromised.

Herpes simplex infections

Infection with herpes simplex is common and usually symptomatic in about 10% of those infected. Herpesvirus type 1 (HSV1) is spread by infected saliva and transmission requires close personal contact. Primary infection may affect the mouth, skin or eye. Herpes type 2 (HSV2) is a genital infection usually spread by sexual contact. Neonatal infections with HSV2 occur during birth from the mother's genital tract and with HSV1 during the post-partum period. Acute gingivostomatitis, keratoconjunctivitis and recurrent cold sores are common manifestations. Severe infections can occur in those with eczema (eczema herpeticum). The most feared complication is HSV1 encephalitis, which if untreated has a mortality rate of 70%. The drug of choice again is acyclovir.

Infectious mononucleosis

Glandular fever is the best-known clinical syndrome caused by Epstein–Barr virus (EBV). It is characterised by systemic somatic complaints consisting primarily of fever and sore throat. There is an exudative tonsillitis, the lymph nodes are enlarged and the spleen is often palpable. A macular rash is often seen particularly if ampicillin has been given. Complications are rare and include splenic rupture, airway obstruction, haemolytic anaemia, aplastic anaemia, myocarditis, interstitial pneumonia and neurological manifestations such as ataxia, peripheral neuropathy and Guillain–Barré and Reye syndromes.

Poliomyelitis

Poliovirus is an enterovirus transmitted by the faecoenteral route. The virus first multiplies in Peyer patches in the small intestine and then (about 10 days later) undergoes a viraemic phase. Most children are asymptomatic though some can have non-specific flu-like symptoms. Some children can have myalgia with meningeal signs but no paralysis. In those children in whom anterior horn cells are destroyed, flaccid paralysis ensues. Life-threatening paralysis of the respiratory muscles occurs in those with high spinal, bulbo-spinal and bulbar poliomyelitis. Recovery is slow and can take as long as 18 months. Any residual paralysis after that is likely to be permanent and affected muscles will undergo atrophy and fibrosis. Immunisation has eradicated the disease in many countries and it is hoped to achieve this worldwide by the year 2000.

Table 56 Clinical categories of paediatric HIV infection

Category	Symptoms
N	Asymptomatic
A	Mildly symptomatic; at least two of:
	Lymphadenopathy
	Hepatomegaly
	Splenomegaly
	Parotitis
	Rash, ear, nose and throat infections
B	Moderately symptomatic:
	Single episode of a severe bacterial infection
	Lymphocytic interstitial pneumonia
	Anaemia, neutropenia, thrombocytopenia
	Cardiomyopathy, nephropathy
	Hepatitis, diarrhoea
	Candidiasis, severe varicella-zoster or herpes simplex virus infection
C	Severely symptomatic (AIDS):
	Two serious bacterial infections
	Encephalopathy
	Wasting syndrome
	Opportunistic infections
	Disseminated mycobacterial disease
	Cancer (Kaposi's sarcoma, lymphoma)

Human immunodeficiency virus

Paediatric acquired immunodeficiency syndrome (AIDS) is caused by the HIV type 1 (HIV-1). Children are infected by vertical transmission, transfusion of contaminated blood products, intravenous drug usage or by sexual transmission. In the UK, almost all children with HIV-1 infection have acquired it from their mothers. Table 56 describes the clinical spectrum of HIV infection in children. The early diagnosis of infection in children born to HIV-positive mothers can be made with the detection of immune complex, dissociated p24 antigenaemia. However, confirmation that infection has not occurred requires a negative antibody test at 18 months, or two negative PCR tests or viral culture after 3 months of age.

Management

Zidovudine (AZT) given perinatally decreases vertical transmission. In infected children, antiretroviral treatment is usually only started once they become symptomatic or there is a rapid fall in the CD4 count. Combinations of AZT and didanosine or AZT and zalcitabine appear to be more effective than AZT alone. Triple therapy with the addition of a protease inhibitor is increasingly being used but there are insufficient data at present to recommend its routine use. Antiretroviral treatment should be monitored clinically and with measurements of the CD4 counts and the viral load as plasma HIV RNA.

10.6 Miscellaneous infections

Malaria

Malaria is endemic in many parts of the world. For prac-

tical purposes malaria may be regarded as two disease entities, the more dangerous being that caused by infection with *Plasmodium falciparum*. The other is caused by *P. vivax*, *P. ovale* or *P. malariae*. The severity of clinical features correlates with the degree of parasitaemia. Malaria is characterised by intermittent fever and a palpable spleen. Cerebral malaria is a life-threatening condition with mortality rates of around 20%.

Management

Along with supportive therapy, specific therapy is provided by chloroquine, and amodiaquine or quinine in those with drug-resistant infections. Chemoprophylaxis should be taken 1 week prior to travelling in an endemic area and continued for 4–6 weeks after returning. Appropriate physical precautions against bites are also an important measure.

Candidal infection

Thrush is a superficial mucosal infection with a *Candida* sp. that affects approximately 2–5% of newborns and is a causative agent of nappy dermatitis. Candidal vulvovaginitis will occur in as many as 75% of pubertal females.

Management

Most candidal infections are superficial and can be treated with topical anti-fungals such as nystatin, clotrimazole or miconazole. Disseminated infection can occur in the immunocompromised child and may require to be treated with fluconazole or amphotericin B.

Mycoplasma infection

Mycoplasma pneumoniae is the only known human

mycoplasmal pathogen. It is transmitted via droplet infection but is not a highly communicable disease. The peak incidence of infection occurs in the school age group (5–15 years). Bronchopneumonia characterised by severe symptoms and a paucity of clinical signs is typical of early disease. Roentgenographic findings are not classical though unilateral dense infiltrates are seen mostly in the lower lobe. Bullous myringitis and infections of the skin, CNS, heart, blood and joints are rare complications. Diagnosis is based on rising titres of cold haemagglutinins and is often associated with a mild haemolytic anaemia that is Coombs positive.

Management

In general, mycoplasmal infection is a mild illness and patients rarely require hospitalisation. Since the organism lacks a cell wall, it is resistant to penicillin and the macrolide antibiotics (i.e. erythromycin, clarithromycin) are the drugs of choice.

Chlamydial infection

Chlamydiae are obligate intracellular bacteria. The recognised human pathogens include *Chlamydia trachomatis*, *C. pneumoniae* (TWAR) and *C. psittaci*. *C. trachomatis* is the causative agent of trachoma and lymphogranuloma venereum (LGV). Trachoma is the most important cause of preventable blindness in the world and is endemic in middle and southeast Asia. *C. trachomatis* is also responsible for a wide range of sexually transmitted infections in adults. Maternal cervical chlamydial infections can result in conjunctivitis in the neonatal and pneumonia in early infantile age groups. The TWAR agent is a major respiratory pathogen in the school-age child. As with *Mycoplasma pneumoniae*, it is known to trigger asthma and exacerbate pulmonary symptoms in those with cystic fibrosis. *C. psittaci* is the aetiological agent in psittacosis. Therapy is by either a macrolide antibiotic or a tetracycline.

Kawasaki disease (mucocutaneous lymph node syndrome)

Kawasaki disease (KD) is an acute self-limiting multisystemic vasculitis of childhood of unknown cause. It is currently believed that an infectious trigger causes it and bacterial superantigens have been implicated. It affects children younger than 10 years, predominantly those younger than 3 years. The course of KD is divided into three clinical phases.

The acute phase is characterised by fever, conjuncti-

val injection, mouth and lip changes, swelling and erythema of the hands and feet, rash, lymphadenopathy, aseptic meningitis, diarrhoea and hepatic dysfunction.

The subacute phase is a period when fever, rash and lymphadenopathy resolve but irritability, anorexia and conjunctival injection persist. Periungual desquamation of the fingers and toes, arthritis and arthralgia, myocardial dysfunction and thrombocytosis occur during this phase, which typically lasts from approximately 10 to 24 days of the illness. Other associated features include aseptic meningitis, hydrops of the gallbladder, otitis media, uveitis and extreme irritability in infants.

The convalescent stage begins when clinical signs disappear and continues until the erythrocyte sedimentation rate returns to normal, usually after 6–8 weeks of onset.

Diagnosis

The diagnosis is made when four of the following five signs or symptoms are present with fever for at least 5 days:

- polymorphous rash
- conjunctival injection
- oral mucosal changes
- cervical lymphadenitis
- erythema, swelling or desquamation of the hands and feet.

No diagnostic test exists, and clinicians must carefully exclude diseases that mimic KD. The differential diagnosis for KD is indicated in Box 33. In addition to the above clinical findings, KD causes aneurysm formation in medium-sized arteries, particularly the coronary arteries. These lesions are found in 25% of patients; they may persist, scar with stenosis or resolve angiographically. Those who develop coronary thrombosis will require more aggressive treatment, including fibrinolytic therapy and angioplasty. Complications include myocardial infarction, which may occur during the acute illness or later, as a result of the coronary abnormalities.

Management

Treatment consists of administering high-dose aspirin and intravenous immunoglobulin during the acute phase (till day 14 of the illness) and low-dose aspirin in the convalescent phase, with the goal of relieving acute illness and minimising sequelae. Although most respond rapidly, almost 10% of children do not improve clinically with treatment.

Self-assessment: questions

Multiple choice questions

1. Isolation is recommended:
   a. Until all lesions are crusted in chickenpox
   b. Until 4th day of rash in measles
   c. Until 9 days after parotitis in mumps
   d. During the entire illness after respiratory syncytial virus infection
   e. Until 5 days of therapy is completed in pertussis

2. The following drugs are useful in the management of acute rheumatic fever:
   a. Phenoxymethylpenicillin (penicillin V)
   b. Benzylpenicillin (penicillin G)
   c. Prednisolone
   d. Ibuprofen
   e. Haloperidol

3. Rifampicin chemoprophylaxis is recommended for:
   a. Children with *Haemophilus influenzae* meningitis at discharge from hospital
   b. All household contacts of those with *H. influenzae* meningitis
   c. Close contacts of those with meningococcal meningitis
   d. Siblings of those with tuberculous meningitis
   e. Close contacts of those with lepromatous leprosy

4. Coagulase-negative staphylococci are:
   a. The commonest cause of nosocomial bacteraemia
   b. The commonest pathogen involved in shunt meningitis
   c. Capable of causing native valve endocarditis
   d. Implicated in spontaneous peritonitis
   e. Best treated with glycopeptide antibiotics

5. Clinical manifestations of gonococcal infection include:
   a. Purulent tonsillopharyngitis
   b. May be completely asymptomatic
   c. Ophthalmitis
   d. Pustular skin lesions
   e. Perihepatitis

6. Viral infections associated with latent infections of the CNS include:
   a. Herpes viruses
   b. Measles
   c. Rubella
   d. Mumps
   e. Influenza

7. Viruses capable of causing anterior horn cell disease include:
   a. Polioviruses
   b. Enterovirus
   c. Varicella
   d. Epstein–Barr virus
   e. Coxsackievirus A and B

8. In HIV infection in children:
   a. Presence of antibody to HIV at 12 months of age is diagnostic
   b. A major cause of death in children is *Pneumocystis carinii* infection
   c. Measles, mumps and rubella vaccine is contraindicated
   d. All infants of HIV-positive mothers will contract the infection
   e. Persistent thrombocytopenia may be the first clinical sign

9. Mosquito-borne illnesses include:
   a. Malaria
   b. Filaria
   c. Tularaemia
   d. Leishmaniasis
   e. Onchocerciasis

10. Parvovirus infections can cause:
    a. Aplastic anaemia
    b. Congenital deformities
    c. 'Slapped cheek' disease
    d. Fetal hydrops
    e. Prodromal high fever prior to the appearance of a rash

11. Primary pulmonary tuberculosis is often characterised by:
    a. A positive Mantoux test
    b. Pleural effusion
    c. Non-specific symptoms
    d. Paroxysmal productive cough
    e. Erythema nodosum

12. The following are examples of inactivated vaccines:
    a. BCG
    b. Yellow fever
    c. Pertussis
    d. Rabies
    e. Oral typhoid vaccine

13. Drugs used in chemoprophylaxis are:
    a. Rifampicin
    b. Chloroquine
    c. Diphenoxylate
    d. Erythromycin
    e. Co-trimoxazole

14. The following are often associated with human herpes virus 6 infections:
    a. Roseola infantum
    b. Febrile seizures
    c. Neutropenia
    d. Gingivostomatitis
    e. Rapid resolution of symptoms with acyclovir

15. The following agents are common causes of exudative tonsillopharyngitis:
    a. Coxsackievirus
    b. Epstein–Barr virus
    c. Beta-haemolytic streptococci
    d. Adenovirus
    e. Corynebacterium

16. Vesicular skin lesions are seen in the following infections:
    a. Varicella
    b. *Pseudomonas aeruginosa*
    c. Human herpesvirus 6
    d. Staphylococcal
    e. Coxsackievirus

17. The following infections are correctly matched with the drug of choice:
    a. Tuberculosis and gentamicin
    b. Mycoplasmal pneumonia and tetracycline
    c. Scabies and miconazole
    d. Pediculosis and malathion
    e. Methicillin-resistant staphylococci and vancomycin

18. Of the commonly seen fungal infections in childhood:
    a. Ringworm is best treated with griseofulvin
    b. Candidal vulvovaginitis is a very common infection
    c. Pulmonary aspergillosis is a problem of the immunosuppressed
    d. HIV infection is the most common predisposing factor for disseminated cryptococcosis
    e. Candidal paronychia is best treated with topical therapy

Case histories

Case history 1

A 3-year-old child is brought to you with a history of fever and a rash that has appeared on her face.

How would you approach the problem?

Case history 2

For the presentations listed below of children with fever, select the most likely cause from the following:

coxsackievirus
streptococci
staphylococci
Pneumococcus sp.
pertussis
Chlamydia
Mycobacteria
herpes simplex virus
Kawasaki disease
Pseudomonas sp.
malaria
Haemophilus influenzae
adenovirus
Epstein–Barr virus.

1. A 5-year-old child presents with fever and an abscess on the sole of his left foot. A thorn penetrated it 7 days ago while out in the garden and since then the foot has become swollen and tender and today the puncture site has been discharging bluish-green pus.
2. A 12-year-old has a 2-week history of fatigue, fever and sore throat. On examination she has cervical lymphadenopathy and splenomegaly. The white cell count is $5 \times 10^9/l$ with many atypical mononuclear cells and the serum aspartate aminotransferase (AST) is 200 U/l.
3. A 3-year-old presents with an acute onset of fever and dysuria. On examination of his urine there is macroscopic haematuria. There is antecedent history of an upper respiratory tract infection 1 week previously. He is otherwise well and normotensive. The full blood count is normal; urine culture is sterile and ASO (anti-streptolysin 'O') and DNAase B titres are not elevated.
4. A 4-year-old presents with fever, puffy eyes and oliguria of 4 days duration. Urine analysis is normal and the chest X-ray shows an enlarged heart.

Short notes

Write short notes on:

1. The presentation and management of a child with scarlet fever
2. How to investigate a child with pyrexia of unknown origin (PUO).

Self-assessment: answers

Multiple choice answers

1. a. **True.** Moist lesions contain active virus.
   b. **True.** Infectivity is from the onset of the prodromal period until the 4th day of the onset of rash.
   c. **True.** Mumps is transmissible from several days before and after the classical swelling(s) appear.
   d. **True.** The most important preventive measure to prevent nosocomial infection is isolation of affected hospitalised children and infants.
   e. **True.** Antibiotics shorten the infectivity period but not the duration of illness.

2. a. **True.** It is used for chemoprophylaxis in those who have suffered an attack of rheumatic fever. It is preferably given life long.
   b. **True.** For those in whom there is a doubt about compliance with oral therapy.
   c. **True.** When there is active carditis, its use may decrease the degree of endocardial damage.
   d. **False.** Relief of pain and inflammation is best done with salicylates.
   e. **True.** This is the drug of choice in those who develop rheumatic chorea.

3. a. **True.** Nasopharyngeal colonisation may not be successfully eradicated otherwise.
   b. **True.** Unvaccinated children under the age of 4 years have a high risk of developing invasive disease.
   c. **True.** In epidemics, the secondary attack rate in household contacts may be as high as 5%.
   d. **False.** Meningitis is not an open infection and is not infectious; however, siblings and other contacts should be screened for tuberculosis (Mantoux and chest X-ray).
   e. **False.** Chemoprophylaxis in close contacts of leprosy has not been shown to be of any benefit.

4. a. **True.** This results from increased usage of percutaneous intravenous devices.
   b. **True.** Signs and symptoms may not be overt and diagnosis delayed.
   c. **True.** Though infection of a prosthetic valve is more common.
   d. **False.** This is associated with *Pneumococcus* spp.
   e. **True.** For example, vancomycin, teicoplanin.

5. a. **False.** Pharyngeal infections are generally asymptomatic.
   b. **True.** About 10% of teenagers with gonococcal vaginitis and most pregnant women are asymptomatic.
   c. **True.** Especially occurs in the unprotected neonate.

   d. **True.** This is seen in the newborn.
   e. **True.** Also known as the Fitz–Hugh–Curtis syndrome.

6. a. **True.** Latent activation of the varicella zoster virus in the geniculate ganglion produces facial palsy, loss of taste, tinnitus, vertigo and hearing loss (Ramsay–Hunt syndrome).
   b. **True.** Subacute sclerosing panencephalitis can occur.
   c. **True.** Progressive rubella panencephalitis can occur.
   d. **False.** It is a cause of acute CNS infections.
   e. **False.**

7. a. **True.** Poliovirus directly affects the anterior horn cells.
   b. **True.** It causes a non-polio paralytic illness.
   c. **False.** Though varicella infection is associated with a cerebellitis.
   d. **False.** This is not a neurotropic virus; it targets B lymphocytes.
   e. **True.** These are enteroviruses like poliovirus and can cause non-polio paralytic illness.

8. a. **False.** Antibody is seen only after 15 months of age.
   b. **True.** It causes a fatal pneumonia.
   c. **False.** Live viral vaccines can be safely given.
   d. **False.** Usually only 20–35% will become infected.
   e. **True.** Isolated anaemia or neutropenia may also occur.

9. a. **True.** Bites from previously infected female anopheline mosquitoes.
   b. **True.** Both anopheline and culicine mosquitoes can infect according to the geographic locales.
   c. **True.** Though it can be transmitted by other vectors as well.
   d. **False.** The vector is a sandfly.
   e. **False.** The vector is a blackfly.

10. a. **True.** It occurs particularly in those with chronic haemolytic anaemias.
    b. **True.** Infection in pregnancy more commonly may result in fetal hydrops, death and miscarriage.
    c. **True.** This is the first stage of the disease.
    d. **True.**
    e. **False.** This seen in exanthem subitum caused by human herpesvirus 6; fever is unusual in parvovirus infections in children.

11. a. **True.** It is usually positive 4–8 weeks after infection.

b. **True**. This follows rupture of a subpleural focus into the pleural cavity.

c. **True**. Symptoms such as fever, malaise and anorexia are often seen.

d. **False**. A productive cough is unusual in primary tuberculosis.

e. **True**. Usually occurs in the first 4–8 weeks of infection.

12. a. **False**. A live attenuated vaccine.

b. **False**. A live attenuated vaccine.

c. **True**. Whole-cell killed vaccines are now being replaced by acellular vaccines in some countries.

d. **True**. Human diploid cell vaccine.

e. **False**. A live attenuated vaccine.

13. a. **True**. It is used for close contacts of those with *H. influenzae* and meningococcal meningitis.

b. **True**. It is used for those travelling to regions with endemic malaria.

c. **False**. This is an anti-diarrhoeal agent.

d. **True**. It is used in non-immunised infants who have been exposed to pertussis.

e. **True**. It is used to prevent *Pneumocystis carinii* infections in the immunocompromised host.

14. a. **True**. This is also known as exanthem subitum.

b. **True**. Febrile seizures can occurs in 15–35% of those with an acute febrile illness caused by HHV-6.

c. **True**. Often occurs with lymphocytosis.

d. **False**. Though it is commonly seen with herpes simplex virus infections.

e. **False**. HHV-6 is only partially sensitive to acyclovir.

15. a. **True**. It causes a condition called herpangina.

b. **True**. It occurs in the majority of infections related to EBV.

c. **True**. This is the commonest bacterial cause.

d. **True**. Acute febrile pharyngitis is the most common adenoviral infection of childhood.

e. **True**. Though the membranous pharyngitis caused by *C. diphtheriae* is better known.

16. a. **True**. The lesions are a hallmark of chickenpox.

b. **True**. It causes bluish fluid-filled vesicles called ecthyma gangrenosum.

c. **False**. HHV-6 causes a macular rash.

d. **True**. Bullous impetigo is fairly common.

e. **True**. The lesions are a component of the hand–foot–mouth syndrome.

17. a. **False**. While *M. tuberculosis* is sensitive to the aminoglycosides, the prolonged use of this group of drugs is not recommended and its use is restricted to organisms shown to be resistant to other drugs.

b. **False**. The use of tetracycline is restricted in

children and erythromycin is the drug of choice in this case.

c. **False**. Miconazole is a topical antifungal and topical malathion is recommended.

d. **True**.

e. **True**. An alternative is teicoplanin.

18. a. **False**. It is best treated with topical antifungals such as clotrimazole and miconazole. Griseofulvin is reserved only for highly refractory or ungual cutaneous mycoses.

b. **True**. It is seen in up to 75%.

c. **True**. It is especially a problem in those with chronic neutropenia receiving a mixture of antibiotics for a length of time.

d. **True**. Though otherwise normal individuals may develop meningitis or pneumonia.

e. **True**.

Case history answers

Case history 1

The diagnosis of an infectious exanthem is frequently considered to be an impossible task, but the truth is that most have common causes and a probing history and judicious physical examination are often all that is required.

General history. First, the child's immunisation history needs verification. In this example, immunisation with MMR should have been completed at this age. Is there a history of contact with infectious diseases within the last few weeks? Remember that incubation periods vary. Enquire whether the child received any antibiotics recently (ampicillin-induced rash in EBV infections?).

History of fever and rash. Which came first, the fever or the rash? Erythema infectiosum is characterised by a rash with no fever, whereas the rash only appears after the fever subsides with exanthem subitum (roseola infantum). What kind of rash is it? Vesicles often herald a varicella infection. What is the distribution? Varicella tends to occur first on the trunk and then spreads centripetally, while measles appears first in the face and nuchal region and then spreads downwards.

Clinical findings. What are the other signs? Is there lymphadenopathy (often seen in rubella); is there a characteristic enanthem (measles); is there tonsillopharyngitis (EBV, measles); is there splenomegaly (EBV, rubella and many viral illnesses)? How ill is the child? In most viral infections, the child will appear relatively well, but in meningococcal disease (where the rash spreads rapidly all over the body) the child is often shocked.

Exclude systemic, non-infectious disease. Also remember that a fever with rash is not always caused by an infection and can be caused by allergic reactions, collagen vascular disorders and certain drugs.

Case history 2

1. *Pseudomonas* sp. While staphylococcal and

Table 57 Investigative work up for PUO

Test	Diagnostic importance
Full blood count	
White cell count	Often elevated in bacterial infections
Platelets	Reduced with hypersplenism; raised with connective tissue disease
Blood smear	Malaria
Blood cultures (aerobic/anaerobic)	
Urine analysis/culture	Urinary tract infection
Tuberculin skin testing	Tuberculosis
X-ray examination	
Chest	
Sinuses, mastoid	
Bones	
Bone marrow examination	
Histology	Malignancies
Culture	Fungi, leishmaniasis, mycobacteria, salmonella
Serology	
Viral titres	Infectious mononucleosis, toxoplasmosis
Autoantibodies	Connective tissue disease
Radioactive scans	Gallium or technetium scans for osteomyelitis, deep-seated abscesses
CT or MRI imaging	
Invasive	
Biopsy	
Endoscopy	

streptococcal infections may also present in this fashion, *Pseudomonas* spp. are common garden commensals and are often found on decaying wood. They produce a green-blue pigment called pyocyanin that gives the pus its characteristic colour.

2. Epstein–Barr virus. While adenovirus and streptococcal infections may present with sore throat, the systemic features are atypical of these infections and the child is in the wrong age group for Kawasaki disease. The atypical large monocytes moreover are typical of the disease and give it the name of infectious mononucleosis.

3. Adenovirus. The most common infectious causes of haematuria are bacterial or viral cystitis and poststreptococcal glomerulonephritis. The last is associated with hypertension, raised streptococcal titres and painless haematuria. In the absence of a bacterial isolate, viral cystitis must be considered and adenovirus 11 is a common culprit.

4. Coxsackievirus. While this child is in the right age group for Kawasaki disease and clearly has congestive cardiac failure, the onset is too acute and no other features of the disease are present. This child probably has viral myocarditis, and coxsackievirus B1–4 are known to cause both myocarditis and pericarditis.

Short notes answers

1. Scarlet fever is caused by an erythrogenic toxic strain of group A, α haemolytic streptococci. After an incubation period of 2–4 days, the child develops tonsillitis, fever, headache and malaise. The rash develops within 12 hours of the onset and rapidly becomes generalised. It consists of a fine punctate erythema that blanches on pressure. The face is spared but the cheeks are flushed and the child is 'scarlet'. The tongue has a thick white coating through which the inflamed papillae project and a white strawberry tongue. By day 4–5 the tongue peels leaving a red strawberry appearance. The skin rash fades after that with desquamation. Treatment with penicillin leads to a rapid recovery but it must be given for 10 days to eradicate the organism.

2. Ordering a large number of tests in every child with PUO is a waste of time and money. Diagnostic tests most likely to provide a prompt and definitive diagnosis should be used. The pace of evaluation should match the seriousness of the illness. Tests may be required more quickly in a seriously ill patient, while in a chronically ill child evaluation may proceed more logically and in an ambulatory setting. A proper clinical history, which will need to be repeated as patients often remember important details on subsequent questioning, and regular thorough physical examination are the cornerstones of diagnosis of PUO. A list of possible investigations are given in Table 57.

Blood disorders and neoplasia

Key points

You should be familiar with:

- The differential diagnosis in a child with anaemia and be able to take a relevant history
- The differential diagnosis and management of persistent bleeding and be able to take a relevant history
- The common malignancies of childhood and appreciate their presenting symptoms and signs
- How to examine for pallor, icterus, lymph nodes and hepatosplenomegaly.

11.1 Development of the haematopoietic system

Developmental haematopoiesis occurs in three anatomic stages: mesoblastic, hepatic and myeloid. Mesoblastic haematopoiesis occurs in extraembryonic structures, principally in the yolk sac and begins in the third week of gestation. By about 6 weeks of gestation, the extraembryonic sites begin to ablate and hepatic haematopoiesis is initiated. By the 10th to 12th week, mesoblastic haematopoiesis ceases and a small amount of haematopoiesis is evident in the bone marrow. The liver remains the predominant organ until the last trimester of pregnancy.

The haemoglobin molecule is a tetramer made up of two polypeptide chains, each chain having an iron-containing haem group attached. The major haemoglobin (Hb) of the normal adult (HbA) is made up of one pair each of α and β polypeptide chains. HbA is, therefore, represented as $\alpha_2\beta_2$. The α and β chains differ in both the number and sequence of amino acids and their synthesis is directed by separate genes. As shown in Table 58 six different haemoglobins can be detected in the blood cells of the embryo, fetus, child and adult. Some HbA can be detected even in the earliest embryos and accordingly antenatal diagnosis of major β-chain haemoglobinopathies such as thalassaemia is possible. Table 59 shows normal haematological values.

11.2 Anaemias

Blood loss

Anaemia is defined as a reduction of the red blood cell (RBC) volume or haemoglobin below the normal range. Anaemias can be classified on the basis of the size of the red blood cells, which may be large (macrocytic), small (microcytic) or normal-sized (normocytic) (Box 34). The normocytic anaemias can be differentiated by the reticulocyte count (immature red cells, normally comprising 1% of total red cells) and the Coombs' test (which

Table 58 Haemoglobins present at different ages

Hb type	Chains	Age at which occurs
Embryonic haemoglobins		
Gower – 1	$\zeta_2\varepsilon_2$	Disappears by 3 months
Gower – 2	$\alpha_2\varepsilon_2$	Disappears by 3 months
Hb Portland	$\zeta_2\gamma_2$	
Foetal haemoglobin		
HbF	$\alpha_2\gamma_2$	Predominant haemoglobin at 8 weeks; 90% of haemoglobin at 6 months and 70% at birth. Less than 2% at 1 year of age and throughout life
Adult haemoglobins		
HbA	$\alpha_2\beta_2$	Detectable early in the fetus and forms 5–10% of haemoglobin at 6 months of gestation and 30% at birth
HbA_2	$\alpha_2\delta_2$	2–3% during adult life, 1:30 ratio of HbA_2:HbA

Table 59 Normal haematological values

	Haemoglobin (g/dl)	MCV (fl)	White cell ($\times 10^9$/l)	Platelets ($\times 10^9$/l)
Cord blood	13.7–20.1	110	9–30	150–450 at all ages
3 months	9.5–14.5	110	6–18	
6 months to				
6 years	10.5–14.0	70–74	6–15	
7–12 yrs	11.0–16.0	76–80	4.5–13.5	
Adult	12.0–18.0	80	5–10	

detects rhesus antibodies on the surface of red cells) (Fig. 65). A decrease in the circulating haemoglobin leads to a decrease in the oxygen-carrying capacity of the blood. Physiological adjustments to the anaemia include increased cardiac output and shunting of blood towards vital organs. The level of 2,3-diphosphoglycerol (2,3-DPG) increases in the red cell, with a resultant 'shift to the right' of the oxygen-dissociation curve and a more complete transfer of oxygen to the tissues. Pallor is manifest in the conjunctiva, mucous membranes and skin when the haemoglobin levels fall to 7–8 g/dl. With increasingly lower levels, weakness, tachypnoea, tachycardia, dyspnoea, cardiac dilatation and ultimately congestive heart failure ensue.

BOX 34
Causes of microcytic and macrocytic anaemias

Microcytic anaemia	Macrocytic anaemia
Iron deficiency	Folic acid deficiency
Thalassaemia syndromes	Vitamin B_{12} deficiency
Lead poisoning	Orotic aciduria
Chronic infections	Liver disease
Sideroblastic	Hypothyroidism
Pulmonary haemosiderosis	Drug-related damage

Anaemia with decreased red cell production

Normally, a drop in the haemoglobin level and the

Fig. 65 Causes and differentiation of the normocytic anaemias.

accompanying 'anoxia' stimulates the production of erythropoietin (Epo). Red cell production by the marrow in response to Epo may expand several fold to compensate for a mild-to-moderate reduction in the red cell lifespan (normally 120 days). In a variety of anaemias, the bone marrow loses its usual capacity for sustained production and expansion of the red blood cell mass. In these instances, there is a decrease in the number of erythrocyte precursors or reticulocytes in the blood. With elevated Epo levels, the absolute number of reticulocytes should rise. A normal or low absolute reticulocyte count in anaemia is indicative of ineffective erythropoiesis or relative bone marrow failure.

Physiological anaemia of infancy

The fetus lives in a relatively hypoxic environment and, therefore, has a higher haemoglobin and haematocrit than older children. From birth to 6–8 weeks, there is a progressive decline in haemoglobin levels, termed the physiological anaemia of infancy. Several factors are operative with the rise in oxygen saturation to 95%. Epo levels drop and it takes a while before renal receptors mature. The fetal RBC has a shorter lifespan (90 days) and the rapid increase in body size also adds to the need for an increase in the RBC production. When the haemoglobin level has fallen to 9–11 g/dl at 2–3 months of age in full-term infants, erythropoiesis resumes. Since iron stores are largely acquired by the fetus in the third trimester, the decline in haemoglobin in preterm infants may be more extreme and rapid. In the latter group, RBC transfusion may be necessary to provide adequate oxygenation. Oral iron will only be useful after 4–8 weeks as Epo is not active till then. In very-low-birth-weight infants, recombinant human Epo (r-HuEpo, epoietin) has been used successfully in conjunction with iron from birth to decrease transfusion requirements.

Iron-deficiency anaemia

Iron-deficiency anaemia is the most common haematological disease of infancy and childhood (Box 35). The newborn infant contains about 0.5 g of iron, whereas the adult content is estimated at about 5 g. Accordingly, to maintain a positive iron balance in childhood, about 1 mg iron must be absorbed each day.

As the high haemoglobin concentration of the newborn falls during the first 2–3 months of life, considerable iron is reclaimed and stored. These reclaimed stores are usually sufficient for blood formation in the first 6–9 months of life. In term infants, anaemia caused solely by inadequate dietary iron is unusual before 4–6 months but becomes common at 9–24 months of age. Thereafter it is relatively uncommon.

BOX 35 Causes of iron-deficiency anaemia	
	Causes
Deficient intake	
Increased demand	Low birth weight, prematurity, congenital heart disease
Increased loss	
Gut	Cow's milk related, Meckel diverticulum, gastro-oesophageal reflux, polyps with bleeding, hookworm infestation
Lung	Pulmonary haemosiderosis
Impaired absorption	Chronic diarrhoea, inflammatory bowel disease

The usual dietary pattern observed in infants with iron-deficiency anaemia is the consumption of large amounts of cow's milk and of foods not supplemented with iron.

Signs and symptoms
Chronic anaemia is remarkably well tolerated with very few symptoms and signs. As the child becomes progressively iron deficient and the haemoglobin drops to below 8.0 g/dl, symptoms such as pica and tiredness may be seen and pallor observed on examination. At haemoglobin levels less than 5 g/dl, the child may be irritable and anorexic and, in addition to pallor, examination may reveal tachycardia, signs of congestive cardiac failure, a flow murmur and koilonychia (spooning of the nails on the fingers and toes). A spleen is palpable in 10–15% of children with iron-deficiency anaemia.

Laboratory diagnosis
Haemoglobinisation of the RBCs is affected and the cell is misshapen (poikilocytosis), small (microcytosis) and pale (hypochromic). The decrease in iron leads to a decrease in serum ferritin and iron with an increase in the iron-binding capacity. This is diagnostic of iron-deficiency anaemia. The absolute reticulocyte count indicates an insufficient response to anaemia, though nucleated RBCs can be seen in the peripheral smear. The white cells are normal but thrombocytosis (600×10^9/l to 1000×10^9/l) or thrombocytopenia may be present. The bone marrow is hypercellular with erythroid hyperplasia. The erythroid precursors (normoblasts), however, have scanty fragmented cytoplasm with poor haemoglobinisation.

Treatment
Treatment is based on dietary regulation and iron supplementation. A decrease in consumption of milk decreases the loss of blood iron from the gut in those with intolerance to cow's milk protein and facilitates the intake and absorption of iron-rich foods. Iron supplementation must be in the ferrous form and the dose should provide 6 mg/kg elemental iron per day. Iron absorption is improved when taken between meals, though this may cause nausea. Parenteral iron (iron dextran) can be used in those intolerant to cow's milk protein but has no therapeutic advantage over oral iron.

The megaloblastic anaemias

The megaloblastic anaemias have in common certain abnormalities of RBC morphology and maturation. Both folic acid and vitamin B_{12} are cofactors required in the synthesis of nucleoproteins and their deficiencies result in defective synthesis of DNA and, to a lesser extent, RNA and protein. The arrest in development or premature death of cells in the marrow results in ineffective erythropoiesis. In the peripheral blood, RBCs are larger (increased mean corpuscular volume (MCV)) and

Table 60 Treatment of folic acid or vitamin B_{12} deficiency

	Normal μg/24 h	Treatment
Folic acid	100	50–100 μg daily for 2 weeks
Vitamin B_{12}	1–5	1 mg once
		1 mg for at least 2 weeks where there is neurological involvement

oval, hypersegmented neutrophils and giant platelets are also seen. In the marrow, macrocytosis is obvious and although the red cells appear to have sufficient haemoglobin they still retain an immature nucleus.

Folates are abundant in green vegetables, fruits and animal organs (e.g. liver, kidney) and are absorbed from the small intestine as pteroylmonoglutamates. Vitamin B_{12} is derived from cobalamins, mainly from animal sources or secondary to production by microorganisms. As vitamin B_{12} is present in many foods, dietary deficiency is rare. It is seen in cases of extreme dietary restrictions (strict vegetarian: 'vegans') where no animal products are consumed. Treatment of folic acid or vitamin B_{12} deficiency is described in Table 60.

Bone marrow failure

Congenital hypoplastic anaemia (Diamond–Blackfan syndrome)
Congenital hypoplastic anaemia is a rare condition presenting between 2 and 6 months of age. One-third of infants have congenital anomalies such as dysmorphic facies or defects of the upper extremities, including triphalangeal thumbs. The children present with macrocytic anaemia, reticulocytopenia and a deficiency or absence of RBC precursors in an otherwise normally cellular bone marrow. Bone marrow cultures show markedly reduced numbers of colony- and blast-forming erythrocytes (CFU-E and BFU-E).

Management. About 50% will respond to long-term corticosteroid therapy and 14% will undergo spontaneous remission. Others are transfusion dependent and death is ultimately related to transfusion-related haemosiderosis.

Transient erythroblastopenia of childhood
Transient erythroblastopenia of childhood (TEC) is a disease of unknown aetiology that occurs between 6 months and 3 years of age. Reticulocytes and erythroid precursors alone are decreased.

Management. Recovery is spontaneous within 1–2 months and treatment is RBC transfusions when anaemia is severe.

Aplastic anaemia
Aplastic anaemia is the failure of the bone marrow to produce all three components of blood, i.e. RBCs, granulocytes and platelets. The causes can be congenital or acquired (Box 36).

Idiopathic development occurs in 70%
Secondary development occurs in response to:
  Drugs: chemotherapeutic agents, chloramphenicol, sulphonamide, phenylbutazone, quinacrine
  Chemicals: DDT, parathione
  Toxins: carbon tetrachloride, toluene, glue
  Irradiation
  Infections: HIV, hepatitis, rubella, cytomegalovirus, parvovirus
  Premalignant conditions: preleukaemia
  Graft-versus-host disease

Congenital anaemias

Fanconi anaemia (FA) is characterised by the progressive onset of bone marrow failure in late childhood. Associated congenital anomalies include increased skin pigmentation, café-au-lait spots, short stature, microcephaly, microphthalmia, abnormalities of the ear, thumb, radius and long bones as well as renal and cardiac anomalies. In 25–50% of patients there is a normal phenotype. Chromosomal studies reveal increased breakages and structural abnormalities. Supportive treatment includes blood component therapy, steroids and androgens. Only allogeneic bone marrow transplantation is curative.

In cases of acquired aplastic anaemia, the aetiology may be a deficiency of pluripotent cells (type I) or suppression of the proliferating stem cells (type II). This suppression may be immune mediated.

The presenting features are usually a gradual onset of anaemia, with pallor, fatigability, weakness and anorexia, thrombocytopenia with petechiae, nose and gastrointestinal bleeding, and granulocytopenia, with an increased susceptibility to infections.

Examination of the bone marrow shows tri-lineage depression or absence of haematopoietic cell precursors. Poor prognostic features include:

- absolute neutrophil count of $<0.5 \times 10^9/1$
- platelet count of $<20 \times 10^9/1$
- <20% of haematopoietic cells in the marrow
- older age
- the presence of haemorrhagic manifestations
- infections.

Management. This is supportive, with blood products and the removal of the offending agent if known. Infections must be treated aggressively and often in an empirical fashion. Methylprednisolone, anti-lymphocyte globulin and cyclosporin A may be effective in those with an immune-mediated suppression of proliferating stem cells. In those refractory to therapy, allogeneic bone marrow transplantation is the only option.

Anaemias with red blood cell destruction

The haemolytic anaemias result from the increased destruction of RBCs. They can arise because of:

- membrane defects
- enzyme deficiencies
- abnormal haemoglobin.

Membrane defects

Membrane defects occur in spherocytosis, elliptocytosis, pyropoikilocytosis, stomatocytosis and paroxysmal nocturnal haemoglobinuria.

Hereditary spherocytosis

Hereditary spherocytosis is an autosomal dominant condition resulting in a defective red cell membrane. The RBC is unable to maintain its biconcave shape, becomes spherical and susceptible to mechanical stress while traversing the spleen and capillaries. The severity of haemolysis varies. Those with severe disease present in the neonatal period with **haemolytic disease of the newborn**. The majority suffer from intermittent jaundice with compensated haemolysis and no anaemia at other times. Most children will have mild-to-moderate splenomegaly. As with any other chronic haemolytic anaemia, a sudden exacerbation may occur through haemolysis or transient marrow aplasia. The latter is often the result of a parvovirus infection. Pigmentary gall stones occur mainly in adults and occasionally in children.

The diagnosis is suspected from the blood film, which shows anaemia and spherocytosis and is confirmed by a negative Coombs' test (Coombs'-positive autoimmune haemolytic anaemia may also show spherocytosis in the peripheral blood) and increased osmotic fragility.

Management. Transfusions should be given for hypoplastic crises and if the anaemia is not compensated. As the erythrocytes are destroyed in the spleen, splenectomy is the treatment of choice. It should be postponed till the child is 5 years old if possible, and pneumococcal vaccine is given prior to splenectomy. Post-splenectomy, penicillin prophylaxis and immunisation with Hib vaccine are continued life-long.

Enzyme deficiencies

Enzyme deficiencies causing RBC destruction include pyruvate kinase, glucose 6-phosphate dehydrogenase (G6PD) and related deficiencies.

Glucose 6-phosphate dehydrogenase

There are over 300 distinct enzyme varieties of G6PD deficiency, an X-linked condition. The commonest are G6PD B$^+$ and the G6PD A$^+$ present in the African-American population.

There are four distinct clinical syndromes based on the type of enzyme defect (Table 61):

- oxidative stress-induced haemolysis (caused by drugs, infection, other illnesses)
- favism (sensitivity to a chemical in beans)
- neonatal jaundice
- chronic congenital haemolytic anaemia.

Table 61 Clinical features of representative variants of glucose 6-phosphate dehydrogenase deficiency

	A⁻	Mediterranean	Canton	Chicago
Ethnic group	African	Greek	Chinese	N. America
Prevalence	Common	Common	Common	Rare
G6PD activity (%)	10–20	0.5	4–24	0.5
Drug- and infection-associated haemolysis	+	+	+	+
Favism	0	++	+	0
Neonatal jaundice	±	++	+++	++
Increased activity in RBC after haemolysis	+	±	+	+
Chronic haemolysis	0	+	0	++
Fall in haemoglobin with haemolysis (g/dl)	2–5	4–10	4–10	Chronically (<10)

The drugs implicated are mainly the sulphonamides and the antimalarials. Favism, as the name implies, is seen in certain individuals who experience haemolysis when exposed to fava (broad) beans (by either ingestion or inhaling the pollen). The diagnosis is established by estimating the G6PD level. This is done a few weeks after the acute haemolytic episode as enzyme levels may be high in young red cells and could result in spurious high levels if tested at the time of presentation.

Management. The prevention of haemolysis is the most important aspect in management. Individuals from high-risk groups should be screened and once identified should be educated to avoid precipitating agents.

Abnormal haemoglobin: the haemoglobinopathies

The sickle cell syndromes

Sickle haemoglobin (HbS) has glutamic acid in position 6 of the β chains instead of valine, a result of a point mutation. When deoxygenated this haemoglobin polymerises to rigid crystal-like rods that give the cell the characteristic sickle shape. This also provides the cell with resistance to parasitisation with *Mycobacterium falciparum* (in malaria) as any infected cell will promptly sickle.

This is an autosomal co-dominant condition. Clinical manifestation usually occurs in later infancy as HbS gradually replaces HbF. The clinical features are usually the result of arterial blockage by sickled cells, with resultant hypoxia and infarction of the affected tissue. Severe symptoms are associated with the homozygous state, sickle cell disease (HbSS) but are also seen with Hb S-β⁰ thalassaemia and HbSC disease.

Acute vasocclusive crises presenting with acute onset of pain are the commonest manifestation. The **hand–foot syndrome** presents as symmetrical swelling of hands and feet owing to ischaemic necrosis of small bones. The **acute chest syndrome** occurs as a result of pulmonary infarction or fat embolisation secondary to infarction elsewhere. Ten per cent of children will have cerebrovascular occlusion. Progressive renal damage is the norm, with diffuse glomerular and tubular fibrosis and occasionally papillary necrosis. **Hypersplenism**

and acute splenic sequestration are more common in infants and young children. In those with a concomitant G6PD deficiency, **haemolytic crises** may occur as well. In common with other congenital haemolytic disorders, life-threatening **aplastic crises** may result from parvovirus infection. Autoinfarction of the spleen occurs by late childhood and these children have increased susceptibility to infections with *Pneumococcus*, *Haemophilus* and *Salmonella* spp. In later life, indolent leg ulcers may pose problems.

The definite diagnosis, distinguishing sickle haemoglobin from the sickle cell variants is made by electrophoresis in an acidic pH and haemoglobin solubility. In high-risk families, antenatal diagnosis is possible.

Management. Almost all children with HbSS will have pain on a nearly daily basis. Paracetamol, anti-inflammatory agents, narcotics and, on occasion, epidural analgesia may be required. In those with a crisis, maintenance of hydration is essential. Blood transfusions are given only when necessary. In those with severe complications, chronic long-term transfusion regimens will avert crises but these children will also require iron chelation to prevent haemosiderosis. As there is functional hyposplenism, prompt treatment of suspected / proven infections is a must as is prophylaxis with penicillin and pneumococcal vaccination. Infarction of the bone also predisposes to osteomyelitis, with *Salmonella* organisms being the commonest pathogen.

The thalassaemia syndromes

Thalassaemia major is an autosomal co-dominant condition. Two sets of genes, located on chromosome 16, code for the α polypeptide chains. The genes for β, γ and δ chains are closely linked on chromosome 11. The underlying genetic defects include total or partial deletions of globin chain genes and nucleotide insertions, substitutions and deletions. A decrease, absence or functionally defective mRNA results and the haemoglobin polypeptide chain synthesis is decreased or suppressed. The abnormal haemoglobin precipitates in the red cell and the abnormal cell is destroyed in the marrow or spleen. Thus the anaemia is a result of inefficient erythropoiesis as well as increased destruction.

Table 62 The thalassaemias

Type of thalassemia	Globin gene expression	Anaemia	Clinical expression	Haemoglobin findings
Beta thalassaemia				
β^0 homozygous	β^0/β^0	Severe	Thalassaemia major	HbF >90%; no HbA
β^+ homozygous	$\beta+/\beta^+$	Moderately severe	Thalassaemia intermedia	HbF 60–80%; HbA 20–40%
β^0 heterozygous	β/β^0	Mild to moderate	Splenomegaly, icterus	Increased HbA$_2$, HbF
β^+ heterozygous	β/β^+	Mild to moderate	Normal	Increased HbA$_2$, HbF
β silent carrier	β/β^+	Normal	Normal	Normal
Alpha thalassaemia				
α silent carrier	$\alpha/\alpha\alpha$	Mild or normal	Normal	Normal
α trait	α/α or $/\alpha\alpha$	Mild or normal	Normal	Newborn: Hb Barts 5–10%
HbH disease	$/\alpha$	Moderate to severe	Thalassaemia intermedia	Hb Barts (γ^4), 20–30%
α hydrops	α^0	Severe	Hydrops	Hb Barts >90%

Homozygous β^0 thalassaemia presents in later infancy as HbF levels decline (Table 62). In the absence of regular blood transfusions, these children become anaemic and develop features of extramedullary haematopoiesis. Massive expansion of the marrow of the face (malar hyperplasia) and skull (frontal bossing) produce the 'chipmunk' facies. Pallor, haemosiderosis and jaundice produce a greenish-brown complexion. The liver and spleen enlarge. As there is a large erythrocyte turnover, with or without transfusion, haemosiderosis occurs, damaging the liver, kidneys, pancreas and heart. As in sickle cell anaemia, indolent leg ulcers may be a problem. Mild forms (Table 62) are often mistaken for iron-deficiency anaemia.

Management. Hypertransfusion protocols aimed at keeping the haemoglobin above 10 g/dl permit normal activity and prevent bone and marrow changes in thalassaemia major. Transfusions are usually necessary once every 4–5 weeks. Regular chelation with desferrioxamine is essential to prevent haemosiderosis. This is usually given as a continuous subcutaneous infusion at night. Splenectomy can be offered to older children with hypersplenism to help to decrease the transfusion requirement. Allogeneic bone marrow transplantation can be offered in severe cases.

11.3 The bleeding child

A series of biochemical and physiological events are initiated to stop the flow of blood when a blood vessel is injured (Fig. 66). The vascular component is involved in constricting the damaged vessel; the platelets plug the defect and the clot is formed and stabilised by plasma coagulation factors. Defects in any one of these components can lead to prolonged bleeding from minor injuries. The common causes are listed in Box 37.

The spontaneous onset of petechiae and bruising in an otherwise well child is a relatively common symptom of childhood.

Henoch–Schönlein purpura

In **Henoch–Schönlein purpura**, there is a characteristic

BOX 37
The common bleeding disorders

Vascular: Henoch-Schönlein purpura
Platelet
  Decreased number: Idiopathic thrombocytopenic purpura (ITP)
  Decreased function: Glanzmann thrombasthenia
Plasma
  Isolated factor defect: haemophilia
  Multiple factor defect: vitamin K deficiency
Multiple factors: disseminated intravascular coagulation

---

distribution of petechiae and bruises over the anterior aspect of the shins, extensor surfaces of the forearms and buttocks. Other symptoms include arthritis (75%), usually polyarticular involving the large joints; gastrointestinal (50%) with colicky abdominal pain, occult or frank haemorrhage and, rarely, intussusception; renal (25–50%) with haematuria, nephrotic syndrome and, rarely, chronic renal failure. The diagnosis is based on the clinical findings as the platelet count is normal. The bleeding is a result of a vasculitis of unknown aetiology. Resolution within a few weeks is the norm though there may be subsequent exacerbations and remissions.

Management
The treatment is supportive for the symptoms of arthritis and abdominal pain. Steroids may be given when there is extensive disease.

Idiopathic thrombocytopenic purpura

Idiopathic thrombocytopenic purpura (ITP) as the name suggests is a disease of unknown aetiology that often presents a few weeks after a viral infection. It presents with spontaneous onset of petechiae and bruising, which have no particular distribution. Mucosal bleeding is not uncommon and nosebleeds may be quite difficult to stop. The platelet count is often less than $20 \times 10^9/l$ (normal $>150 \times 10^9/l$) and nearly all children have increased levels of platelet-bound IgG.

The diagnosis is based on the clinical features and

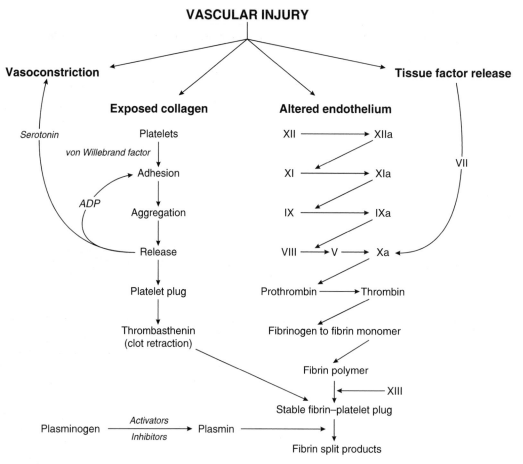

Fig. 66 The coagulation cascade.

platelet count. In 90% the disease will spontaneously remit within 3 months. Only children with platelet counts of less than $20 \times 10^9/l$ and mucous membrane bleeding require treatment.

Management

Therapy is with a course of corticosteroids or, when the bleeding is problematic or refractory, intravenous immunoglobulin. In those children where the condition persists for longer than 6 months, splenectomy will allow the platelet count to rise.

Marrow failure

Marrow failure syndromes including aplastic anaemia and acute leukaemia can also present with a history of bleeding. In these cases, the blood count will reveal pancytopenia.

Platelet/coagulation factor defects

While platelet deficiency/dysfunction presents as petechiae, bruising and mucosal bleeds, coagulation

Table 63 The coagulation factors

International numbers	Synonyms	Description
I	Fibrinogen	Congenital deficiency: afibrinogenaemia
II	Prothrombin	Congenital deficiency is known
III	Thromboplastin	
IV	Calcium	
V	Labile factor, proaccelerin	Congenital deficiency: parahaemophilia, Owren disease
VI	Activated labile factor, accelerin	Same as factor V
VII	Stable factor, proconvertin, SPCA	Congenital deficiency is known
VIII	Antihaemophilic factor	Congenital deficiency: haemophilia A
IX	Christmas factor, plasma thromboplastin component (PTC)	Congenital deficiency: haemophilia B
X	Stuart–Power factor	Congenital deficiency is known
XI	Plasma thromboplastin antecedent (PTA)	Congenital deficiency is known
XII	Hageman factor	Asymptomatic congenital deficiency
XIII	Fibrin-stabilising factor	Congenital deficiency is known

Table 64 The diagnosis of bleeding disorders

Disorder	Inheritance	Prothrombin time	Activated partial thromboplastin time	Platelets	Bleeding time	Specific test
Haemophilia A (factor VIII)	XR	N	E	N	N	Factor VIII
von Willebrand's disease	AD	N	E/N	N	E/N	von Willebrand factor antigen or ristocetin cofactor activity Factor VIII
Haemophilia B (factor IX)	XR	N	E	N	N	Factor IX
Haemophilia C (factor XI)	AD	N	E	N	N	Factor XI
Vitamin K-dependent factors (II, VII, IX and X) (>50% reduction in factors)	AR	E	E	N	N	
Idopathic thrombocytopenic purpura		N	N	D	E	
Glanzmann		N	N	N	E	

XR, sex-linked recessive; AD, autosomal dominant; AR, autosomal recessive; N, normal; E, elevated; D, decreased.

factor deficiencies tend to present with deep-seated and joint bleeds. The coagulation factors are shown in Table 63 and their pathway of activation in Figure 66. A careful history is essential in children with bleeding disorders. The initial screening tests must include a platelet count, prothrombin time, the partial thromboplastin test, bleeding time and, where relevant, levels of factor VIII and IX.

Haemophilia

The dramatic effect of haemorrhages in the European dynasties and the devastating role of therapeutic concentrates in the transmission of AIDS have made **haemophilia A** an object of great medical and public scrutiny. The gene coding for factor VIII lies on the tip of the long arm of chromosome X. In one-third of patients with haemophilia, there is a recent mutation and there is no family history. Clinically indistinguishable but rarer is **haemophilia B** (Christmas disease) which is caused by factor IX deficiency and is also transmitted on the X-chromosome.

Factor VIII circulates in the plasma in a non-covalent complex with von Willebrand factor (vWF). vWF enhances factor VIII synthesis, protects it from proteolysis and concentrates it at sites of active haemostasis. The diagnosis of haemophilia is suspected whenever unusual bleeding is encountered in a boy. As shown in Table 64 the suspicion is supported by the presence of an abnormal activated partial thromboplastin time (APTT) with a normal prothrombin time and a normal platelet count. Factor assay is required to confirm the diagnosis and distinguish factor IX and XI deficiency. It is essential to distinguish patients with severe haemophilia A (<1% of factor VIII) from patients who have moderate (1–4%) or mild (5–25%) disease. Mild or moderate haemophilia is rarely complicated by spontaneous haemarthroses. The hallmark of severe disease is the occurrence of apparently unprovoked bleeding into joints when the child begins to walk. Untreated,

haemarthroses are painful and result in limitation of joint mobility. The inflammatory response to an intra-articular bleed leads to synovitis and ultimately permanent joint damage. Bleeding also occurs at other sites, for example into muscles or as intracranial haemorrhages.

Patients with **von Willebrand's disease** also have factor VIII deficiency as an indirect consequence of a qualitative or quantitative change in the vWF. There are at least four different varieties, and inheritance is either autosomal dominant or recessive. The diagnosis is usually confirmed by measuring the vWF antigen or ristocetin cofactor activity. The latter measures the ability of the vWF to support platelet aggregation in the presence of ristocetin.

Management

The advent of factor VIII replacement revolutionised the management of children with haemophilia A until the AIDS epidemic. Highly refined viral inactivation techniques and recombinantly synthesised factor VIII have now decreased the risk of transfusion-related virus transmission. Desmopressin (DDAVP) increases the plasma levels of factor VIII and vWF and can be used for the non-transfusional treatment of patients with mild or moderate haemophilia and von Willebrand's disease. Tranexamic acid can also be used to stabilise the clot. Factor replacement is necessary for those with severe haemophilia and an on-going bleed. For those with minor bleeds, the replacement is aimed to achieve an increment of factor VIII of about 15%; for haemarthroses replacement is aimed at maintaining levels at 50% till resolution of symptoms. For surgery and intracranial bleeds, levels of 100% may be required.

Certain countries have successfully introduced a prophylactic regimen for severe haemophiliacs. The infusion of factor VIII three times a week can prevent spontaneous haemarthroses. However, the financial implications of such a programme are considerable.

About 10–20% of children with haemophilia unfortunately develop antibodies to factor VIII. The management of these children is complex and includes the use of porcine factor VIII, prothrombin complex concentrates and factor VII infusions (which bypass the need for factor VIII) and, in severe cases, removal of the inhibitor by exchange plasmapheresis or the use of protein A–sepharose columns.

11.4 The neoplastic disorders

Cancer is a rare disease of childhood with an incidence of approximately 1.4 per 10 000 total population. The malignancies of childhood tend to be different from those that occur in adults (Fig. 67). They usually originate in a primitive cell, are aggressive and metastasise early. However, great strides have been made with childhood cancers and in many cases it is possible to achieve a cure.

Overall, the prognosis for childhood cancer has improved since the mid-1970s. More importantly, the majority of children cured can be expected to lead normal lives, hold jobs and raise a family.

Approach to therapy

The improved survival rates in childhood cancers has been made possible by the development of specialised

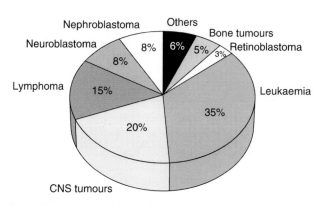

Fig. 67 The common childhood malignancies.

paediatric oncology units. A wide range of health professionals used to dealing with the problems of a child with cancer should be based in these centres, which can offer a multidisciplinary approach. The treatment of most childhood malignancies is multimodal, using a combination of chemotherapy, radiotherapy and surgery. In most cases, an indwelling central venous line is inserted to facilitate management. Various drugs act at different sites in the cell and also at different times in the cell cycle (Fig. 68). Combination chemotherapy (using drugs with different mechanisms of action at the same time) ensures that the malignant cell is targeted in more than one fashion. Ideally, this enables cancer cells to be attacked at different phases of the cell cycle, avoids the toxicity that would occur from the dose required by

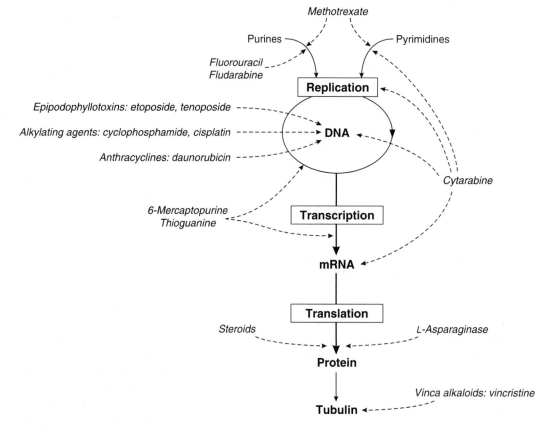

Fig. 68 Sites of action of common chemotherapeutic agents.

a single agent and prevents the emergence of a drug-resistant clone. In practice all these targets are not always achieved.

Side-effects

Side-effects of these drugs are varied and common. In general most of the drugs cause bone marrow suppression, alopecia and mucositis. Therefore, all children receiving chemotherapy pass through a neutropenic period during which they are prone to infections. These can be bacterial, fungal or viral. The empirical treatment with broad-spectrum antibiotics in children with febrile neutropenia has been effective in decreasing mortality and morbidity. In children with acute lymphoblastic leukaemia, who are immunosuppressed for prolonged periods of time, prophylactic co-trimoxazole has reduced the incidence of *Pneumocystis carinii* infection. Long-term toxicities include anthracycline-induced cardiotoxicity and epipodophyllotoxin-induced secondary leukaemias. Radiation may damage the pituitary or the gonads, leading to endocrine deficiency and infertility.

Acute leukaemia

The commonest malignancy of childhood is **acute lymphoblastic leukaemia (ALL)**. The incidence peaks in the 2–6-year age group, unlike **acute myeloid leukaemia (AML)**, which is relatively more common in infancy. The presenting symptoms for both ALL and AML are very similar. A previously well child presents with a history of fever and malaise of a few weeks' duration with pallor and easy bruising or bleeding. Physical examination reveals a pale child with petechiae and bruises and mild-to-moderate enlargement of the lymph nodes, liver and spleen. The blood count usually shows a pancytopenia, though the white cell count (WCC) may be elevated, and often reveals the presence of peripheral immature white cells, referred to as 'blasts'. The diagnosis is confirmed by a bone marrow aspiration. The cerebrospinal fluid is examined to look for CNS disease.

The morphological appearance of the blasts are classified according to the FAB (French–American–British) classification: lymphoblasts are classified as L1, L2 or L3. AML are classified from M0 to M7. Further characterisation of the malignant clone is done by immunophenotyping. This is based on the identification of cells by cell surface molecules that are detected by specific monoclonal antibodies and numbered according to the cluster of differentiation (CD). The commonest ALL is of B cell origin and is usually CD10 positive and is often referred to as common-ALL. T cell leukaemias tend to present with mediastinal masses, high WCCs and CNS involvement at diagnosis.

Management of ALL

In the 1970s, survival in children with ALL was less than

Fig. 69 Actuarial survival curves showing improvement in survival for childhood ALL and AML.

1%. With modern methods of management it is now as high as 70% (Fig. 69). Initial treatment entails the induction of remission, usually using a combination of steroids and two other drugs (e.g. L-asparaginase and vincristine) given over a 4-week period. This is followed by intensification chemotherapy where a different combination of drugs (e.g. etoposide, cytarabine, thioguanine and daunorubicin) are given over a short period of time, usually 5 days. The next phase of treatment is designed to target the CNS. In those at a high risk of CNS disease (WCC >50 × 10⁹/l) or with CNS disease at presentation, either cranial radiation or three pulses of high-dose intravenous methotrexate can be used. In those at low risk (WCC <50 × 10⁹/l) a series of intrathecal methotrexate injections are sufficient. The current United Kingdom Children's Cancer Study Group protocol (Medical Research Council, UKALL 97) also includes a second intensification block. The cornerstone of treatment is to maintain remission. Continuation therapy in UKALL 97 consists of daily oral 6-mercaptopurine, weekly methotrexate and a monthly pulse of steroids and vincristine. CNS-directed therapy is continued with intrathecal methotrexate every 3 months for a total period of 24 months from diagnosis. The risk of relapse is highest in the first 24 months after stopping therapy and virtually negligible 60 months after stopping therapy. The prognostic factors in ALL are given in Table 65.

Table 65 Prognostic factors in ALL

Factor	Good prognosis	Poor prognosis
Age at diagnosis (years)	2–10	<1 or >12
Sex	Female	Male
Presenting WCC	$<50 \times 10^9/l$	$>50 \times 10^9/l$
Immunophenotype	CD10 positive (pre-B cell)	T cell
Cytogenetics	Hyperdiploidy	t(4;11), t(9;22), hypodiploid

Management of AML

Children with AML are treated for a shorter duration but with very intensive pulses of therapy. In the period since the mid-1980s this approach has resulted in a greater than 50% survival (Fig. 69).

Chronic myeloid leukaemia

Chronic myeloid leukaemia is a rare cancer of childhood and is generally curable only by an allogeneic bone marrow transplant. This route can be used with moderate success in those with poor prognosis or relapsed disease.

The lymphomas

The lymphomas include **Hodgkin's disease** (HD) and **non-Hodgkin's lymphoma** (NHL). NHL is more common in the UK and tends to be of T cell, B cell or large cell origin. Lymphomas present as localised enlargement of lymph nodes or other reticuloendothelial organs. T cell disease usually presents with dyspnoea resulting from mediastinal compression caused by involvement of the thymus and mediastinal nodes and/or pleural effusion. In severe cases, this may result in superior vena caval obstruction. Large cell lymphomas tend to present with peripheral tissue masses in the skin and bone or cutaneous infiltration. **Burkitt's lymphoma** usually presents with a mass in the jaw and is endemic in Africa. Sporadic B cell NHL tumours often present as an intra-abdominal mass, occasionally with associated malabsorption or intussusception. In all cases, there may be additional involvement of the bone marrow. The treatment for T cell malignancies is similar to that for ALL. B cell and large cell disease are treated with short pulses of intensive therapy with no continuation therapy.

Management

HD in childhood is commonly of either the nodular sclerosing or lymphocyte predominant type. Therapeutic modalities for children are not greatly different from those used in adults and consist of combination therapy and/or localised radiotherapy. The precise regimen used depends on the histological grade and extent (i.e. stage) of disease (Fig. 70 and Tables 66 and 67).

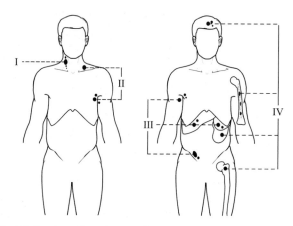

Fig. 70 Staging of lymphomas. Stage I, single node/clump in one anatomical drainage site; stage II, two or more nodes in two sites on the same side of the diaphragm; stage III, two or more nodes on opposite sides of the diaphragm and hepatospenomegaly; stage IV, extranodal sites including brain, bone, bone marrow and kidneys.

Table 66 Clinical staging of Hodgkin's disease

Stage	Extent
I	Involvement of a single lymph node (I) or a single extralymphatic organ or site (I$_E$)
II	Involvement of two or more lymph node regions on the same side of the diaphragm (II) or localised involvement of an extralymphatic organ or site and one or more lymph node regions on the same side of the diaphragm (II$_E$)
III	Involvement of lymph nodes on both sides of the diaphragm (III), which may be accompanied by splenic involvement (III$_S$) or by localised involvement of an extralymphatic organ or site (III$_E$) or both (III$_{SE}$)
IV	Diffuse or disseminated involvement of one or more extralymphatic organs or tissues with or without lymph node involvement

The presence or fever, drenching night sweats, or unexplained loss of weight is denoted by the suffix B, all others by the suffix A.

Table 67 Clinical staging of non-Hodgkin's lymphoma

Stage	Extent
I	Single tumour or single anatomic area, excluding mediastinum or abdomen
II	Single tumour with regional node involvement on same side of the diaphragm; primary gastrointestinal tumour with or without mesenteric node involvement and grossly completely resectable
III	On both sides of the diaphragm; primary intrathoracic tumour; unresectable abdominal disease; paraspinal and epidural tumours
IV	Any of the above with initial CNS or bone marrow involvement

CNS tumours

CNS tumours form a heterogeneous group of conditions. Two-thirds of brain tumours in childhood occur in the posterior cranial fossa. The growing tumour interferes with the CSF pathway and impairs the function of the cerebellum. The presenting symptoms are, therefore, those of raised intracranial pressure, including **lethargy**, **headaches** and early morning **vomiting**, which may be

Fig. 71 CT brain scan showing contrast enhancing medulloblastoma in posterior fossa.

Fig. 72 Abdominal neuroblastoma, resulting in a large, firm irregular mass extending from right flank beyond the midline, abdominal distension with an umbilical hernia, and bilateral periorbital metastases with bruising ('panda eyes').

projectile in nature. Cerebellar dysfunction is manifest by **altered gait** (ataxia), occasionally diplopia and nystagmus. **Papilloedema** is a late clinical finding. Any child who presents with these symptoms and signs should be considered to have a posterior fossa mass and a CT scan of the head should be performed. The tumour can be benign (cerebellar astrocytoma) or malignant (medulloblastoma). Other brain tumours include pinealomas, gliomas, malignant astrocytomas, etc. These tend to present with isolated cranial nerve palsies and long tract signs.

Management

Therapy includes surgical removal if possible, radiation and chemotherapy. Medulloblastomas seed early along the spine and in general the prognosis for malignant CNS tumours is poor, only about 20–30% surviving at 5 years.

Neuroblastoma

Neuroblastoma is of neuroectodermal origin and usually arises in the abdomen (65%), especially from the adrenal gland (35%) and often crosses the midline (Fig. 72). It typically presents in a young child or infant as an abdominal mass. Metastatic disease at diagnosis is usual, the skeletal system and bone marrow being the most common sites. The primary tumour can present in a wide variety of tissues, as paraspinal (dumb-bell) tumours and in skin. It also occurs as rare but well-described paraneoplastic phenomena, such as the opsoclonus–myoclonus syndrome, and as intractable diarrhoea. The diagnosis is based on histopathology, as in other solid tumours. Additionally, 90–95% of the tumours synthesise sufficient catecholamines to result in increased urinary excretion. Poor prognosis is seen in stage IV disease, the loss of the small arm of chromosome 1 and the amplification of the gene N-*myc* in tumour cells.

Management

Therapy for advanced-stage disease centres around platinum compounds in high-dose therapy with autolo-

gous bone marrow/peripheral blood stem cells rescue. Refractory cases have been treated palliatively with radioactive iodine in the compound [^{131}I]-labelled MIBG. Therapeutic progress remains moderate in this disease with survival at 25–30% for advanced-stage disease.

Nephroblastoma

Nephroblastoma is also called Wilms' tumour and arises from the kidney. It generally presents as an asymptomatic abdominal mass that rarely crosses the midline and is occasionally associated with haematuria. A CT scan will show a large mass, usually encapsulated, distorting a thin rim of normal renal tissue (Fig. 73). The tumour tends to invade the renal vein and inferior vena cava and metastasises to the lung. Associated features include aniridia, genitourinary abnormalities (WAGR syndrome), nephrotic syndrome (Denys–Drash), hemihypertrophy and the Beckwith–Wiedemann syndrome. Histology is diagnostic and will classify the tumour into a favourable or unfavourable (undifferentiated) type.

Management

Treatment is based on surgery and chemotherapy (vincristine alone or in combination with actinomycin and adriamycin in advanced disease), with radiotherapy to pulmonary metastases and to the abdomen in tumours that have seeded into the peritoneal cavity. For stage I

Fig. 73 CT scan showing left-sided Wilms' tumour.

(localised disease), prognosis is >95% and for stage IV (disseminated disease) about 50–60%.

Bone tumours

The two most common primary tumours of bone are Ewing's tumour (ET) and osteogenic sarcoma. ET is of neuroectodermal origin and often arises in the rib, pelvis, femur, tibia, fibula or ankle bones. Bulky tumours and intrathoracic or pelvic tumours carry a bad prognosis. Combination chemotherapy using ifosfamide/cyclophosphamide is used to shrink the tumour, which is then excised with a wide margin. Amputation of the affected bone or limb may be necessary. Where surgery is not feasible, local radiotherapy is used.

Osteogenic sarcoma often occurs at the upper end of the tibia (Fig. 74), lower end of the femur and pelvis.

Fig. 74 Osteosarcoma involving the upper tibial metaphysis.

Treatment includes surgical removal of the bone, whenever possible, and high-dose chemotherapy.

Other tumours

Rhabdomyosarcoma, as the name implies, is an undifferentiated soft-tissue tumour arising from primitive striated muscle tissue. It can arise in the pelvis, orbit, limbs and bladder. It tends to be locally invasive but can also metastasise to other tissues, mainly the lung and bone. Therapy is similar to that for Ewing tumour.

Self-assessment: questions

Multiple choice questions

1. The differential diagnosis of a child with hypochromic microcytic anaemia includes:
   a. Lead poisoning
   b. Pulmonary haemosiderosis
   c. Zinc deficiency
   d. Thalassaemia trait
   e. Sideroblastic anaemia

2. The following statements describe oral iron therapy in a child with iron deficiency:
   a. Subjective improvement can occur within 24 hours
   b. Reticulocytosis peaks 3 weeks after starting iron
   c. It may cause a temporary staining of the teeth
   d. Iron absorption is improved by drinking tea
   e. The haemoglobin level will return to normal within a month

3. The following are causes of folic acid deficiency:
   a. Tetrahydrofolate synthetase deficiency
   b. Orotic aciduria
   c. Surgical resection of the small intestine
   d. Pregnancy
   e. Treatment of epilepsy with phenytoin

4. The following are features of vitamin B_{12}:
   a. Its absorption is dependent on intrinsic factor, secreted by the duodenum
   b. The bound vitamin is absorbed in the distal ileum
   c. Deficiency may result in hyperpigmentation
   d. Deficiency is also associated with neuronal degeneration
   e. The congenital absence of transcobalamin I leads to vitamin B_{12} deficiency

5. The following agents may precipitate a haemolytic crisis in those with glucose 6-phosphate dehydrogenase deficiency:
   a. Co-trimoxazole
   b. Aspirin
   c. Naphthalene
   d. Cheese
   e. Port or red wine

6. Pancytopenia can be seen in:
   a. Sickle cell disease
   b. Aplastic anaemia
   c. Leukaemia
   d. Neuroblastoma
   e. Idiopathic thrombocytopenic purpura

7. The following are features of bleeding disorders:
   a. The bleeding time is normal when the platelet count is normal
   b. The failure of the activated partial thromboplastin time (APTT) to correct after the addition of normal plasma indicates the presence of a circulating inhibitor
   c. The prothrombin time (PT) is prolonged in a child with haemophilia C
   d. Factor XIII deficiency is characterised by an abnormal prothrombin and APTT
   e. Fibrinogen deficiency can be corrected by the use of fresh frozen plasma

8. Thrombocytopenia is a feature of:
   a. Wiskott–Aldrich syndrome
   b. Hypersplenism
   c. Kasabach–Meritt syndrome
   d. Aspirin ingestion
   e. Henoch–Schönlein purpura

9. The following associations are characteristic of childhood malignancies:
   a. Nephroblastoma and raised urinary catecholamines
   b. Acute myeloid leukaemia and bleeding gums
   c. Ewing sarcoma and an 'onion peel' appearance on X-ray film
   d. An abdominal neuroblastoma tumour that crosses the midline
   e. Cerebellar astrocytoma and spinal metastases

10. Recognised side-effects of cytotoxic agents include:
    a. Cardiomyopathy after vincristine
    b. Peripheral neuropathy after anthracyclines
    c. Mucosal ulceration after methotrexate
    d. Deafness after carboplatin
    e. Anaphylaxis after asparaginase

11. The following congenital conditions and associated malignant diseases are correctly matched:
    a. Neurofibromatosis and gliomas
    b. Ataxia telangiectasia and lymphoma
    c. Down syndrome and neuroblastoma
    d. Beckwith–Wiedemann and nephroblastoma
    e. Tuberous sclerosis and medulloblastoma

12. The following describe neutrophils:
    a. Neutrophilia may occur with glucocorticoid administration
    b. A shift to the left may be seen in severe infections
    c. A deficiency is characteristic of the Schwachmann syndrome
    d. Severe neutropenia is usually treated with granulocyte infusion
    e. Leukaemoid reaction can be differentiated from leukaemia by the nitro blue tetrazolium test.

13. The following describe autoimmune haemolytic anaemias:
    a. They are usually characterised by a reticulocytopenia
    b. Thrombocytopenia is common
    c. Drugs such as penicillin are aetiological agents
    d. Steroids are the mainstay of therapy
    e. The Coombs' test is positive

14. The following are recognised associations:
    a. Acute haemolysis with the use of anti-malarials
    b. Hookworm infection and megaloblastic anaemia
    c. Chronic haemolytic anaemia and folate deficiency
    d. Autoimmune haemolytic anaemia and severe bacteria infections
    e. Aplastic anaemia and the use of oral chloramphenicol

Short notes

Write short notes on:

1. Bone marrow transplantation
2. Complications of congenital haemolytic anaemia.

Viva voce question

A 17-month-old boy is brought to you with a history of pica, listlessness and failure to thrive. His mother comments that his stomach looks full and she feels that he looks pale. In view of these symptoms, what questions would you ask of the mother and describe your management.

Case history question

> A 6-year-old child diagnosed to have acute lymphoblastic leukaemia 3 weeks ago is being discharged from the ward. He has had a central venous line inserted and he is due to complete his last week of therapy at his local hospital. At discharge his FBC is as follows: Hb 9.3 g/dl; WCC 1.8×10^9/l, with an absolute neutrophil count of 0.4 and platelets of 73×10^9/l. He is due to return to you in 10 days time to start the next phase of treatment.

Discuss how you will arrange the discharge.

Self-assessment: answers

Multiple choice answers

1. a. **True**. The red cells may also have basophilic stippling.
   b. **True**. It is associated with haemoptysis.
   c. **True**. It may result in an iron-deficiency state.
   d. **True**. It is the most common differential diagnosis for iron-deficiency anaemia.
   e. **True**. It is diagnosed by the presence of ringed sideroblasts in a marrow aspirate.

2. a. **True**. For example, an improvement in mood and appetite.
   b. **False**. Reticulocytosis peaks at 5–7 days.
   c. **True**. It will disappear after stopping the medication.
   d. **False**. It can decrease iron availability and absorption.
   e. **True**. It may do so even earlier.

3. a. **False**. It is caused by dihydrofolate reductase deficiency.
   b. **False**. It results in megaloblastic anaemia independent of folic acid deficiency.
   c. **True**. Resection results in decreased absorption of folic acid.
   d. **True**. Malabsorption can occur.
   e. **True**. Though the deficiency rarely results in a clinically significant megaloblastic anaemia.

4. a. **False**. Intrinsic factor and R proteins, required for the absorption of vitamin B_{12} are produced in the stomach.
   b. **True**. A B_{12} deficiency can occur if the terminal ileum has been resected.
   c. **True**. Glossitis and neurological manifestations can also occur.
   d. **True**. It may occur in the absence of overt anaemia.
   e. **False**. Transcobalamin II is the physiologically important transporter.

5. a. **True**. Drugs that have oxidant properties such as sulphonamides, aspirin and antimalarials precipitate haemolysis in these individuals.
   b. **True**. Aspirin is an oxidant drug.
   c. **True**.
   d. **False**.
   e. **False**.

6. a. **True**. Aplastic crises are often associated with parvovirus infections.
   b. **True**. Pancytopenia defines tri-lineage deficiency in the peripheral blood.
   c. **True**. Marrow suppression results from malignant infiltration.

d. **True**. Marrow infiltration suppresses cell production.
   e. **False**. There is only a decrease in the platelet count, which occurs because of peripheral destruction.

7. a. **False**. In Glanzmann disease (thrombasthenia) where there is a platelet function defect, the platelet count is normal but the bleeding time is prolonged.
   b. **True**. The addition of normal plasma should correct for the presence of any deficient factors; an inability to do so suggests the presence of a circulating inhibitor.
   c. **False**. Factor XI as well as VIII and IX deficiencies are phase I disorders and characterised by an abnormal APTT and normal PT.
   d. **False**. The fibrin stabilising factor deficiency is characterised by normal PT and APTT and an abnormal clot solubility in 5 M urea.
   e. **True**. Though fibrinogen concentrates or cryoprecipitate is a more substantial source.

8. a. **True**. Thrombocytopenia, atopic dermatitis and immunodeficiency occur.
   b. **True**. Consumption of cells can also lead to pancytopenia.
   c. **True**. Rapidly enlarging haemangioma, thrombocytopenia and acute or chronic consumption coagulopathy occur.
   d. **False**. Though aspirin can prevent platelet adhesion.
   e. **False**. This is a vasculitis without a thrombocytopenia.

9. a. **False**. This is seen in 90–95% of neuroblastomas.
   b. **True**. It is commonly seen in M3 and M4 types of AML.
   c. **True**. It is caused by repeated periosteal lifting and new bone formation.
   d. **True**. Unlike nephroblastoma, which usually does not cross the midline.
   e. **False**. This is a benign tumour. Medulloblastoma tends to spread down the spinal axis.

10. a. **False**. Peripheral neuropathy occurs after vincristine and cardiomyopathy after anthracyclines.
    b. **False**. Cardiomyopathy is a side-effect of anthracyclines.
    c. **True**. Marrow depression also occurs.
    d. **True**. Renal toxicity also occurs.

e. **True**. There is also local reaction and hypercoagulable conditions.

11. a. **True**. As well as acute myeloid leukaemia.
    b. **True**. Either B cell or T cell.
    c. **False**. Leukaemia is more common in this condition.
    d. **True**. Usually due to deletions of chromosome 11p15.
    e. **False**. Gliomas, rhabdomyomas.

12. a. **True**. Lymphopenia also occurs.
    b. **True**. Particularly apparent in the neonatal period.
    c. **True**. Dwarfism, neutropenia and pancreatic insufficiency occur.
    d. **False**. Though granulocyte colony-stimulating factor (G-CSF) may be useful.
    e. **True**. Normal neutrophils contain superoxide, which will turn the normally yellow nitro blue tetrazolium to blue and appears as insoluble dark blue pigments on normal neutrophils.

13. a. **True**. As more immature red cells escape into the circulation to compensate for the haemolysis.
    b. **False**. Only rarely is immune thrombocytopenia associated with haemolytic anaemia (Evans syndrome).
    c. **True**. Though the most common cause is primary autoimmune haemolytic anaemia, which is idiopathic in nature.
    d. **True**. Red cell transfusion may be necessary; if no compatible blood can be found then the least incompatible should be given.
    e. **True**. It is also called the direct antiglobulin test (DAT), which identifies antibodies and complement components on the surface of circulating erythrocytes.

14. a. **True**. This occurs in individuals with glucose 6-phosphate dehydrogenase deficiency.
    b. **False**. Iron deficiency occurs and hence microcytic anaemia, though fish tapeworm (diphyllobothriasis) infestations colonise the lower intestine and may produce megaloblastic anaemia through B_{12} deficiency.
    c. **True**. There is increased red cell turnover.
    d. **False**.
    e. **True**. This is thought to be an idiosyncratic reaction.

Short notes answers

1. Bone marrow transplantation (BMT) is the infusion of donor marrow or stem cells into a recipient.

   Sources of haematopoietic stem cells for transplantation:

   - allogeneic BMT using HLA-matched sibling
   - allogeneic BMT using HLA, DR-matched or

partially mismatched family members (other than sibling donors) or unrelated donors
- syngeneic BMT from an identical twin
- autologous BMT: the patient's own marrow is cryopreserved and then re-infused (purged or unpurged) after high-dose chemotherapy and/or radiation therapy to treat the underlying malignancy
- peripheral blood stem cells: the number of circulating stem cells can be vastly increased before apheresis with haematopoietic growth factors such as the granulocyte colony stimulating factor (G-CSF)
- umbilical blood stem cells from an unrelated donor
- fetal liver stem cells from an unrelated donor.

In all cases, the marrow is infused back by a peripheral/central vein. Pluripotential stem cells settle in the marrow stroma, proliferate and repopulate the ablated bone marrow.

Principles of therapy. The philosophy with allogeneic or syngeneic transplantation is to replace the host immune–reticuloendothelial system, which is presumably diseased, with that of the donor. To facilitate this, the recipient is heavily immunosuppressed and receives marrow-ablating therapy (either drugs such as cyclophosphamide or busulphan or total body irradiation). In those with leukaemia, the donor immune system then eradicates the leukaemic cells (graft-versus-leukaemia effect). The use of peripheral stem cells is becoming an increasingly popular source of pluripotential stem cells. The relative immunological naiveté and the high numbers of pluripotential cells in cord blood make this an attractive source of stem cells in those patients without a matched sibling donor.

Indications for BMT:

- malignancy: acute lymphoblastic leukaemia in second or third remission, acute myeloid leukaemia in first or second remission, chronic myeloid leukaemia
- non-malignant conditions: congenital immunodeficiencies (e.g severe combined immunodeficiency (SCID)), inherited metabolic disorders (e.g. Gaucher disease, Lesch–Nyhan, etc.), haematological disorders (e.g. thalassaemia, Fanconi's anaemia, congenital neutropenia, etc.).

Acute complications:

- infections as a result of immunosuppression and prolonged period of neutropenia
- acute graft-versus-host disease
- veno-occlusive disease.

Chronic complications:

- chronic graft-versus-host disease
- growth failure
- multiple endocrine problems
- second malignancies
- sterility.

2. Complications of congenital haemolytic anaemia include:

    1. Haemolytic crises leading to a sudden drop in haemoglobin and hyperbilirubinaemia. Seen in patients with G6PD deficiency, sickle cell disease, spherocytosis and thalassaemia
    2. Erythroblastopenic crises resulting in a drop in haemoglobin and reticulocyte count and associated with parvovirus B19 infection. This is seen in sickle disease, spherocytosis and thalassaemia
    3. Vaso-occlusive crises occur in sickle cell and HbSC disease
    4. Splenic sequestration crises are typically seen in sickle cell disease and may be fatal
    5. Hyperhaemolytic crises are usually seen when sickle cell disease is present in conjunction with G6PD deficiency
    6. Organ dysfunction affecting the brain and lungs (sickle cell disease owing to infarction) or liver, heart, pancreas, kidneys endocrine glands, bone, etc. caused by infarction or iron deposition (haemosiderosis) in haemolytic anaemias requiring frequent transfusion, especially with thalassaemia
    7. Gall stones
    8. Hypersplenism in spherocytosis, thalassaemia
    9. Hyposplenism caused by autoinfarction in sickle cell disease
    10. Infections: osteomyelitis in infarcted bone (sickle)
    11. Leg ulcers
    12. Folate deficiency caused by increased red cell turnover.

Viva voce answer

The most common cause for these symptoms is iron-deficiency anaemia. In a child with anaemia, the history is often diagnostic. A broad guideline is given below.

Birth history. Was the child born prematurely or with low birth weight? This could be a contributing factor. Was there prolonged neonatal jaundice suggestive of congenital haemolytic anaemias?

Diet history. Was he breast fed? Artificially fed? Was weaning carried out appropriately and if he required vitamin and mineral supplements did he receive them?

Family history. Is there a family history of anaemia or jaundice? What is the ethnic origin of the child?

Recent history. Is the child on any medication or 'fad' feeds that could precipitate a haemolysis?

System review. Are there any sources of obvious blood loss, i.e. blood in the stools or urine, a previous bout of pneumonia (pulmonary haemosiderosis)? Is there any neurological involvement (megaloblastic anaemia)?

Examination. The child should be examined for pallor and icterus (conjunctiva, oral mucosa, fingernails and palms). Palpate the abdomen gently as a just palpable spleen in children tends to be quite soft and easily missed. The additional presence of mucosal ulcers (neutropenia), petechiae (thrombocytopenia) and lymph node enlargement will suggest that the diagnosis is more sinister. In chronic iron deficiency, the fingernails may be concave (koilonychia) and a blue line on the gums is occasionally seen in lead poisoning. Megaloblastic anaemia is often associated with hyperpigmentation, particularly of the buccal mucosa.

Investigation. The diagnosis is confirmed by examination of the blood film and reticulocyte count (Fig. 65).

Management. Treatment of even severe iron deficiency is successful with oral iron given over a period of 3 months.

Case history answer

You are expected to categorise and explain all the aspects of discharging a child with a chronic illness back to the community.

Predischarge. Has the decision to discharge been discussed with the parents, medical staff, social worker, home-care nurse and other members of the team? Are the parents aware of what to anticipate? Has the ward prescription (TTA) note been done and the medications explained to the parents?

Home environment. Has transport been booked to take the family home? Is the home environment suitable for an immunocompromised child with a central line? Are there many stairs to climb? Is there a telephone? Should the housing association be approached for new housing?

Support for the family. Are the family members coping? Do they need financial help, counselling or to be put in touch with helper groups? Are the instructions for medications clearly written? Who is going to flush the line, the parents or the community nurse? Do they know what to do if the child is unwell and how to contact the medical staff at the hospital?

Community care. Have the social workers and the community-care team been informed about the child's discharge? Does the community nurse know if the line needs to be flushed, if blood samples are to be taken or medications need to be administered? Does the school need a letter? Is respite care needed?

Follow-up. Have the general practitioner and the local referring hospital been contacted? Does the local hospital have details of the treatment the child is on (e.g steroids) and what medicines they require to give? Do they also know who to contact in case of a problem? Do the parents know when and where they are expected to come when they return in 10 days' time?

General surgery, orthopaedics and ears, nose and throat

Key points

You should have an understanding of:

- Symptoms suggestive of surgical disease
- Basic surgical resuscitative measures
- The operative approach for common surgical problems
- Postoperative management.

12.1 Introduction

Although paediatric surgery is a highly specialised field, some surgical problems are sufficiently common that a basic awareness of their presenting symptoms and signs is required. Furthermore, preoperative resuscitation and postoperative management should form part of the undergraduate's armamentarium. Indeed, significant morbidity in surgical patients results from delayed diagnoses, disregard of surgery-related complications and ignorance in postoperative care.

Orthopaedic disorders and ear, nose and throat (ENT) disorders may also require surgical intervention.

12.2 Congenital surgical abnormalities

Many congenital anomalies requiring surgical repair are detected on routine antenatal ultrasound screening. If so, arrangements should be made for the delivery to occur in a specialist centre with facilities for neonatal surgery and neonatal intensive care.

Gastrointestinal atresia

Gastrointestinal obstruction is a common surgical problem, particularly in the newborn. The symptoms and signs vary depending on the site of obstruction: upper gastrointestinal lesions present with early onset of vomiting, which is usually bile stained, whereas lower lesions result in abdominal distension and constipation and then vomiting. Indeed, **bile-stained vomiting** must be taken to represent gastrointestinal obstruction until

proven otherwise. Abdominal tenderness and bowel signs may be difficult to assess, especially in neonates.

Oesophageal atresia

Failure of cannalisation of the oesophagus and connection with the stomach results in high gastrointestinal obstruction in 1 in 4000 live births. In 87% of cases with oesophageal atresia, a tracheo-oesophageal fistula (TOF) connects the distal, blind-ending oesophagus and the trachea (Fig. 75). Air is, therefore, able to enter the stomach, producing a characteristic X-ray appearance with a blind, upper oesophagus and a large gastric gas bubble. Up to 50% of patients with tracheo-oesophageal (TE) abnormalities will have other anomalies involving the vertebrae, anus, cardiovascular system, renal system and radii (VACTER), and these must be investigated appropriately in all patients.

All types of oesophageal atresia, barring the H-type, present in the newborn period. The H-type variant presents with recurrent aspiration and chest infections in later infancy and childhood.

Polyhydramnios usually develops antenatally. Neonates present shortly after birth with increased frothy secretions, choking and cyanosis on feeding. Failure to pass a nasogastric tube (NGT) into the stomach suggests the diagnosis. The baby should be nursed prone as there is a high risk of aspiration, all feeds withheld, a large-bore NGT positioned in the upper oesophagus and placed on continuous suction. Intravenous fluids and, if aspiration is suspected, broad-spectrum antibiotics are commenced and the infant cross matched. Urgent surgery involves closure of the fistula and re-anastamosis of the oesophageal ends. Occasionally, a segment of small bowel is required to bridge the gap. Oral feeds are generally tolerated after about 10 days. Late complications include tracheomalacia, gastro-oesophageal reflux and oesophageal stenosis. The prognosis depends on the preoperative condition and the severity of associated anomalies.

Duodenal atresia

Duodenal atresia arises in 1 in 10 000 births: 30% of cases occur in children with Down syndrome, but it is common in association with other anomalies of the gas-

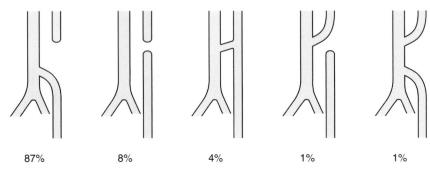

| 87% | 8% | 4% | 1% | 1% |

Fig. 75 Oesophageal atresia with tracheo-oesophageal fistula.

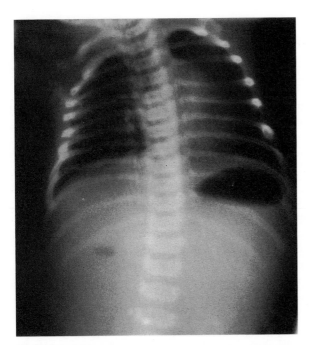

Fig. 76 X-ray showing double bubble appearance of duodenal atresia.

trointestinal tract (e.g. malrotation, oesophageal and anal atresia) and cardiovascular and renal systems. Failure of cannalisation of the bowel after the solid phase of development results in a short, obstructing membrane, long fibrous cord or even complete separation of the bowel ends. Rarely, this lesion is caused by obstructing Ladd's bands or an annular pancreas.

Atresia of the second or third part of the duodenum results in high gastrointestinal obstruction, and polyhydramnios is a feature in 50% of children. Characteristically, vomiting on the first day of life is associated with little abdominal distension. The vomit is usually bile stained since the obstruction is often distal to the opening of the common bile duct. An X-ray film shows air in the stomach and upper part of the duodenum, producing the characteristic 'double bubble' appearance in an otherwise gasless abdomen (Fig. 76). The patient should be stabilised with an NGT to decompress the stomach and intravenous nutritional support, and any associated abnormalities are treated. End-to-

end repair of the duodenum is usually possible in the first instance; resection is necessary with long fibrous cords. Malrotation must be reversed, Ladd bands divided and a duodenoduodenostomy fashioned with an annular pancreas.

Small-bowel atresia

Non-development and incomplete cannalisation of the small bowel may follow ischaemia in utero and may affect one or several sections of the small bowel. Obstruction may result from a discrete membrane, fibrous cord or complete separation of the small bowel and may occur in one or multiple sites. Jejunoileal atresia presents with bile-stained vomiting, abdominal distension and failure to pass meconium. Distended bowel loops are evident on a plain X-ray film and fluid levels on a lateral decubitus film. Contrast studies will delineate the level of obstruction. An NGT should be passed and left on free drainage, and antibiotic prophylaxis and intravenous hydration commenced. Surgical correction is planned when the condition is stable and involves resection of non-viable bowel and, ideally, end-to-end anastomosis in the first instance. Following multiple resections and when bowel distension is severe, a defunctioning ileostomy with distal mucus fistula is preferable, with reversal of the stoma 3 to 4 months later (Fig. 77).

Meconium ileus

Up to a sixth of patients who develop meconium ileus will have cystic fibrosis. Pellets of viscid meconium obstruct the colon and terminal ileum in utero. Dilatation of the proximal bowel may precede perforation and meconium peritonitis. Symptoms and signs similar to small-bowel atresia develop shortly after birth. Plain abdominal films show a hazy, ground glass appearance caused by inspissated meconium containing trapped air bubbles, usually in the right lower quadrant. Patchy calcification is evident in those where peritonitis has occurred, whereas dilated loops on an erect film lack fluid levels owing to the viscid contents. Gentle enemas (e.g. gastrografin with detergent) every 8–12 hours may reduce the impaction in 50% of patients.

Fig. 77 Primary ileostomy and late correction in small-bowel atresia.

Otherwise, an ileostomy is fashioned through which soft catheters are passed and the bowel irrigated at regular intervals using a mucolytic agent (e.g. acetylcysteine). Bowel resection is required with ischaemic complications and meconium peritonitis. Nutritional support, often in the form of total parenteral nutrition, is necessary for many of these patients, especially when there is a delay in establishing oral feeds.

Anal atresia

Anal atresia is a manifestation of maldevelopment of the cloaca. Hence, an imperforate anus is often associated with lower urogenital defects, especially a fistula to the perineum, urethra, bladder or female vestibule. Additionally, anal atresia may be associated with urological malformations, sacral agenesis, other bowel atresias and heart defects. The diagnosis relies on the absence of an anal orifice on routine examination at birth and failure to pass meconium. The level of the atresia and presence of a fistula should be determined preoperatively. After the first 24 hours, the infant is placed prone for half an hour with the buttocks supported over a small towel. A radio-opaque marker is placed on the anal dimple and a lateral X-ray film taken. If the distance between the rectal gas shadow and the marker is greater than 1 cm, this is suggestive of a high atresia and an indication for a colostomy. Low lesions and those where the anal sphincter is intact (as suggested by a well-formed perineal crease and anal dimple) are repaired by a simple pull through operation (anoplasty). Many will require further treatment to relieve a variable degree of constipation. Lesions above the pelvic muscular sling usually require a defunctioning colostomy and late correction. These, especially if associated with a rectovesical fistula and sacral agenesis, have a guarded prognosis for future bowel continence.

Biliary atresia

Failure of cannalisation or progressive obliteration of the intra- and/or extrahepatic biliary tubules results in biliary atresia in 1 in 10 000 live births. Up to 85% involve the entire extrahepatic ducts, making surgical correction difficult. Biliary atresia is the most important cause of obstructed hyperbilirubinaemia in the newborn, presenting with persistent conjugated hyperbilirubinaemia, pale stools and dark urine, hepatomegaly and failure to thrive. The prognosis improves with earlier diagnosis and is poor if treatment is commenced after the first 6 weeks of life. The diagnosis is suggested by biochemical evidence of an obstructed jaundice. Biliary atresia must be differentiated from other causes of cholestatic jaundice and neonatal hepatitis. Ultrasonography should exclude a choledochal cyst and other causes of extrahepatic biliary obstruction. Biliary atresia is more likely than neonatal hepatitis if the stools are persistently acholic (pale) and there is no bile on aspiration of duodenal contents.

Furthermore, hepatobiliary scintigraphy should demonstrate preserved uptake of isotope tracer by the functioning hepatocytes but absent excretion into the bowel. With hepatitis, uptake is sluggish but excretion does eventually occur. Ultimately, the diagnosis is confirmed by demonstrating an absence of biliary cannaliculae, bile plugs and fibrosis on liver biopsy. In contrast, with neonatal hepatitis there is widespread disruption of the lobular architecture, focal necrosis and an intense inflammatory response.

Correctable lesions (e.g. choledochal cyst) should be resected. For biliary duct atresia, a hepatoportoenterostomy (Kasai procedure) is performed, preferably before the eighth week of life, when there is a 90% chance of establishing adequate biliary flow. The operation entails the anastomosis of a loop of small bowel to the porta hepatis, thereby re-routing biliary drainage from residual, small cannaliculae into the bowel.

Ascending cholangitis is a serious complication following this procedure and must be suspected and treated with broad-spectrum antibiotics whenever a fever and increasing jaundice develop. Despite palliation by the Kasai procedure, chronic hepatic inflammation results in cirrhosis and portal hypertension. Ultimately, liver transplantation is the best long-term option for many of these patients.

Malrotation and volvulus

Infants whose bowel has not developed along the usual embryonic 'anticlockwise' pattern develop bowel malrotation. This predisposes the bowel to twisting on its own axis, constricting the lumen and compromising its blood supply. In most cases, the caecum lies in a subhepatic position and the superior mesenteric artery is tethered along a narrow stalk, predisposing to a midgut volvulus. The condition usually manifests acutely in infancy when signs of bowel obstruction are associated with a rapid deterioration in clinical state (Fig. 78). Surgery to release the volvulus, resect necrotic tissue and fix the remaining bowel in its correct alignment is life saving and should not be delayed. Occasionally, malrotation presents subacutely in preschool children who fail to thrive and develop intermittent bouts of abdominal pain, distension and vomiting caused by recurrent subacute bowel obstruction. The malrotation can be confirmed by contrast studies of the small bowel, prior to corrective surgery.

Hirschsprung's disease

Hirschsprung's disease occurs in 1 in 5000 live births and is more common in boys (4:1). It is the most common cause of lower intestinal obstruction in the neonate and is occasionally associated with other anomalies (e.g. Down syndrome, heart disease). Failure of neuroblast migration from proximal to distal bowel results in an absence of ganglion cells in the submucosa, absent Meissner and Auerbach plexi, and hypertrophied nerve

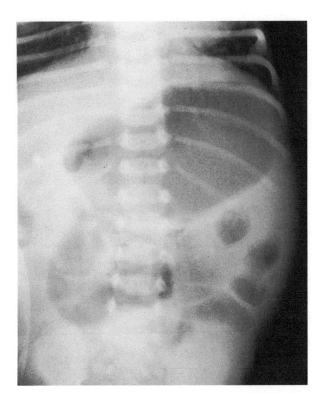

Fig. 78 X-ray showing dilated bowel loops and fluid levels due to volvulus.

Fig. 79 Congenital diaphragmatic hernia. (a) Clinical appearance with cyanosis, respiratory distress and scaphoid abdomen. (b) Radiological appearance with bowel loops in thorax, mediastinal shift and a gasless abdomen.

bundles with increased levels of acetylcholinesterase beyond the submucosa. The aganglionic segment commences at the internal anal sphincter and progresses proximally for a variable distance. It is limited to the rectosigmoid in 75% of patients but, in 10%, it affects the entire colon. A gradual increase in neurones is seen in a transition zone that varies in length until normal histological appearances prevail.

Hirschsprung's disease should be considered in term babies who fail to pass meconium within 48 hours of birth. Patients usually present in the neonatal period with abdominal distension, which often precedes vomiting. Explosive, foul motions may follow a per rectum examination, which may confirm a 'tight' lower rectal segment. If undiagnosed, stasis of bowel contents and mucosal disruption increases the risk of enterocolitis and septicaemia. Occasionally Hirschsprung's disease is diagnosed in older children following prolonged, severe constipation and, rarely, is a cause of failure to thrive owing to an associated protein-losing enteropathy.

Confirmation of the diagnosis relies on a lower bowel contrast study showing a microcolon of variable length, rectal manometry (if available) and a punch biopsy of the lower rectum. At operation, several biopsies should be sent for frozen section and the resection margin performed at the site of normal and not transition bowel. Short-segment Hirschsprung's disease (i.e. not extending beyond the descending colon) has an excellent prognosis. Those with long-segment disease, particularly those with total colonic Hirschsprung, have a poor

prognosis for long-term continence. Rectal pouch refashioning procedures have been designed following total colectomy but the improvement in loose stool and excessive stool frequency is often short lived.

Hernias

Diaphragmatic hernia

In up to 1 in 4000 births, absence or a defect of the diaphragm allows the abdominal contents to herniate into the thoracic cavity. Although this may occur through the oesophageal hiatus (hiatal hernia) and behind the sternum (Morgagni hernia), it is usually in the left posterolateral position (Bochdalek hernia) (Fig. 79.) The last is always associated with malrotation and often found in the presence of cardiovascular, neurological, gastrointestinal and major karyotypic abnormalities. The hernial mass prevents adequate lung development on the ipsilateral side and, if there is significant mediastinal shift, pulmonary hypoplasia is also significant contralaterally.

The diagnosis is generally made on antenatal ultrasound screening. The infant is breathless and cyanosed at birth and deteriorates if resuscitated by means of face mask oxygen alone. This inevitably allows air into the stomach and bowel, much of which is compressing the lungs, thereby further aggravating the degree of respiratory embarrassment. Such infants should be intubated immediately and ventilated, a large bore NGT passed and the stomach contents aspirated. Once stabilised after 12–24 hours, the diaphragm is repaired surgically, sometimes with a prosthetic patch in those with a large defect.

Diaphragmatic hernia is associated with a significant morbidity and mortality of about 40% in the early neonatal period, mainly because of the severe degree of pulmonary hypoplasia and hypertension. This invariably necessitates a prolonged period of conventional ventilatory support. Currently, research is centred around the feasibility of extracorporeal membrane oxygenation (ECMO) and fetal surgery for this condition, although the benefit of this approach is, as yet, unknown. Long-term survivors have an increased risk of reactive airways disease, developmental delay, gastro-oesophageal reflux, nutritional problems and failure to thrive.

Inguinal hernia

Inguinal hernia is seen in almost 2% of children, making this the most common lesion requiring operation in childhood. It occurs in about 30% of premature infants and in most presents before the age of 6 months. The majority occur in boys (4:1) and are almost invariably indirect in type and right sided; only 10% are bilateral. Inguinal hernias arise following persistence of the processus vaginalis, a primitive protrusion of the peritoneum through which the testes descend into the inguinal canal.

Inguinal hernias are commonly associated with undescended testes in males. They generally present as an intermittent lump in the groin, scrotum or labia majora, especially during straining or crying. Incarceration develops in 10% of children but can be reduced after sedation and gentle palpation in the majority. Incarceration should be followed by hernia repair within 48 hours. The risk of strangulation is much greater in the small newborn and in the first year of life, and is suspected if vomiting and abdominal distension develop in the presence of a tender, non-reducible mass. In neonates, surgical repair is best performed prior to discharge from hospital, whereas in the infant age group, repair should be effected electively soon after diagnosis. There is less urgency in older children, where the abdominal defect is wide and the hernia is rarely complicated by bowel obstruction. Any associated anomaly such as undescended testes should be addressed concurrently. The operative complication rate and recurrence risk for inguinal repair are 1% and 4%, respectively.

Hydrocoele

Although not strictly hernias, hydrocoeles are commonly associated with inguinal hernias especially in neonates. They arise when persistence of the processus allows fluid to accumulate in the scrotal sac. The anomaly is usually bilateral and produces painless, cystic swellings that transilluminate brilliantly, sometimes with testicular shadows visible within. Most will resolve spontaneously. Surgery is only indicated when hydrocoeles persist beyond 12 months and involves ligation of the patent processus vaginalis.

Gastroschisis

Gastroschisis describes herniation of loops of bowel not encased within a sac of Wharton's jelly through a defect in the abdominal wall usually to the right of the umbilicus (Fig. 80a). The diagnosis is usually made on antena-

a   b

Fig. 80 (a) Congenital gastroschisis: herniation of naked bowel, sometimes strangulated, in an otherwise normal infant. (b) Exomphalos: bowel plus abdominal viscera herniate in a sac of Wharton's jelly; other anomalies may coexist.

tal ultrasound and naked bowel loops are seen extruding through the abdominal wall at birth. The newborn must be resuscitated, and not fed; an NGT is passed and intravenous fluids commenced. The bowel is wrapped in warm plastic film to prevent heat loss and excessive drying prior to surgery. Surgery may necessitate bowel resection if the extruded loops undergo external volvulus and ischaemia. Problems may be encountered on attempting to reinsert the bowel into a relatively small, underdeveloped abdominal cavity, and a staged closure procedure is required.

Exomphalos

With exomphalos (omphalocoele), abdominal contents including bowel and viscera such as liver and spleen herniate through the umbilicus in a sac of Wharton's jelly (Fig. 80b). This occurs in approximately 1 in 5000 births. This defect, unlike gastroschisis, may be associated with abnormalities of the karyotype as well as congenital anomalies of the cardiovascular, urogenital and neurological systems. The association of exomphalos with macroglossia, gigantism and neonatal hypoglycaemia constitute features of the Beckwith–Wiedemann syndrome.

Fig. 81 Intravenous pyelogram showing hydronephrosis and a duplex left-sided collecting system.

Neurological abnormalities

Neural tube defects and hydrocephalus

These are discussed in Chapter 6.

Craniosynostosis

The premature fusion of one or more cranial sutures results in an abnormally shaped head and, in some cases, increased intracranial pressure. Craniosynostosis may occur as part of a multiple malformation syndrome, often with autosomal dominant inheritance, e.g. Crouzon syndrome (with proptosis and conductive hearing loss) and Apert syndrome (with syndactyly). The management involves complex, combined faciomaxillary and neurosurgical repair.

Urogenital abnormalities

The primitive kidney develops from the mesonephric duct and migrates upwards along the posterior abdominal wall to lie in the paravertebral gutter beneath the overhanging lower ribs. Defects in this embryological process result in congenital anomalies of the renal tracts and are very common both in isolation and in association with anomalies of other major systems, including the heart, brain, gastrointestinal tract and skeleton. In the **prune-belly syndrome**, renal anomalies are associated with poor renal function and absent abdominal musculature and undescended testes. This condition, like many severe congenital renal anomalies, results in oligohydramnios and secondary pulmonary hypoplasia.

Hydronephrosis

Obstruction at the pelviureteric (PUJ) or vesicoureteric junction (VUJ), ureters and urethra result in retrograde pressure and dilatation of the urinary tract. Renal pelvic dilatation (hydronephrosis) may be seen on antenatal ultrasound scan, and if severe, may be associated with renal dysfunction. Attempts to alleviate the pressure by the insertion of drains antenatally have produced disappointing results and postnatal procedures are favoured. Postnatal serial ultrasound scans are performed to monitor the progression of the hydronephrosis; micturating cystoureterograms (MCUG) to assess ureteric reflux and a DTPA (diethylenetriamine pentaacetic acid) or MAG3 isotope excretion scan to assess renal function.

Early surgery is indicated if there is bilateral disease, severe reflux and renal dysfunction. Nephrosotomy drainage is beneficial in the short term, pyeloplasty for PUJ obstruction and ureteric reimplantation for VUJ obstruction. The outcome is related to the degree of obstruction and extent of renal parenchymal dysfunction, especially if both kidneys are involved.

Fig. 82 X-ray showing dilated bowel loop with clear 'cut off' suggestive of intussusception.

Duplex system and ureterocoele

A duplex system generally involves a second ureter draining an abnormal, often obstructed, upper pole renal moiety and connecting lower down than the normal ureter into the bladder or reproductive organs (Fig. 81). If renal function is satisfactory, the ureter should be reimplanted, although in most cases a nephroureterectomy is necessary. Cystic dilatation of the lower ureter produces a ureterocoele, commonly associated with duplex systems, and which almost invariably results in ureteric obstruction.

Treatment involves excision and ureteric reimplantation in all but the smallest lesions.

Posterior urethral valves

Posterior urethral valves are congenital valves that lie within the posterior urethra in boys and result in severe obstruction with subsequent dilatation of the renal tracts. They are a cause of renal failure in infancy and early intervention is essential. The diagnosis is confirmed by MCUG and during cystoscopy, when ablation/resection of the valves can be carried out. The prognosis is worse in those with deranged renal function, ureteric reflux and urinary infection. A third of patients go on to develop end-stage renal failure and require renal transplantation.

Ambiguous genitalia

The surgical treatment of ambiguous genitalia is covered in Chapter 8.

12.3 Acquired surgical abnormalities

Obstructive gastrointestinal lesions

Pyloric stenosis

Pyloric stenosis involves hypertrophic enlargement of the gastric pylorus, resulting in high gastrointestinal obstruction. It typically presents with vomiting and weight loss in males (especially first born and with a family history) at around the age of 3–6 weeks. Non-bilious vomiting occurs soon after feeds and becomes progressively more forceful until it is dramatically 'projectile'. Infants are immediately hungry after vomiting. Clinical signs include visible peristalsis from left to right across the upper abdomen, wasting and dehydration in severe disease. A pyloric 'tumour' the size of an olive may be palpable while the infant is being fed (i.e. during a test meal), and the thickened gastric wall can be confirmed by ultrasound scanning. Hypochloraemic metabolic alkalosis may be present because of loss of chloride and hydrogen ions from the stomach. Hypokalaemia may follow compensatory exchange of potassium ions for hydrogen ions in the kidneys. Management involves rehydration with dextrose–saline and potassium supplementation. This is usually sufficient to revert the alkalosis prior to surgical Ramstedt's pyloromyotomy.

Hernias

Epigastric and **umbilical** hernias are usually small (less than 1 cm) and resolve spontaneously as the child grows, negating the need for surgical intervention. They are invariably present after repair of an exomphalos and require simple closure with adjoining of the rectus abdominis muscles at the age of 2–4 years. **Inguinal** hernias are discussed above.

Intussusception

The majority of intussusception arises in infants, mostly boys, aged between 3 months and 3 years and generally does not have an underlying abnormality in the bowel. In a few cases, a bowel polyp, Meckel diverticulum, inflammatory mass (e.g. Peyer patch), haematoma (e.g. with Henoch–Schönlein purpura), or lymphomatous mass presents a focus for gastrointestinal peristalsis to 'push the bowel along' as the inner intussusceptum. The latter is often composed of terminal ileum and ascending colon and is often held up in the outer intussuscipiens at the level of the transverse colon. Eventually stretching of the adjoining mesentery and associated oedema compromise the bowel's blood supply and mucosal sloughing ensues. Hence, an initial history of recurrent paroxysmal abdominal pain, often with pallor, screaming and drawing up of the lower limbs, is followed by a deterioration in the general condition and 'redcurrant jelly' stools. The stools contains mucus, mucosa and blood and imply mucosal sloughing as a result of bowel ischaemia. Hopefully, the diagnosis is suspected earlier on the basis of a good history and the finding of a sausage-shaped mass, usually in the epigastric region. The mass may vary in size and position, is ill defined in between spasms and may be more readily palpated by simultaneous abdominal and rectal examination. A plain abdominal X-ray film may show a dilated bowel shadow with a clear 'cut-off' in the region of the splenic or hepatic flexures (Fig. 82), whereas the double ring appearance of intussusceptum within intussuscipiens is evident on ultrasound. However, the latter investigation is usually waived and the diagnosis confirmed on a contrast enema. In experienced hands, this is best performed using air as the contrast medium, going on to attempt to reduce the intussusception by pressure-regulated air insufflation. This is contraindicated in those where significant bowel ischaemia or perforation is suspected, when urgent surgery should follow resuscitation. Any gangrenous portions and leading focus will need to be resected/biopsied, the intussusception undone and the residual bowel re-anastomosed.

Despite a small risk of recurrence (10% with hydrostatic and 2% with surgical reduction), the prognosis is excellent provided the diagnosis is suspected and treatment commenced before gangrene is established. If untreated, this condition is usually fatal.

Meckel diverticulum

Meckel diverticulum is a small bowel outcrop formed as a remnant of the omphalomesenteric (yolk) sac. It usually measures 3–6 cm and is positioned on the antimesenteric border, 50 cm proximal to the caecum. It is usually an incidental finding at laparotomy. In the majority of symptomatic cases, the diverticulum contains ectopic gastric mucosa that secretes acid, resulting in ulceration of the surrounding ileal mucosa and painless rectal bleeding, manifest as brick-red stools. Meckel diverticulum may result in an intussusception and may occasionally become inflamed, presenting in a similar fashion to acute appendicitis. Where the diverticulum is attached to the abdominal wall by a fibrous band, a volvulus and bowel obstruction may ensue. These patients will present with acute or subacute abdominal pain, sometimes localised to the periumbilical region, and vomiting. Acute attacks cannot be differentiated from acute appendicitis and the diagnosis is often confirmed at surgery. When Meckel diverticulum is suspected in patients with subacute symptoms, the diverticulum can be demonstrated by intravenous injection of a technetium-99m pertechnetate (^{99m}Tc)-labelled tracer, which is taken up by the ectopic gastric mucosa producing a

'hot spot' on imaging. Treatment involves surgical resection of the diverticulum.

Inflammatory gastrointestinal conditions

Appendicitis

Appendicitis remains the most common ailment requiring surgery in childhood. It arises through inflammation of the redundant appendix, possibly after blockage of the lumen by a faecolith, occasionally a tumour, foreign body, infection (Salmonella, Shigella, Ascaris spp.) or abnormal mucus (e.g. cystic fibrosis). If untreated, venous congestion gives way to bacterial invasion, abscess formation and mucosal ischaemia, with eventual perforation and peritonitis. Because of the difficulty of making the correct diagnosis in childhood, perforation occurs in up to 70% of those aged less than 4 years, compared with 30% in adolescents. Patients usually present with a 24–36-hour history of central abdominal pain, low-grade fever, nausea and vomiting. The last follows the pain and is usually infrequent. Diarrhoea, if present, is generally unimpressive. As the inflammation extends to the appendiceal peritoneum, the pain is localised to McBurney's point, two-thirds distance between the umbilicus and right anterior superior iliac spine. Maximal tenderness with rebound is found on examination in this area. If these signs are absent, it is prudent to perform a per rectal examination to exclude tenderness in the right pararectal area, suggestive of a retrocaecal inflamed appendix. Systemic debility together with generalised abdominal pain, rebound and guarding are suggestive of peritonitis. Symptoms and signs are localised to the left side in those with situs inversus. Investigations are useful to eliminate other conditions in the differential diagnosis (Table 68) but are unnecessary if the clinical diagnosis is not in doubt.

Management
Acute appendicitis is associated with a mortality of about 0.5%, mainly through missed or delayed diagnosis, resulting in perforation and infection.

Treatment consists of preoperative resuscitation with fluids and analgesia followed by an appendicectomy. Routine preoperative antibiotics reduce postoperative wound infection. Broad-spectrum cover is required for those with an abscess or perforation.

Inflammatory bowel disease

Ideally surgery is avoided in children with inflammatory bowel disease. It is sometimes necessary to treat localised areas of severe inflammation, bleeding, constriction and chronic fistulation in **Crohn disease**. However, the risk of recurrence is almost 50% within 5 years of surgery and surgery may potentiate fistulation, stricture and adhesion formation. Resection should be kept to a minimum to avoid a short-bowel syndrome.

Table 68 Differential diagnosis in acute appendicitis

Diagnosis	Symptoms and signs	Investigation
Infection		
Urinary tract	Urinary symptoms	Urinalysis
Gastrointestinal (e.g. *Salmonella*, *Campylobacter*, *Shigella*, *Yersinia*, *Ascaris* spp.)	Vomiting before pain Diarrhoea dominant	Stool, blood culture
Inflammatory conditions		
Mesenteric adenitis	Prodrome, pain not localised	
Henoch–Schönlein purpura	Skin, joint problems	Urinalysis, full blood count normal
Crohn's, ulcerative colitis	Pain, diarrhoea, weight loss	Contrast meal, biopsy
Chemotherapy typhilitis	Drug history, diarrhoea	Neutropenic
Surgical disorders		
Torsion, undescended testis	Testes absent	Abdominal ultrasound scan
Intussusception	Paroxysmal pain, mass	X-ray, contrast enema
Meckel diverticulum	Similar symptoms, signs	^{99m}Tc-labelled tracer scan
Constipation	Infrequent, firm stool	Examination per rectum, plain abdominal X-ray

Associated abscesses often need surgical drainage in both Crohn's disease and **ulcerative colitis**. In the latter, an acute deterioration in the general condition associated with increased loose bloody stool, abdominal pain, distension and diminished bowel sounds may herald **toxic megacolon**. Failure to respond rapidly to conservative management involving intravenous hydration, analgesia, broad-spectrum antibiotics and anti-inflammatory agents is an indication for an emergency total colectomy.

Urological abnormalities

Obstructive lesions

Acquired hydronephrosis, PUJ and VUJ obstruction require similar treatment to the congenital lesions (see above). Subsequent ureteric stenosis following previous surgery may be alleviated by pyeloplasty techniques employed during cystoscopy. Polyps and tumours, usually botyroid sarcomas in children, may be found in the bladder and require resection and appropriate chemotherapy.

Urinary calculi

Urinary calculi develop in patients with abnormal urine or those with abnormal urinary tracts, especially if this is associated with urinary stasis and recurrent infection. Stones often result in frank or microscopic haematuria, bouts of recurrent renal colic, symptoms of an associated urinary tract infection and occasionally acute ureteric obstruction. Stones are usually demonstrated on ultra-

sound imaging and, if calcified, on plain abdominal X-ray film. If found, a full assessment of the urinary tracts is necessary to rule out stasis, obstruction or infection. A screen of the serum and urine will exclude a metabolic disorder predisposing to stone formation (Box 38).

Management
Many calculi, both intrarenal (e.g. nephrocalcinosis) and those lying within the collecting system, are small and require medical management aimed at the underlying metabolic disorder and control of infection. Larger calculi (e.g. staghorn calculi) are typically associated with infection, especially caused by *Proteus* species. Treatment is directed at ensuring a constant diuresis and appropriate urine pH to prevent stone precipitation. Occasionally open surgery is required for those stones resulting in severe bleeding, obstruction or recurrent infection. For appropriately sized and positioned stones, lithotripsy can be used.

Abnormalities of the reproductive organs

Testes

Undescended testes

Undescended testes are found in about 1% of boys, usually during routine examination. Bilateral undescended testes occur in 25% of affected individuals and may be associated with dysmorphic syndromes and karyotypic abnormalities. Undescended testes may arise because of incomplete descent along the normal tract, usually as a

---

BOX 38
Causes of urinary calculi

Abnormal urine and serum

Excess salts: hypercalcaemia, hypercalciuria, hyperphosphaturia
Organic acids: hyperuricaemia, hyperoxaluria
Amino acids: xanthinuria, cystinuria

Abnormal urinary tract

Recurrent infection
Pelviureteric or vesicoureteric junction obstruction
Duplex systems
Renal tubular acidosis

result of a short spermatic cord. Alternatively, maldescent of the gonad results in the testes lying in an ectopic position. Some testes are particularly retractile and it is important to palpate with warm hands, locating and 'fixing' one side first, before searching for the missing organ throughout the inguinal region down to the scrotum. If located, a gentle attempt should be made to determine the extent to which the testes can be milked into the scrotum. Ultrasound scanning may locate missing/abdominal testes. Testes lying outside the scrotum will not function normally and, if bilateral, carry a high risk of infertility. In addition, intra-abdominal testes have a 30-fold increased risk of malignant change (usually seminoma) after the third decade of life. Hence, orchidopexy, whereby the testis is untethered and fixed in the scrotum, should be performed between the age of 1 and 2 years. Any associated inguinal hernia and hydrocoele should be treated simultaneously.

Testicular torsion

Testicular torsion arises when the testis twists on its vascular pedicle, producing venous congestion and local ischaemia. The condition presents with acute pain and local swelling in preschool and school-age boys. Examination confirms a tender, swollen scrotal mass associated with bluish discoloration. The testis is often not palpable within the swelling, which does not transilluminate.

Management
Treatment entails analgesia followed by urgent surgical untwisting of the affected organ. In view of the risk of recurrence bilaterally, orchidopexy (fixation) of *both* testes in the scrotum is performed. Surgery within 6 hours of torsion carries a 90% chance of testicular salvage but a good outcome is unlikely with prolonged delay. Torsion in neonates usually results in infarction and later involution with loss of the testis. Supportive treatment is appropriate in the first instance, with prosthetic implants later in life and, for those with bilateral infarction, testosterone replacement.

Malignant swelling

Malignant testicular swelling is usually caused by leukaemic–lymphomatous infiltration, rarely by primary testicular teratomas. While biopsy is required in the first instance, total excision is indicated for a primary tumour, followed by chemoradiotherapy as appropriate.

Penis

Hypospadias, present in 0.2% of newborns, arises when the meatus opens somewhere along the ventral aspect of the penile shaft. Most are glandular and of little consequence; more severe forms result in penile curvature (chordee). Up to 10% are associated with undescended testes and inguinal hernias and, as with those patients

with hypospadias resulting in ambiguous genitalia, require karyotype analysis. Treatment entails expert plastic repair to achieve a normal appearance, voiding and sexual function.

Female reproductive tract

Imperforate hymen presents with primary amenorrhoea and requires simple dissection and release of intravaginal contents. All forms of **ovarian cancer** are extremely rare in childhood and include leukaemic infiltration, teratoma and dysgerminoma. The prognosis is generally poor except with highly differentiated multicystic teratoma, which is cured by total resection.

12.4 Orthopaedic disorders

Congenital abnormalities

Congenital dislocation of the hip (CDH)

Congenital dislocation of the hip (CDH) has a variable presentation and is probably better termed as developmental dysplasia of the hip, to reflect its many facets. The disorder is related to ligament laxity, breech delivery and neuromuscular disease and has a multifactorial pattern of inheritance. Although unstable (clicky) hips are seen in 1% of all newborns, true dislocation affects 1 in 1000 live-born infants and is more common in girls (9:1). **Subluxatable** hips lie 'loose' and the femoral head slides in the acetabulum. **Subluxated** hips lie away from the floor of the acetabulum. **Dislocatable** hips can be manually displaced from the acetabulum with a palpable clunk. The hip is considered to be dislocated when the femoral head lies outside the acetabulum. The diagnosis of CDH is made by routine physical examination of the newborn, as shown in Figure 83.

Beyond 2–3 months, the characteristic instability of the joints may be lost and there is more likely to be limited abduction of the hip and asymmetrical skin folds. Persistent dislocation and late-onset subluxations are associated with permanent dysplastic changes at the hip, an unstable waddling gait and a positive Trendelenburg test (Fig. 84).

The place of radiology in the diagnosis of CDH is controversial and currently ultrasound is proving to be more valuable than X-ray as it is able to reveal the cartilaginous areas of the joints and dynamic instability during movement of the hip.

Treatment should be started at once. The hips are held in at least 90° flexion and 60° abduction using a device (e.g. Malmö splint or Pavlik harness). Dislocations resistant to conservative management are treated with adductor tenotomies and closed reduction and a hip spica. Abnormalities persisting beyond 18 months of age are difficult to manage and may require open reduction with realigning derotation osteotomies and possibly acetabular angulation.

Fig. 83 Clinical manoeuvres to detect CDH in the neonatal period. (a) The Ortolani manoeuvre is a reduction manoeuvre to place a hip back into the normal position. The hip is abducted slightly, then with the index and long fingers over the greater trochanter the thigh is raised to gently reduce the hip. (b) The Barlow provocative test detects whether the hip is subluxatable or dislocatable. The thumb is placed on the inner aspect of the thigh near the lesser trochanter. The hip is adducted and longitudinal pressure is exerted on the thigh with the thumb pushing it towards the table. In both instances the other hand is used to stabilise the pelvis.

Talipes varus and valgus

Club foot may be caused by neuromuscular imbalance of the lower foot, sometimes vertical malposition of the talus. It arises in 0.1% of predominantly male births and is bilateral in 50% of patients. Club foot can produce inward, medial deviation of the forefoot (talipes equino varus, TEV), or abduction at the ankle with external, lat- eral deviation of the forefoot (talipes calcaneo valgus, TCV, Fig. 85). Although these anomalies may be features of a generalised dysmorphic syndrome, they are usually isolated findings. The severity of the condition is assessed on clinical appearance and the ease by which the foot can be brought into the normal position by sim- ple manipulation. Minor problems resolve with physio- therapy and positioning exercises, which can be taught

Fig. 84 Trendelenburg's test. Bearing weight on the normal left leg (a) causes the pelvis to tilt up with elevation of the opposite leg. Standing on the right leg (b) with the unstable hip causes the pelvis to tilt down and the buttock to fall; compensatory scoliosis.

Fig. 85 (a) Congenital talipes equino varus and (b) calcaneo valgus.

to the parents. Severe deviation may require serial orthopaedic manipulation, malleable splints, plaster casts and, if there is no improvement by 3 months, refashioning surgical procedures before normal alignment is achieved.

Skeletal dysplasias

There are a multitude of congenital and hereditary conditions that result in abnormal bone and skeletal development. Although many of the conditions listed in Table 69 are extremely rare, others are sufficiently common to present in most paediatric and orthopaedic practices.

Osteogenesis imperfecta
Osteogenesis imperfecta results from abnormal bony moulding and ossification giving rise to brittle bones. The severe dominant variants are associated with multiple fractures in utero and may be lethal, especially when multiple rib fractures result in a collapsed thorax and significant pulmonary hypoplasia. Recessive forms are more benign, presenting with recurrent fractures after minor trauma and are associated with blue sclerae.

Treatment involves reduction of the fractures and genetic counselling.

Achondroplasia
Achondroplasia is the most common short-limb syndrome, affecting 1 in 2000 live births. It is dominantly inherited although 80% of new cases are spontaneous mutations. It results in characteristic short limb bones and abnormalities in moulding of the bones at the base of the skull. Subluxation of the cervical atlanto-axial joint makes intubation and manipulation under general anaesthetic potentially hazardous. Other forms of short-limb skeletal dysplasias are rare and often lethal, especially when associated with significant involvement of the thoracic cage.

Skeletal malformations

Scoliosis
Scoliosis is usually a primary, idiopathic condition that is slightly more common but often more severe in girls. Occasionally, scoliosis is secondary to a fixed abnormality in the vertebral column (e.g. hemivertebra, skeletal dysplasia), neuromuscular disease, neurocutaneous syndrome and ligamentous laxity (e.g. Marfan syndrome). Functional scoliosis occurs secondary to disproportionate spasm following a neuromuscular disorder involving the vertebral column and spinal nerves (Box 39).

A full examination is essential to exclude any associated abnormality. The back is examined from behind for

Table 69 Skeletal dysplasia and malformations

Disorders	Inheritance	Description
Generalised disorders		
Osteogenesis imperfecta	AD, AR	Brittle bones, fractures, blue sclerae
Multiple exostosis (diaphyseal aclasis)	AD	Disfiguring bony outgrowths
Multiple enchondromata (Ollier disease)	SP	Intraosseous expanding chondromas
Osteopetrosis (Albers–Schönberg disease)	AR	Dense, brittle, marble bones; loss of bone marrow
Short-limb syndromes		
Achondroplasia	AD	Short limbs, large head
Thanatophoric dwarfism	SP	Short limbs, thoracic hypoplasia
Jeune syndrome	AR	Asphyxiating thoracic dystrophy
Isolated patchy disorders		
Fibrous dysplasia (McCune–Albright syndrome)	SP	Patchy hyperpigmentation, patchy fibrous bony disorganisation

AD, autosomal dominant; AR, autosomal recessive; SP, sporadic inheritance.

BOX 39
Causes of scoliosis

Primary scoliosis

Idiopathic scoliosis
Congenital scoliosis
Hemivertebra, unsegmented vertebrae
Spina bifida
As part of syndromes (VATER, neurofibromatosis, Marfan, Klippel–Feil, Sprengel)

Secondary scoliosis

Neuromuscular scoliosis
Cerebral palsy
Muscular dystrophy
Spinal muscular atrophy
Compensatory scoliosis
Muscular strain
Osteomyelitis in vertebrae
Spinal, extraspinal tumour
Lower limb, pelvic discrepancy

symmetry and curvature after correction for any discrepancy in the pelvis, hips and lower limb lengths. Both lateral (scoliosis) and anterior (kyphosis) displacement should be assessed as the patient stands and bends forward. Serial standing X-ray films will confirm and monitor the progression of the curve. The risk of progression is greatest in premenarchal girls with a curve greater than 20°. Often those between 25° and 45° are managed with orthotic devices (e.g. Milwaukee brace), whereas greater curves require surgery, generally entailing posterior spinal fusion with a prosthetic support (e.g. Harrington rod).

Sprengel shoulder

Sprengel shoulder involves a high riding and underdeveloped scapula (usually unilaterally) that requires orthopaedic reconstructive surgery.

Asymmetric limb shortening

Asymmetric limb shortening may be associated with various syndromes (e.g. Russell–Silver), unilateral underdevelopment and limb ischaemia. It may be treated with limb-lengthening procedures.

Acquired inflammatory conditions

Infective osteomyelitis and arthritis

Osteomyelitis

Osteomyelitis is almost exclusively caused by bacterial organisms except in utero, when osteitis secondary to rubella and cytomegalovirus occurs. Staphylococcal species are the usual infecting organisms although tuberculous osteomyelitis is still seen, even in developed countries (Table 70). This deep-seated infection is not only a feature of neonates and the immunosuppressed but is also seen in otherwise normal children who are not at particular risk of infection. Bacteraemia, often without clinical manifestations, results in the 'seeding' of micro-organisms in bone where an indolent abscess develops. A 'spiking' fever with general malaise is usually associated with local erythema, swelling, tenderness over the affected bone and limitation of movement (pseudoparalysis) because of pain. Neurological signs may arise following spinal compression in those with spinal osteomyelitis and vertebral collapse.

Investigations confirm the site and extent of infection and identify the organism. The white cell count and erythrocyte sedimentation rate (ESR) are usually raised. *Several* blood cultures must be taken, preferably during temperature spikes when the microbiological yield is likely to be greatest. At times, especially in those partially treated with oral antibiotics, microbiological confirmation is only successful on culture of a biopsy specimen. X-ray films are usually unremarkable in the early stages of infection but after 2 weeks show bony irregularities, rarefaction, cystic changes and, eventually, a periosteal reaction with sclerosis and increased ossification. An isotope-labelled scan employing technetium-99m will show an area of increased uptake ('hot spot') and is essential in children with a high swinging fever and evidence of bacterial sepsis but without an obvious focus.

Treatment entails combination antibiotics given for 6 weeks and administered via the intravenous route for at least 10 to 14 days. Neonates should be given combination antibiotics to cover *Staphylococcus aureus* and group B streptococci plus Gram-negative coliforms (e.g. methicillin and an aminoglycoside). Children under 5 years are covered for *S. aureus* and *Haemophilus influenzae* type b with cefuroxime or ceftriaxone. Older children with proven *S. aureus* infection receive flucloxacillin and fusidic acid. Large collections of pus require drainage. Those with sickle cell disease should be given flucloxacillin plus an aminoglycoside, whereas clindamycin is effective against anaerobes. Tuberculous osteomyelitis necessitates triple therapy with rifampicin, isoniazid and ethambutol.

Subacute infection may become walled off by sclerosis, resulting in a localised abscess (Brodie abscess), typically in the upper tibia. Chronic osteomyelitis that persists for months despite adequate antibiotics results in marked radiological changes, with widespread bone disruption and necrosis, ossification layering beneath the periosteum (involucrum), cystic cavities and sclerot-

Table 70 Infecting organisms in osteomyelitis

Organism	Patients	Sites	Comments
Staphylococcus aureus	All groups	Any	Commonest organism
Haemophilus influenzae type b	<3 years	Any	Becoming rare
Group B streptococci	Neonates	Any	
Coliforms	Neonates	Any	
Neisseria sp.	Neonates	Any	Also sexually active
Streptococcal spp.	All groups	Any, foot	
Gram-negative bacilli	All groups	Any	
Pseudomonas spp.	All groups	Foot	Also immunoparesis
Salmonella spp.	Sickle cell disease	Any, vertebrae	
Brucella spp.	Older children	Any, vertebrae	
Anaerobes	After bites, trauma	Local bones	
Mycobacteria (TB)	Older children	Any, spine	Also immunoparesis
Fungi	Neonates	Any	Also immunoparesis

ic necrotic bony fragments (sequestrum). Surgical reconstruction with bone graft augmentation may be necessary, especially in those with an adjoining septic arthritis and development of a Charcot joint. Children with recurrent or multifocal osteomyelitis, especially involving atypical organisms, must be investigated for an underlying immunoparesis.

Septic arthritis

Septic arthritis is often caused by similar organisms to osteomyelitis (Table 70) with *S. aureus* being the most common agent in neonates and children over the age of 5 years and, until the advent of Hib vaccine, *H. influenzae* in those aged 2 months to 5 years. Up to 30% have an associated osteomyelitis. Patients present with a fever, swelling, erythema, warmth, pain and limitation of movement in the affected joint, which assumes a position that offers maximal pain relief (antalgic posture). Management is similar to osteomyelitis. Blood cultures are positive in 35% of patients, whereas diagnostic arthrocentesis reveals a positive growth in 75% of infections. The joint must be aspirated and immobilised in its functional position for 72 hours before physiotherapy is started to prevent permanent contractures and arthrodesis.

Inflammatory arthritis

Transient arthralgia

Transient arthralgia is relatively common in childhood and presents with pain and local limitation of movement following a viral upper respiratory tract infection (URTI). It usually affects the hips and is the most likely cause of an irritable hip. A non-deforming, self-limiting **reactive arthritis** may follow gastrointestinal illnesses, especially those caused by salmonella, shigella, campylobacter and yersinia. Joint pain, swelling and restricted movement usually involve the larger joints (e.g. knee, ankle) and may be associated with impressive sterile effusions that require drainage.

Treatment includes analgesia, anti-inflammatory agents e.g. non-steroidal anti-inflammatory drugs (NSAIDs), physiotherapy and mobilisation as early as possible.

Arthritis and arthralgia are common manifestations of other conditions in childhood, including inflammatory bowel disease, psoriasis, Reiter disease, systemic lupus erythematosus (SLE) and the vasculitides. The last include a number of rare inflammatory conditions, including Kawasaki disease, polyarteritis nodosa and Henoch–Schönlein purpura.

Rheumatoid conditions

Rheumatoid conditions in childhood are rare. Rheumatoid factor (RF)-positive **polyarticular juvenile chronic rheumatoid arthritis** (JCA) is similar to the multiarticular condition seen in adulthood and usually affects girls (80%). The small joints of the hands and feet are predominantly involved; patients presenting with

stiffness and joint pain, particularly in the morning. Chronic, progressive joint deformity develops in 60% of affected patients. RF-negative polyarticular JCA tends to present earlier in childhood, is generally mild and is rarely associated with complications such as pericardial, pleural and peritoneal involvement and rheumatoid nodules. **Pauciarticular arthritis** is usually RF negative and generally involves less than four large joints. **Systemically presenting rheumatoid disease** (Still's disease) is largely associated with extra-articular manifestations. It presents with a fever of unknown origin, together with erythematous rashes, generalised lymphadenopathy, mild hepatosplenomegaly and, occasionally, rheumatoid nodules. Joint involvement is late or initially unimpressive, though up to 25% go on to develop chronic, debilitating arthritis.

Investigations often confirm anaemia with a raised white cell count, sometimes with a striking neutrophilia, raised platelet count, elevated ESR, acute-phase reactants (such as C-reactive protein (CRP)) and complement levels (C3, C4). In childhood, RF and anti-nuclear antigen (ANA) are generally negative.

First-line management includes control of the temperature and the use of anti-inflammatory agents such as aspirin and NSAIDs. Disease-modifying drugs such as gold salts, D-penicillamine and methotrexate are all associated with serious side-effects and their use must be monitored carefully in a specialist centre. Steroids are only indicated for severe, unresponsive systemic disease and iridocyclitis. Initial protection of any affected joints should be followed by disciplined physiotherapy, occupational therapy and early mobilisation. The use of special splints can greatly improve function, and orthopaedic procedures are applied to treat severe joint deformities.

Ischaemia and apophysitis

Irritable hip

The irritable hip is caused by local painful inflammation in the hip(s) and presents with a limp. It is generally seen in boys aged 3–8 years and may be secondary to a self-limiting, transient synovitis following a viral URTI or local jarring trauma after a fall. Pain and a limp are associated with limitation in abduction and internal rotation. Investigations including X-rays should be normal.

Treatment is conservative, with analgesia and bed rest, preferably for 7 days.

With similar symptoms in the 5–10 age group, the possibility of **Perthes disease** must be considered. This is presumably caused by compromise of the delicate blood supply to the growing femoral head, resulting in ischaemic necrosis. Degenerative fragmentation produces distinctive radiological changes, including flattening of the femoral head, sclerosis with cystic changes in both the femoral head and acetabulum, and widening of the femoral metaphysis (Fig. 86). The con-

Fig. 86 (a) Perthes disease. Destruction of the femoral head with sclerosis, cystic changes and metaphyseal widening. Note similar changes in acetabulum. (b) Slipped upper femoral epiphysis with posterior, downward displacement of the femoral head.

dition usually affects boys (5:1) and is bilateral in 20%. Analgesia should be combined with strict bed rest and abduction stretching exercises until symptoms resolve and regeneration is evident on X-ray film. Although most will recover fully, in others destruction of the femoral head is permanent. This is more likely the greater the degree of initial fragmentation and in those aged 10 years or more, when prolonged bed rest with hip traction is indicated. Containment of the femoral head is achieved with the use of an abduction cast/orthosis though results are better with surgical osteotomy. In severe cases, femoral osteotomy is combined with the insertion of pins to fix the femoral head in the acetabulum, thereby stabilising the situation until regeneration occurs. Osteoarthritis of the affected joint is a late complication.

Slipped upper femoral epiphysis

Slipped upper femoral epiphysis (SUFE) affects mostly overweight boys above the age of 10 years. The condition is usually chronic with symptoms of pain and a limp for several months. Occasionally slippage is acute, patients presenting with severe pain and inability to bear weight. There is external rotation of the affected limb with loss of internal rotation, flexion and abduction at the hip. Evidence of posterior displacement of the femoral head is seen on anteroposterior and lateral X-ray films of the hips (Fig. 86b). If analgesia, bed rest and hip traction do not suffice, pinning of the femoral head (epiphysiodesis) in order to prevent further slippage is indicated. The possibility of coexisting hypothyroidism and pituitary disease must be excluded. Severe

cases will result in osteoarthritis of the hip joint in early adulthood.

Trauma

Fractures

Fractures are extremely common in active children, especially boys. They should be suspected, looked for on X-ray and reduced with appropriate strapping or plaster. Most fractures in childhood involve self-resolving greenstick fractures. However, fractures may be associated with serious complications, especially following major, multiple trauma, as seen with road traffic accidents or a fall from height. In this instance, the whole child must be examined thoroughly, the general condition stabilised and organ and soft tissue injuries addressed. The risk of infection with compound fractures is great and these must be treated aggressively with intravenous antibiotics. Air embolism may complicate open, compound fractures involving the long bones. Non-fusion and pseudoarthrosis may require re-fracturing and pinning under general anaesthetic.

Soft tissue injuries

The multitraumatised child with injury to several major organs presents a major challenge to the paediatric resuscitative team. A thorough detailed assessment of the child must be performed and repeated as the condition alters. The key to management is identifying all the problems and correcting these in order of urgency.

Intravenous access and blood sampling for cross-match are a priority. Major, life-threatening problems such as cardiorespiratory failure (e.g. caused by a pneumothorax and tamponade), organ lacerations, transected blood vessels, etc. must be corrected urgently. Non-life-threatening injuries (e.g. skin lacerations) and fractures can be addressed once the patient's condition is relatively stable. Support of the cardiorespiratory, renal and liver function should accompany attention to normalising haematological and metabolic indices.

12.5 Disorders of the ears, nose and throat

Congenital anomalies

Cleft lip and palate

Cleft lip and palate are relatively common abnormalities, with an incidence of about 1 in 1000. They may be isolated or form part of a generalised chromosomal abnormality (e.g. trisomy 13) or syndrome (e.g. Stickler syndrome, in association with eye abnormalities). The clefts may be unilateral or bilateral, partial or complete (Fig. 87). They are usually clinically obvious although small clefts of the uvula may be missed unless a careful examination is made.

Management is best undertaken by an experienced multidisciplinary team. The cleft palate may disrupt feeding, a problem that can be circumvented with the use of special teats. The aesthetically more distressing cleft lip is corrected around the age of 3–6 months. Repair of the palate is delayed to allow for maximal growth, and is carried out once phonation becomes a necessity, usually around 10–15 months. Pharyngoplasty

and surgery for midfacial hypoplasia may be required later in childhood.

Pierre–Robin sequence

The combination of a complete cleft palate with a small lower jaw (micrognathia) results in a major handicap with regard to sucking and feeding. These children are nursed in the prone position on custom-designed frames and require expert nursing care to supervise their feeds. The cleft palate is corrected as soon as possible, care being taken not to disrupt the development of the midface, further compromising the defect.

Abnormalities above the glottis

Congenital abnormalities above the glottis include a cleft glottis and laryngeal web. They present with stridor from birth and are diagnosed by microlaryngo-bronchoscopy (MLB). Repair is carried out as early as possible and follow-up maintained to ensure that stenosis does not develop.

Abnormalities below the glottis

Larnygotracheomalacia is caused by congenital weakness in the laryngeal and tracheal walls, which partially collapse on inspiration. This is the most common cause of neonatal stridor and, in the vast majority, resolves spontaneously as the child grows. Those with severe stridor and airway obstruction requiring repeated intubation may require surgical tracheal reinforcement.

Acquired infective lesions

Infections of the upper airways are discussed in Chapter 3.

Unilateral cleft lip   Bilateral cleft lip   Midline cleft palate

Fig. 87 Clinical appearance of cleft lip and cleft palate.

Problems with foreign bodies

Foreign body inhalation

The possibility of foreign body inhalation is obvious in those who choke and collapse while eating. In many cases, inhalation of a peanut or similar object follows attempts to swallow these once thrown in the air and then caught 'on the wing'. Temporary airway obstruction results in a minor choking or spluttering episode, which is relieved as the foreign object is displaced distally further down the airway. Later, progressive signs of respiratory distress, breathlessness, cyanosis and fever develop as distal obstruction and incipient pneumonia ensue. An early plain chest X-ray film *taken on expiration* may show early air trapping owing to a ball valve effect; later films generally show an area of collapse/consolidation. Most inhaled objects contain organic matter and are not radio-opaque. Once stabilised the child should undergo endoscopic examination under anaesthesia and the foreign body should be removed. Antibiotic cover is advisable for almost all cases.

Foreign body insertion

Children have a predilection for inserting objects such as beads, pencils and rubber erasers into the external auditory meatus or nostrils. If lodged tightly these require expert removal by the ENT surgeon if further trauma and infection to the area are to be avoided.

Self-assessment: questions

Multiple choice questions

1. The following statements describe bowel obstruction:
   a. Vomiting is a feature of upper but not lower gastrointestinal obstruction
   b. Abdominal distension is the most reliable indicator of bowel obstruction
   c. Oesophageal atresia is rarely associated with a tracheo-oesophageal fistula
   d. Duodenal atresia is often seen in children with Down syndrome
   e. High anal atresia has a poor prognosis for future bowel continence

2. The following statements are true:
   a. Gastroschisis is usually an isolated defect
   b. Exomphalos is a feature of Beckwith syndrome
   c. Diaphragmatic hernias are generally left sided
   d. Diaphragmatic hernia is usually associated with pulmonary hypoplasia
   e. Diaphragmatic hernia is usually an isolated defect

3. With regard to neural tube defects:
   a. The incidence of spina bifida is reduced by folic acid in the last trimester
   b. A rise in maternal α-fetoprotein may suggest the presence of a neural tube defect
   c. Open lesions should be closed surgically without delay to avoid infection
   d. Hydrocephalus is a good prognostic feature in association with spina bifida
   e. Neonatal hydrocephalus usually follows a congenital not an acquired defect

4. Hirschsprung disease is characterised by the following:
   a. Bowel obstruction, sometimes from birth
   b. Male preponderance
   c. Normal distribution of neural ganglia in severely affected bowel
   d. A rat-tail appearance on barium enema
   e. Short-segment disease involving the ascending colon

5. The following statements are correct:
   a. Dandy Walker cysts result in hydrocephalus through abnormalities in the IIIrd ventricle
   b. Hydrocephalus may follow decreased absorption of CSF
   c. Hydronephrosis may be detected antenatally
   d. Posterior urethral valves are associated with ureteric reflux in most patients
   e. Surgery for ambiguous genitalia is determined by the patient's karyotype

6. The following statements are correct:
   a. Malrotation arises because of a clockwise twist of the bowel
   b. The inferior mesenteric artery is usually constricted during midgut volvulus
   c. Diaphragmatic hernia is invariably associated with malrotation
   d. Incarceration is more common in infants and neonates
   e. Inguinal hernias are usually direct in type

7. Surgical management of urinary tract obstruction entails:
   a. Resection of posterior urethral valves not before the age of 1 year
   b. Routine antenatal insertion of nephrostomy drains for those with hydronephrosis
   c. Preoperative micturating cystoureterogram for those with megaureters
   d. DTPA scans in children below 1 year with urinary obstruction
   e. Resection and ureteric re-implantation with ureterocoeles

8. The following statement are correct:
   a. Congenital dislocation of the hip is more common in girls
   b. Most 'clicky hips' resolve by 6 weeks
   c. Talipes equinovarus is generally associated with karyotypic abnormalities
   d. Achondroplasia is inherited in a recessive fashion
   e. Slipped upper femoral epiphyses may be associated with abnormalities in growth hormone

9. The following are associated with an increased risk of scoliosis:
   a. Hemivertebrae
   b. Paraspinal, tuberculous abscess
   c. Spinal dysraphism
   d. Congenital dystrophy
   e. Tuberous sclerosis

10. The following statements are correct:
    a. A cleft lip is of greater consequence than a cleft palate
    b. Testicular torsion in the neonate has a good prognosis
    c. Orchidopexy should be performed bilaterally
    d. Meckel diverticulum is found on the mesenteric border
    e. Meckel diverticulum is easily differentiated from acute appendicitis

Short notes

Write short notes on the following:

1. The management of a 6-week-old infant with 10% dehydration caused by a pyloric stenosis that has been confirmed on test feed and ultrasound
2. The investigative approach with a 4-year-old boy who presents with acute pain in the hip
3. The main types and key features of juvenile chronic rheumatoid arthritis
4. The investigation of a 10-year-old child who develops frank haematuria and passes a stone per urethra.

Viva voce question

An 10-month-old infant had bacterial meningitis as a neonate and now has a ventriculoperitoneal shunt for postmeningitis hydrocephalus. He presents to casualty with a 24-hour history of increasing lethargy and vomiting. In view of the possible causes for these symptoms, what questions would you ask of his mother; describe your management.

Self-assessment: answers

Multiple choice answers

1. a. **False**. It is a feature of both, although vomiting occurs earlier in upper rather than lower gastrointestinal obstruction.
   b. **False**. Bile-stained vomiting is the most important sign.
   c. **False**. A fistula is present in the huge majority of patients.
   d. **True**. This is the most common congenital abnormality of the bowel in Down syndrome, although it also occurs in newborns without trisomy 21.
   e. **True**. Especially if the atresia extends well above the pelvic levator sling and is associated with sacral abnormalities and fistulae.

2. a. **True**.
   b. **True**. Other features are macroglossia, gigantism (EMG syndrome), organomegaly and neonatal hypoglycaemia.
   c. **True**. Mostly occurs through the left foramen of Bochdalek.
   d. **True**. This arises through pulmonary compression by the bowel in utero and is a major determinant of outcome.
   e. **True**. However, it is sometimes associated with anomalies of the heart and bowel including tracheo-oesophageal atresia and fistula.

3. a. **False**. Folic acid is given before conception and during early pregnancy.
   b. **True**. Especially with open lesions such as myelomeningocoeles, encephalocoeles and anencephaly.
   c. **True**. The risk of ascending infection leading to encephalitis is very high with open neural tube defects leaking CSF.
   d. **False**. The opposite is true.
   e. **False**. It usually follows intraventricular haemorrhage or infection.

4. a. **True**. Although a physical barrier is not present, the inability of the bowel to undergo normal peristalsis results in a functional obstruction compounded by severe constipation.
   b. **True**. Although *total colonic* disease is more common in females.
   c. **False**. There is a total absence of neural ganglia.
   d. **True**. This describes the radiological appearance of the transition zone, tapering from dilated upper bowel to small-bore aganglionic bowel below.
   e. **False**. Short-segment disease does not extend beyond the descending colon.

5. a. **False**. Abnormalities are in the IVth ventricle.
   b. **True**. Obstruction of the arachnoid granulations after intraventricular haemorrhage prevents CSF absorption.
   c. **True**. By antenatal ultrasound scanning.
   d. **True**. It occurs in two-thirds of patients.
   e. **False**. The male phenotype may be impossible to achieve despite a 46XY karyotype.

6. a. **False**. The twist is anticlockwise.
   b. **False**. The superior mesenteric artery is constricted.
   c. **True**. With a diaphragmatic hernia, the bowel would not have had the opportunity to rotate anticlockwise and assume its normal position.
   d. **True**. Hence, inguinal hernias must be repaired *before* discharge from neonatal units.
   e. **False**. They are usually indirect.

7. a. **False**. Resection should occur as soon as possible after birth.
   b. **False**. This approach is not effective.
   c. **True**. MCUG will assess the degree of reflux.
   d. **False**. This will assess renal function but after 1 year of age.
   e. **True**. Ureterocoeles are associated with ureteric reflux and obstruction that will not resolve without surgery.

8. a. **True**. There is a 4:1 preponderance.
   b. **True**. Most hip 'clicks' without overt dislocation are simply the result of ligamentous stretching.
   c. **False**. It is usually an isolated defect.
   d. **False**. It is a dominant condition.
   e. **True**. Other features are obesity and hypothyroidism.

9. a. **True**. This occurs in primary, structural scoliosis.
   b. **True**. This is secondary scoliosis.
   c. **True**. Spina bifida.
   d. **True**. Myopathies and dystrophies are commonly complicated by progressive scoliosis, which should be looked for on routine examination and spinal X-ray films.
   e. **True**. Although tuberous sclerosis is a neurocutaneous condition, scoliosis is more common in neurofibromatosis.

10. a. **False**. A cleft palate results in feeding problems.
    b. **False**. Most will infarct.
    c. **True**. This is because of the risk of contralateral torsion.
    d. **False**. It is found on the anti-mesenteric border.
    e. **False**. Presentation is usually identical.

Short notes answers

1. The infant should be rehydrated, stabilised by correction of the alkalosis, hypochloraemia and hypokalaemia, and prepared for surgery:

   a. Establish intravenous access
   b. Obtain samples for acid–base status, bicarbonate, chloride and potassium ion levels and cross-match
   c. Record pulse, blood pressure, urine output
   d. Commence rehydration using 0.45–0.9% saline with 5–10% dextrose
   e. Add potassium at 3–4 mmol/kg per day (NB: maintenance 2 mmol/kg per day)
   f. Arrange preoperative anaesthetic review
   g. Organise surgical pyloromyotomy
   h. Monitor with apnoea alarm postoperatively because of the increased risk of apnoeas.

2. The most likely cause would be minor ligamentous strain caused by trauma or transient inflammatory arthralgia. An ischaemic insult (e.g. Perthes disease) is common in this age group, whereas slipped upper femoral epiphysis is unusual. Pauciarticular juvenile arthritis rarely involves a single hip joint, whereas serious infection (e.g. osteomyelitis), tumour and a haematoma are rare. Hence, a clear history of any preceding events including trauma, symptoms of infection (especially upper respiratory and gastrointestinal), a family history of arthritis and bleeding diathesis, and drug history must be sought. Examination should focus on evidence of infection, fever, trauma, generalised lymphadenopathy and signs of arthropathy elsewhere. A full assessment of the affected joint should confirm tenderness and limitation in movement. Investigations include a full blood count with differential, erythrocyte sedimentation rate and anteroposterior and lateral X-ray of the hip in the first instance. Several blood cultures must be taken if there is a high temperature. A clotting screen is essential if a diathesis is suspected, rheumatoid factor and antinuclear antibody for rheumatoid disease, and CT scan with biopsy if a tumour is a possibility following the X-rays.

3. The key differences between the three main types of juvenile chronic rheumatoid arthritis are listed in Table 71.

4. Investigation is directed at excluding an abnormal urinary tract and abnormal urine, which could result in an increased propensity for stone formation. Hence comprehensive imaging of the renal tracts is required. A plain abdominal X-ray will detect nephrocalcinosis and radiolucent stones, i.e. those containing calcium and cystine. Ultrasound demonstrates dilatation and congenital/developmental abnormalities of the renal systems, whereas an intravenous urogram may be useful to show stasis, obstruction and filling defects caused by calculi. A micturating cystourethrogram excludes any associated reflux, and functional isotope scanning demonstrates differential renal function (DMSA) and obstruction (DTPA or MAG3).

   The urine should be tested for infection and cultures organised. Serum abnormalities such as hypercalcaemia, hyperphosphataemia and hyperuricaemia can result in urinary stones and should be excluded. Serum and urine pH and acid–base balance must be evaluated if renal tubular acidosis is suspected. In addition the 24-hour urine calcium excretion and calcium:creatinine ratio are required in cases of hypercalciuria. Urinary oxalate, xanthine, cystine and uric acid levels can be measured and many of these amino acids form crystals in the urine that can be visualised on polarising microscopy.

Viva voce answer

The differential diagnosis includes shunt infection and malfunction owing to blockage or mechanical breakage. Malfunction would result in raised intracranial pressure. Hence, the following questions are important:

- Does the child have a temperature, sweats, red painful swelling over the shunt? – indicative of infection
- Does he seem particularly irritable? Do the vomiting and lethargy show a diurnal variation (e.g. worse in

Table 71 Juvenile chronic arthritis (JCA): types and major manifestations

| | Polyarticular | | Pauciarticular | | Systemic onset |
	RF⁻	RF⁺	Type I	Type II	
JCA (%)	25	10	35	10	20
Female : male ratio	9:1	4:1	4:1	1:9	4:1
Onset (year)	Any	>8	4–10	>8	Any
Joints	Multiple	Multiple	<4	<4	Variable
Sacroiliitis	No	Rare	No	Yes	No
Iridocyclitis	Rare	No	30%	10%	No
Chronicity (%)	10	>50	20	<10	25
RF (%)	–	100	–	–	–
ANA (%)	25	75	90	0	0
HLA	NS	DR4	DR5,6,8	B27	NS

RF, rheumatoid factor; ANA, anti-nuclear antibody; HLA, histocompatibility antigen; NS, non-specific.

the morning)? – symptoms of raised intracranial pressure.

A full examination is required to exclude any other cause for these symptoms (e.g. acute tonsillitis). The shunt system must be examined for signs of sepsis along the tract (i.e. swelling, erythema, tenderness, discharge), as well as for signs of blockage or shunt breakage (i.e. tense, unyielding reservoir, palpable kinks or gaps along the shunt tubing). Investigation should include an assessment of the white cell count, acute

inflammatory indices (e.g. erythrocyte sedimentation rate) and blood cultures. An X-ray of the shunt system and review by the neurosurgical team are required before a sample of CSF is taken for microscopy and culture. Fractured or displaced shunts require surgical replacement. Infected shunts must be removed and prolonged intravenous antibiotics given until the CSF is sterile and a new shunt inserted. In the interim, raised intracranial pressure must be controlled by the insertion of a temporary, exteriorised shunt system.

Behavioural disorders, social paediatrics and injuries

Key points

You should have a basic knowledge of:

- Behavioural disorders of childhood
- The impact of social factors on child health
- How to deal with the injured child
- How to identify and manage the abused child
- The basic management of accidental poisoning.

13.1 Introduction

An ever increasing workload in paediatric health services is devoted to disease and problems stemming from social deprivation. In underdeveloped nations 'social paediatrics' is largely related to widespread poverty, starvation, overcrowding, infectious diseases and child labour. In developed countries, social deprivation is primarily concentrated in inner cities where poverty, poor family structure and criminal activities, often related to illicit drug abuse and associated crime, abound. It is a sad indictment of 'modern society' that child abuse in various forms is an all too common problem, presenting with depressing regularity. Furthermore, this problem is likely to continue to increase as the family unit continues to disintegrate, leaving young, unsupported single parents to cope with the rigours of everyday life as well as young children. The situation is compounded by the intermittent presence of non-biological parents, often the abusers, and a lifestyle complicated by financial deficiencies, unemployment, drugs, parental ill-health and depression. All too often social services are poorly funded or inadequate to meet the increasing demands of deprived children. Indeed, in many countries worldwide, social services are rudimentary at best if not totally non-existent.

13.2 Behavioural disorders

Normal behavioural patterns

Habits

Thumb sucking is seen in almost all children and may persist for several years, eventually petering out during the early school period. Only 10% still suck their thumbs at 5 years of age. This habit commonly recurs in those children who regress for whatever reason, especially during a serious prolonged illness. **Repetitive mannerisms** such as finger clicking and guttural noises are voluntary movements usually seen in boys and exacerbated during times of stress. They are used to irritate parents and usually disappear when the child is gainfully distracted.

Breath holding

The voluntary cessation of breathing in a child who becomes deeply cyanosed can be a frightening experience for the uninitiated. This behavioural tactic is generally the culmination of a bout of crying or a tantrum, following an attempt at disciplining a stubborn child aged 6 months to 2.5 years. Forced expiration and apnoea follow a cry. Breath holding usually stops once cyanosis is established and is followed by further howling or sobbing. Some children hold their breath to the point of syncope, sometimes with brief tonic–clonic jerks, after which breathing resumes, cyanosis disappears and recovery ensues. Management is aimed at ensuring the diagnosis by taking a graphic history of the 'episodes', confirming normality on examination and reassuring the parents. Tacit ignoring of the episodes is the best ploy but, in practice, is easier said than done!

Tantrums

Children learn acceptable behaviour by testing the limits of adult tolerance. If thwarted, they may opt for an extreme form of attention seeking whereby they fly into an uncontrolled, sustained rage. Such temper tantrums are more likely during periods of fear, pain and illness. They generally arise in children aged 1–4 years. Recurrent tantrums persisting beyond 5 years, especially those exceeding 15 minutes more than three times a day, may imply an underlying neurodevelopmental disorder. Parents should handle these episodes with a firm disciplinary approach, care being taken to avoid conflicting, inconsistent and reinforcing messages. Corporal punishment is rarely better than non-corporal punitive measures. Nevertheless, it has not been shown to cause any long-term sequelae and controlled, consistent corporal punishment can be a useful measure if kept as a last resort.

Abnormal behaviour

Enuresis

Daytime bladder control commences by 18 months onwards and nappies are no longer required during the day by approximately 2–3 years and at night by 3–5 years. Indeed only 7% of boys (and less for girls) bedwet at 5 years of age. Up to 75% of affected children have never been dry (primary enuresis), whereas 25% regress after at least a year of dryness (secondary enuresis). The majority result from minor inadequacies in toilet training, with over- or underemphasis on rigid bladder control imposed on the child. These problems resolve spontaneously and require little investigation other than to rule out urinary tract infection. Others, especially secondary enuretics, experience underlying psychological stress and the possibility of family discord, bereavement, socio-economic disadvantage and problems at school should be explored. The prognosis is good, once the stressful trigger is eliminated. Organic causes are rare but continuous day and night-time dribbling is suggestive of an ectopic ureter. The enuretic child should be made to feel involved in treatment, which is directed at achieving an empty bladder at bedtime. This involves avoiding drinks 2–3 hours before bedtime, voiding before going to bed and again when woken when the parents retire. These practices, when coupled with star charts and a reward for dry nights providing positive reinforcement, are usually successful in 80% of children.

The definitive treatment for enuresis is through the use of conditioning alarms (bell or buzzer). These work by alerting the child as soon as dribbling commences, thereby waking the child who can then empty their bladder. Drug therapy, including imipramine and desmopressin nasal spray (DDAVP), is useful for more resistant cases but generally only offers temporary relief.

Encopresis

Encopresis describes the lack of bowel control either during the day or night beyond the age of 3 years. It generally affects 1% of boys and, like enuresis, may be primary or secondary. Many of these boys are emotionally disturbed and suffer with associated constipation and overflow. The latter must be controlled and a programme of toilet training commenced within the framework of child and family psychotherapy.

Sleep disorders

Minor sleep disturbances are commonplace and usually secondary to anxiety in the child such as a fear of school and parental conflict. **Nightmares** are terrifying dreams that are remembered and result in waking, usually occurring in anxious schoolgirls. **Night terrors** are more common in boys, may be associated with sleepwalking and result in an anxiety state that wakens the child who, nevertheless, cannot recall the dream. Establishing a period of calm before bedtime (e.g. quiet reading of favourite book) may be effective therapy. Calm reassurance is usually all that is required following the event. Occasionally light night-time sedation is required but addictive agents such as tricyclics and benzodiazepines should be avoided.

Eating problems

Feeding problems in infancy

Possetting, the regurgitation of small amounts of milk, is normal in infants below the age of 6 months when gastro-oesophageal reflux is common. When severe, repeated 'winding', placing the infant on the right side after a feed, milk thickeners and, occasionally, a prokinetic agent (e.g. cisapride) can be tried. **Underfeeding** results in irritability and poor weight gain whereas **overfeeding** is characterised by recurrent vomiting with excessive weight gain. Both are usually secondary to inadequate maternal skills and are easily corrected with sympathetic counselling.

Stool frequency is variable and true **constipation** is characterised by firm stool that is difficult to pass. Anal fissures and strictures should be excluded on examination. Constipation is almost exclusive to infants receiving formula milk, and a careful review of the correct reconstitution and volume content of the milk is indicated. Increasing the amount of fluid in the milk is often sufficient in the first few months, followed by increasing fibre later on. Suppositories and mild enemas are sometimes necessary for short periods.

Colic arises in infants before the age of 3 months. It results in paroxysms of abdominal pain manifest as inconsolable crying for several hours, often with striking regularity each evening. It follows intestinal distension owing to swallowed air but is rarely secondary to overfeeding, intestinal fermentation of excess carbohydrate and maternal stress. A careful examination is mandatory to rule out serious pathology. Simple advice regarding over/underfeeding, regular 'winding' and reassurance is usually all that is required. Paracetamol and various anticolic medications can be tried: most have little impact on the course of events. In severe cases where family anxiety is intolerable, a mild sedative can be given to settle the child.

Pica

The ingestion of non-nutrient substances including dirt and faeces is common in young children. Persistence of this behaviour beyond the age of 2 years is suggestive of mental retardation, psychological maladjustment and severe family discord and requires investigation. Children who regularly indulge in pica are at an increased risk of parasitic infection and lead poisoning.

Anorexia nervosa

Anorexia nervosa affects 1 in 300 teenage girls; the girls have an abnormal body image, intense fear of obesity and strive to lose weight by any means. Affected girls are very intense, preoccupied with eating and become emaciated. Hypotension, bradycardia, poor temperature control and amenorrhoea are common clinical findings, while evidence of hypothalamic–pituitary–ovarian axis and bone marrow failure are seen on investigation. Death from electrolyte disturbance, arrhythmias and heart failure occurs in 10%. Stepwise nutritional rehabilitation and correction of electrolyte disturbances are combined with psychotherapy and, if indicated, treatment of depression.

Bulimia

Girls with bulimia also have an abnormal body image and fear of obesity. They strive to lose weight by bingeing, followed by self-induced emetic purges, intermittent restricted diets and excessive use of laxatives. The treatment for this disorder is similar to that of anorexia nervosa.

Learning and cognitive behavioural disorders

Attention deficit disorders

Attention deficit disorder (ADD) is seen in about 4% of school-age children and is the most common cause of academic underachievement. ADD is characterised by poor concentration skills, impulsivity and, in some cases, hyperactivity and behavioural problems. These children are generally fidgety, impatient, noisy and sometimes aggressive. As a result, they have difficulty learning and making friends. Treatment involves a multidisciplinary approach involving medical, psychological and educational services. Disciplining such children can be extremely frustrating and exhausting, and parents should be encouraged to reinforce acceptable behaviour while patiently ignoring misbehaviour. The help of a specialised child psychologist and self-help groups is often invaluable. Tricyclic antidepressants and psychostimulants (e.g. methylphenidate, dextroamphetamines) can be used with careful supervision, especially in those with severe hyperactivity. Dietary manipulation and vitamin supplements are ineffective.

Autism

Autism is characterised by poor verbal and non-verbal skills and a low concentration span, together with repetitive ritualistic behaviour that, if interrupted, often precipitates a tantrum. Patients lack empathy, fail to make friends, adhere to stereotyped, solitary play and indulge in verbal repetition (echolalia). Autistic features may follow neurological injury, though the aetiology is usually unknown. Management entails speech therapy and behaviour modification using psychological conditioning programmes. Neuroleptics play a useful role in those with aggressive tendencies and dangerous behaviour. The prognosis is better for those with less destructive behaviour, reasonable intelligence and language development.

13.3 Psychiatric disorders

Neuroses

Anxiety states

Anxiety following a worrying life event is relatively common in childhood and generally resolves with sympathetic counselling. Anxieties related to specific situations (phobias) are less common and require

behavioural therapy. School phobia may be a manifestation of underlying depression or problems at school.

Depression

Depression manifests as apathy, inactivity, anorexia and failure to thrive in preschool children, and tearfulness, withdrawal, eating, clinging and behavioural disorders in school children. Depression is most common in adolescent girls, who may report fatigue, feelings of sadness, worthlessness and suicidal intentions. The last merits emergency admission to a paediatric psychiatric unit where expert counselling together with appropriate antidepressants (e.g. tricyclics, serotonin-reuptake blockers) can be provided. The prognosis is worse with no clear precipitating insult (which can be eliminated), associated psychotic features, psychomotor retardation and a positive family history. The risk of relapse during childhood is high and many of these children continue to suffer with depression in adulthood.

Psychoses

Manic depressive psychoses

Depressive symptoms together with hallucinations and delusions (often paranoid) are indicative of a psychotic bipolar disorder. Bouts of depression alternate with periods of excessive, unfocused activity, sometimes with inappropriate euphoria (mania). This condition is rare and best treated with lithium carbonate.

Schizophrenia

Schizophrenia is rarely seen in childhood. It manifests with thought disorders, chaotic thought processes, flattened affect, paranoid delusions, hallucinations, poor integration in society and disastrous interpersonal relationships. Many go on to suffer with schizophrenia in adulthood. Neuroleptics must be combined with multidisciplinary behavioural therapy if these children are to integrate successfully in a normal childhood environment.

Suicide and parasuicide

Parasuicide

Parasuicide is the unsuccessful attempt at killing oneself. It occurs in 1% of adolescents, is more common in girls and is often announced beforehand as a cri de coeur. The ingestion of tablets is the preferred method. All attempts at suicide, however innocuous, must be considered seriously and require admission to hospital. A trained psychiatrist must review all patients prior to discharge. The seriousness of intent can be gauged by the probability of rescue when viewed from the child's point of view. All patients should be given follow-up counselling and all precipitating factors in the patient's psychosocial background explored. Any conflict, anger and resentment in the family must be addressed.

Suicide

In some developed countries, suicide is the second most common cause of death in adolescents. It is more common in white males, especially in those who carefully pre-plan the attempt (e.g. with suicide notes, etc.) rather than those who have a sudden impulse to inflict self-harm. The increasing incidence of suicide is related to increasing substance abuse, increasing marital breakdown, depression, social isolation and availability of weapons. Violent methods are more common in boys, whereas drug overdose is the preferred method in girls. A reduction in the alarming increase in suicides will only follow radical changes in modern lifestyles. Nevertheless, up to 40% of successful suicides follow a previous attempt so that the importance of heeding any cri de coeur cannot be stressed enough.

13.4 Social paediatrics

The social impact of a modern society

The **family unit** consisting of two parents and close relatives living within the same household or nearby is fast disappearing. As a result, many children are brought up by a single, unsupported parent who herself/himself may be very young. This, in itself, may not result in any problems and is preferable to living with squabbling parents whose relationship is beyond salvage. The situation may be compounded by distant, inaccessible friends and relatives, unstable relationships with intermittent partners who are not the biological parent, unemployment and financial hardship. Little familiarity with indifferent neighbours increases social isolation. The strain within such a disjointed framework can be considerable and increases the risk of failure to cope, substance abuse, depression and child abuse. Furthermore, modern mobile society incurs multiple house moves through job changes, divorce and remarriage. These impose involuntary readjustments in the children with regard to the family, friendships, schooling and the community. These problems are particularly severe for migrants moving from one society to another with a completely different culture and language.

Social services for children

In many countries social services are rudimentary at best, non-existent at worst. Developed countries have social workers especially devoted to tend the needs of children. Their work includes providing financial support, allowances, provision of adequate housing, fostering services, investigation and management of child abuse. They are aided by several child-support agencies

Table 72 Use of illicit substances in adolescents in developed countries

Illicit substance	Trend	Male:female ratio
Alcohol	Increasing/steady	Approaching 1:1
Smoking	Increasing in girls	Approaching 1:1
Illicit drugs		
Marijuana	Decreasing	Both
Cocaine	Levelling off	Male > female
Crack cocaine	Increasing	Male > female
Ecstasy	Increasing	Both
Heroin	Steady	Male > female
Non-prescription drugs		
Stimulants/steroids	Steady/declining	Male > female
Diet pills	Steady	Females

and adoption services and work in close collaboration with drug abuse agencies and the Police Child Protection Unit.

Illicit substance abuse

The widespread availability of illicit substances combined with peer pressure, adolescent 'escapism and exploratory urges' results in the worrying statistics listed in Table 72. Up to 70% of teenagers drink alcohol regularly, 5% on a daily basis. Thirty per cent smoke tobacco daily and though the trend is declining in males, the opposite is true for females. Marijuana was extremely popular until recently and although its use is declining, that of crack cocaine and ecstasy is increasing. Intravenous heroin addicts still number approximately 1% of adolescents (4% for inhaled heroin), whereas 4% of adolescents admit to taking anabolic steroids, 15% non-prescription stimulants and 30% of females have a lifetime prevalence of taking diet pills.

Drug addicts are often unemployable or disinterested and turn to crime or prostitution in order to finance their habit. Consequently, drug-related crime is one of the greatest problems in large cities. 'Kicking the habit' once established is considerably more difficult than avoiding it in the first place. Prevention is best achieved through widespread education on the risks involved, together with limiting drug availability. The acute management involves detoxification specific for each individual substance, followed by long-term psychosocial support.

13.5 Accidental injury

Burns

Scalds are typically seen in children below the age of 4 years and are the cause in 85% of admissions following burn injury. **Flame, chemical** and **electrical burns** make up the remaining 15%. Prevention is extremely important. Adherence to strict laws pertaining to non-flammable clothing, upholstery, toys and water heating settings is responsible for the reduction in fatalities.

Table 73 Classification of burns

Type of burn	Symptoms, signs	Outcome
First degree: epidermis only	Pain, erythema	Healing without scars
Second degree: epidermis and dermis	Very painful, blisters	May heal with scars, moderate fluid loss
Third degree: full thickness	Painless, little bleeding	Contractures, scars, severe fluid imbalance, require grafting

Indeed, most burn patients survive the ordeal; death usually follows severe smoke inhalation and cerebral anoxia. The site and depth of the burn(s) should be documented (Table 73) and the extent of the affected areas calculated as a percentage of the body surface area (SA) from designated paediatric 'burn charts'. Burn patients should be examined for other injuries, evidence of respiratory embarrassment and signs of shock, especially likely with more than 15% burns. Resuscitation should include the safeguard of the airway with intubation and artificial ventilation if necessary, and establishment of good venous access.

Rehydration is commenced at 4 ml/kg body weight for every per cent SA burnt, with half this requirement being replaced in the first 8 hours. Electrolyte imbalance, hypoalbuminaemia and anaemia must all be corrected while adequate analgesia with opiates is provided. Burnt areas must be covered with sterile dressings and kept clean with a topical bacteriostatic agent. Dead tissue is debrided and large denuded areas grafted by a team specialised in this work. Nutritional support, if necessary with total parenteral nutrition, is essential to minimise the catabolic effects of a major burn and encourage healing. Antibiotics are not started unless there is clear evidence of infection or with subsequent fever and positive cultures. Psychological support may be necessary for those with disfiguring injuries, especially to the face.

Smoke inhalation results in pulmonary epithelial sloughing, alveolar destruction, oedema, degradation of surfactant and atelectasis. Mortality is as high as 50% in severe incidents and survival depends on intensive-care support of the airway and lungs with artificial ventilation and, with upper airway burn involvement, a tracheostomy.

Accidental ingestion

Accidental ingestion of medication or toxic agents is usually seen in children aged less than 6 years; older children, especially teenagers, often overdose intentionally. The precise agent(s), amount(s) ingested and time lapse since ingestion must be ascertained. Unless very familiar with the substance involved, immediate telephone contact with the nearest **poison centre** will establish the potential toxicity and urgency of the situation. If in doubt all children must be admitted for 24 hours for observation. Those in a critical state require resuscitation and transfer to a life-support unit. A few agents have an **antidote** (Table 74); otherwise general support-

Table 74 Specific treatment/antidote for ingested substances

Ingested agent	Antidote/treatment
Carbon monoxide	Oxygen
Cyanide	Sodium nitrite + thiosulphate, or hydroxycobalamin + thiosulphate
Iron	Desferoxamine
Nitrobenzene	Methylene blue
Opiates	Naloxone
Organophosphates	Atropine
Paracetamol	N-Acetylcysteine

ive measures are instigated. These include intravenous access, maintenance of blood pressure with fluid and, if necessary, inotropic support.

Induced emesis with ipecac has a poor recovery rate of ingested material, is useless at 4 or more hours after ingestion and is contraindicated in those less than 6 months of age or if comatose. The airway should always be protected by placing the child in the left lateral position.

Gastric lavage is rarely used in children and is only effective if attempted within an hour of ingestion.

Activated charcoal placed or swallowed into the stomach prevents further absorption of many agents.

Forced diuresis is only indicated in specific forms of poisoning.

Haemodialysis is ineffective in many instances because of volume of distribution and poor clearance rates of most drugs.

Specific poisoning

Paracetamol overdose results in nausea and vomiting followed by abdominal pain and liver dysfunction by 48 hours. The liver dysfunction peaks at around 80 hours before resolving slowly. Serum paracetamol levels should be measured at 4 hours postingestion and compared with standard nomograms, administering N-acetylcysteine if the level is elevated above the 'treatment' line. Liver function including prothrombin time must be assessed daily.

Salicylates in overdose cause hyperventilation, vomiting, tinnitus and lethargy. Respiratory alkalosis is replaced, after an initial 12-hour phase, by hypokalaemia, lactic acidosis and progressive dehydration. The peak plasma level is best ascertained in a sample taken 6 hours after ingestion and compared with a nomogram. Dehydration and acid–base and electrolyte imbalance should be corrected by administering appropriate fluid, bicarbonate and potassium. Forced diuresis may compound pulmonary oedema and, like haemodialysis, is reserved for severe toxicity not responsive to alkalinisation and rehydration.

Iron ingestion in excess results in gastrointestinal irritation with pain, vomiting and diarrhoea (sometimes with blood), followed by apparent recovery after about 6 hours, only to be replaced by hypoglycaemia, acidosis and potentially fatal liver failure between 2 and 4 days later. Pyloric stenosis may follow local mucosal damage and is manifest 3 weeks after the event. Total serum iron levels are elevated and exceed the total iron-binding capacity. Forced emesis, lavage and charcoal are seldom effective. Treatment is largely supportive together with intravenous desferrioxamine and haemodialysis if renal failure complicates the overdose.

Antidepressants are widely prescribed for adult patients and, unfortunately, are frequently found and ingested by children. **Tricyclic** antidepressant ingestion results in tachycardia, dry mucous membranes, drowsiness and hypertension, followed later by hypotension. Arrhythmias, convulsions and coma may lead to death. Forced emesis is contraindicated though activated charcoal may be useful in reducing absorption. Patients should be admitted with ECG monitoring. Acidosis is corrected with bicarbonate, seizures with diazepam and phenytoin and arrhythmias with lignocaine (lidocaine). Renal dialysis is rarely effective.

Acids and alkalis both cause local damage to the gastrointestinal tract. Alkaline agents cause oesophageal necrosis and strictures while acids irritate the oesophagus and gastric pylorus causing necrosis, perforation and late strictures. Oral irritation is associated with drooling and dysphagia. If tolerated, water and milk should be drunk in the first instance. Endoscopy should be attempted 24 hours later. Clear, neutral fluids are continued until all symptoms abate. There is no place for ingested acid or alkaline antidotes.

13.6 Non-accidental injury

Suspicion of non-accidental injury

In the majority of cases, accidents are bona fide resulting from the everyday rough and tumble of childhood. The onus is on the examining doctor to first suspect, then investigate an injury as *non-accidental* (NAI). A sensible approach is required to avoid overdiagnosis and unnecessary emotional trauma to the family, while ensuring no case is missed. The benefit of doubt must always be given to the *child*. Inconsistencies in the history, implausible explanations, outright untruths and delay in presentation raise the possibility of NAI. A forever-changing history is a hallmark of NAI, the perpetrators embarking on a 'fishing expedition' whereby several explanations are offered in the hope that one will be

accepted. A non-committal approach should be adopted, allowing the history to be delivered at will with few leading questions. Suspicious findings on examination include multiple injuries, often of differing age, injuries incompatible with the history obtained and injuries that could only result from excessive force being applied to the child (e.g. whip marks). The injury must be assessed in the context of the history and age of the child: hence, a fracture of the humerus may be explicable in a boisterous 6 year old falling off a fence but is highly suspicious in a 4-month-old infant.

Whenever suspected, the child should be examined fully and any suspicious areas investigated (e.g. X-ray examination of swollen limbs). The child should be admitted, any injuries attended to and investigated as appropriate. It is well to remember that many of these cases will end up in a court of law. Hence, it is of paramount importance that detailed notes are made, including drawings of any injuries with measurements, discoloration and estimated age clearly documented. Investigations should, whenever possible, be kept to a minimum in order to avoid further trauma to the child. A platelet count and clotting profile is necessary in those with bruises/haematomas (if only for legal reasons), and a skeletal survey in children presenting with fractures. Skull X-ray and a CT scan of the brain are indicated following non-accidental head injury.

Overt cases of child abuse are, in some ways, easier to manage. There is no doubt that the child must be kept in a place of safety, in most cases an acute hospital ward. Social services must be informed as soon as possible and, in cases of grievous harm or death, the police are also contacted. If the child's carers refuse admission, an emergency magistrate's order can be obtained to appoint the child a ward of court. The magistrate will then instruct where the child as well as any other sibling at risk is nursed (e.g. ward, temporary foster home). It is not the remit of the medical professionals to be judgmental. They should concentrate on treating and safeguarding the child while referring the case to the relevant authorities whose job it is to direct allegations, accusations and arrests.

Many cases of suspected abuse are less clear cut. Although there may be an inconsistent history and unusual injuries, these may not be tantamount to flagrant abuse. Reference to the local children's *At Risk Register* and discussion with social services may heighten one's suspicions if previous concerns have already been noted. If in doubt, it is best to admit the child and observe and/or investigate over the subsequent few days. A **case conference** attended by all relevant personnel (e.g. medical, nursing, social services, police, school and legal representatives) should review all cases of NAI/suspected abuse. During the conference, decisions regarding the placement of the child (e.g. back home, foster home), the addition of the child's name on the *At Risk Register* and prosecution must be taken. Most children are returned to their biological parents for whom

Fig. 88 Clinical manifestations of non-accidental injury. A, multiple bruises, lacerations of different ages; B, bite mark; C, cigarette burns; D, immersion burn injury; E, retinal haemorrhages; F, old rib fractures with callus formation; G, severe emaciation following neglect; H, whip marks; I, depressed skull fracture with haematoma; J, spiral long bone fracture.

social service support is organised. Varying degrees of supervision can be imposed by law, depending on the severity of each case.

Specific forms of child abuse

Child abuse can take many forms and produce a range of clinical manifestations of non-accidental injury (Fig. 88).

Burns

Accidental burns are common in children. However, scalds affecting the buttocks, lower back, posterior aspects of the lower limbs and feet suggest an **immersion** injury (Fig. 88d). Likewise small, multiple, ring or target-like burns suggest **cigarette burn** injuries (Fig. 88c) and, like clearly demarcated burns from a hot iron, are highly suspicious.

Bruises

Bruises of varying sizes and ages on the shins of active schoolboys are of no consequence. However, similar bruises distributed over other parts of the body including the trunk and head, especially if associated with other injuries, should alert one to the possibility of repeated battering (Fig. 88a). It is important to age the bruises (preferably photograph the lesions) and attempt to account for each lesion from the history. Small mirror-image bruises arranged in a semicircular pattern suggest **bite marks** (Fig. 88b), whereas multiple linear, criss-cross bruising and lacerations indicate a **whipping** injury (Fig. 88h). **Haematomas** often accompany bruises: they should be aged, measured and, if large and associated with significant pain and limitation of movement, may herald an underlying fracture.

Fractures

Except in those with osteogenesis imperfecta or with a

history of major trauma (e.g. a road traffic accident), **multiple fractures** are always suspicious. This is especially so if the fractures are old, of different ages and in characteristic sites, e.g. rib, skull and spiral fractures of long bones (Fig. 88f, i, j).

Head injuries

The most common and potentially lethal NAI of the head in small babies without adequate head control involves intracerebral haemorrhage and oedema following a **shaking** injury. **Depressed skull fractures** (Fig. 88i) are seen in older children and present with inconsolable crying, swelling, bruising over the site of trauma, and coma in those with significant underlying brain damage.

Munchausen syndrome by proxy

Munchausen syndrome by proxy is a much publicised but rare form of child abuse that occurs when a psychiatrically unwell guardian, almost always the mother, falsifies illness in her child. This may involve the fabrication of symptoms and signs, the actual causation of illness by exposure of the child to toxins, and alteration of laboratory results. These individuals obtain gratification through the attention focused on themselves as a result of their child's illness. Many such parents have had some medical or nursing background and can be extremely clever at disguising the fictitious nature of their child's illness. The abused children are invariably too young to implicate their mother as the true offender. They may present with quite bizarre features that, as with smothering and intentional poisoning, may persist in hospital. However, an improvement in symptoms and signs may follow a period of planned, close observation without the mother present and may clinch what can be a very difficult diagnosis to prove. The parent should be seen by a sympathetic physician and the child social and legal services alerted.

Emotional deprivation and neglect

Child abuse emanating from chronic physical and emotional neglect may present with non-organic failure to thrive (Fig. 88g) and short stature. These children are often unkempt. Their chronic exposure to an inappropriate mother–child relationship and inattention results in behavioural abnormalities such as apathy, frozen watchfulness, food obsession and autoerotic activity, as well as delayed developmental milestones. However, the last improves on admission to hospital where the child's initial aloof nature gives way to a ravenous appetite, overclinging behaviour and need for comfort. A history of rejection, neglect and NAI in their mother is common.

Sexual abuse

Sexual abuse constitutes any activity with a child below the age of consent that is carried out for the gratification of the adult. In the majority of cases, the offender is usually a male family member or friend known to the child. Sexual abuse constitutes approximately 15% of child abuse and is reported in 1–2 of every 1000 children. The increased incidence since the 1970s is partly the result of increased reporting. However, given that 20% of adult females and 5% of males admit to being abused as children, this incidence is still an underestimate of the true size of the problem.

Sexual abuse is an extremely delicate paediatric problem and can only be dealt with by experienced, sympathetic professionals. Occasionally a distressed child presents in a dishevelled state, partially clothed with evidence of a recent assault amounting to rape or sodomy (usually by a stranger). More often (especially with family perpetrators), there is no associated violence and the possibility of sexual abuse is raised by a chance comment or abnormal or inappropriate sexualised or seductive behaviour. Abused victims may develop non-specific manifestations such as enuresis, poor school performance, truancy, depression, tantrums and sleep and eating disorders. Perineal discomfort, erythema and discharge may be absent or non-specific.

Experienced interviewers should obtain the history with representatives of the medical, social, legal and police services present unobtrusively. A video recording can help to limit the number of traumatic interviews. Any suspected or alleged case of a penetrating assault should be examined with a view to excluding other physical injuries. In a girl, unless there are signs of severe bleeding or peritonitis, examination of the genitalia must be left to the gynaecology–paediatric–forensic team and, if necessary, carried out under general anaesthesia. Lacerations, scratch marks, bruises, tears of the hymen must be documented and, whenever possible, photographed. Samples for culture, semen analysis and blood typing should be obtained. Injuries should be dealt with and any bleeding staunched. Involvement of an experienced child counsellor and careful follow-up is required to address any psychoemotional sequelae.

Child exploitation

Child labour was commonplace in Victorian times but, sadly, this together with slavery, prostitution and involvement in pornographic practices remain ways in which adults exploit children even today. These problems are more prevalent but certainly not exclusive to developing countries. Their long-term eradication will only become a reality with improved respect for human rights worldwide, international cooperation between police forces and stricter penalties for offenders.

Self-assessment: questions

Multiple choice questions

1. The following statements describe behavioural disorders:
   a. Thumb sucking at 3 years is indicative of a psychosocial disorder
   b. Breath holding does not result in seizure activity
   c. Severe tantrums are best managed by intense psychotherapy
   d. Overfeeding suggests a problem with mothering rather than the child
   e. Pica is pathognomonic of iron-deficiency anaemia

2. With regard to anorexia and bulimia nervosa:
   a. Anorexia is more common in girls, bulimia in boys
   b. Patients are usually happy-go-lucky extroverts who forget to eat
   c. Amenorrhoea is a common complication
   d. Death occurs in 1% of patients
   e. Misuse of laxatives is a common association

3. The following constitute appropriate therapy:
   a. Dietary manipulation for attention deficit disorders
   b. Psychological conditioning for autism
   c. Behavioural therapy for school phobia
   d. Major psychotropics for anxiety-related depression
   e. Lithium for manic psychosis

4. With regard to illicit substance abuse:
   a. Abuse generally starts in late school-age children
   b. The use of crack cocaine is on the increase
   c. Smoking is decreasing in both sexes
   d. Drug abuse is the major cause of crime in teenagers and young adults
   e. Drug taking is the commonest cause of HIV infection in children

5. The following statements describe accidental ingestion:
   a. It usually occurs in school-age children
   b. It is rarely fatal
   c. Most cases should be managed at home
   d. Forced emesis is indicated except in comatose patients
   e. Haemodialysis is a useful last resort in severe cases

6. The following increase the risk of child abuse:
   a. The presence of a live-in, non-biological father
   b. Social deprivation
   c. Parents who were abused as children
   d. Specific cultural or racial origins
   e. Prematurity

Case histories

Case history 1

A 4-month-old boy is brought to casualty by his 18-year-old mother who noted a swelling of his right elbow over the preceding 24 hours. Examination confirms marked swelling of the elbow, overlying green-brown discoloration and painful limitation of movement. The boyfriend felt that the child had caught his arm between the cot sides.

How would you manage this case?

Case history 2

A baby is born at 37 weeks of gestation to a young woman who was on a registered drug-abuse programme with the local social services and taking a regular supply of methadone. She had suffered repeated beatings from her violent boyfriend, who had disappeared early during the pregnancy. She attended all antenatal clinics, had stopped smoking tobacco but was still on methadone at the time of birth. At 12 hours of age the infant was noted to be jittery with a shrill cry.

1. What is the most likely cause for this baby's symptoms?
2. What other clinical manifestations may develop over the next few hours?
3. What treatment is indicated?

The child remains very jittery over the next 36 hours and has at least two brief, generalised convulsions. Following a thorough examination you are confident that the general clinical condition has not deteriorated but order some investigations.

4. What investigations would be appropriate at this point?

The child is eventually discharged (without any medication) and followed up regularly in the outpatient department.

5. What steps would you take prior to discharge?

6. What may have accounted for the apparent change in mothering skills?

7. What action would you take following the last clinic visit?

After a 3-month period of excellent progress, the mother and child start to default from clinic appointments. After several attempts, the social services are finally able to visit and note that the mother looked dishevelled and had several bruises on her arms as well as a black eye. She claimed to have tripped and fallen downstairs. She is coaxed to attend the next paediatric clinic. During the visit it is obvious that the child had not been bathed for several days, had a severe nappy rash and had lost weight.

Short notes

Write short notes on truancy.

Self-assessment: answers

Multiple choice answers

1. a. **False**. It is a normal behavioural pattern at this age.
    b. **False**. It may result in hypoxia-related seizures.
    c. **False**. The best ploy is to ignore the episodes.
    d. **True**. It is usually simple overanxiety.
    e. **False**. Though it may be associated with iron deficiency.

2. a. **False**. Both are far more common in girls.
    b. **False**. Patients are usually introverted, shy, anxious types.
    c. **True**. Both primary and secondary amenorrhoea occur.
    d. **False**. Death occurs in 10%.
    e. **True**. Laxatives are used in an attempt to purge the body of 'excess calories' from the lower end.

3. a. **False**. This is an ineffective approach.
    b. **True**. This forms the basis of autistic rehabilitation programmes.
    c. **True**. Therapy is used to help to re-learn appropriate behaviour and suppress the phobia.
    d. **False**. These are rarely required; counselling, reassurance and simple anxiolytics generally suffice.
    e. **True**. As for therapy in adults.

4. a. **False**. Teenagers are the usual starting group.
    b. **True**. Cocaine is becoming more popular and widely available.
    c. **False**. Smoking is increasing in girls.
    d. **True**. Most crime in adolescents centres around illegal activities in order to fund an illicit drug habit.
    e. **False**. Perinatal transmission accounts for most cases of AIDS in childhood; an ever decreasing number acquired the disease from contaminated blood products received during the period 1970–1986. Household contacts of HIV-positive parents have very little or no risk of contamination. Sexual and drug-related transmission is becoming more common but presents in late adolescence and early adult life.

5. a. **False**. It is more usual in preschool children.
    b. **True**. Most are innocuous and simply require observation.
    c. **False**. Almost all should be admitted for overnight observation.
    d. **False**. Emesis is often unsafe and rarely effective.
    e. **False**. Few ingested agents are effectively removed by dialysis.

6. a. **True**. He is usually (although not invariably) the abuser.
    b. **True**. This compounds a poor social framework and is a scenario that encourages child abuse.
    c. **True**. It is a sad fact that abused parents are more likely to abuse their own children.
    d. **False**. Abuse knows no cultural barriers.
    e. **True**. This is a well-documented statistic.

Case history answers

Case history 1

The findings suggest a significant injury to the elbow with the development of a haematoma and the possibility of an underlying fracture. The first stage in management is to confirm the extent of the injury, reduce any fractures, relieve a haemarthrosis and provide adequate analgesia. An X-ray of the elbow joint and orthopaedic opinion are indicated in the first instance. There are a number of discrepancies in the story: a 4-month-old cannot sustain such an injury simply by getting caught in cot sides and the age of the bruising is inconsistent with the history. Indeed, as seen in Table 75, green-brown discoloration arises after 7–10 days. Therefore, this case is suspicious and must be assumed to be one of child abuse. The infant must be admitted to the ward (place of safety), all injuries carefully documented (and photographed) and a skeletal survey plus clotting screen performed. The social services must be contacted, the *Child Abuse Register* consulted, the Police Child Protection Unit informed and a case conference organised. Clear decisions regarding placement of the child, supervision of the family and further investigation into the case must be taken before discharge can be contemplated.

Case history 2

1. The most likely diagnosis is neonatal withdrawal syndrome following methadone use by the mother. Withdrawal occurs in around 50% of babies whose mothers take methadone during pregnancy, especially if taken within 24 hours of parturition.

Table 75 Guide for 'dating' bruises

Day	Colour
1	Red
3	Blue
5	Purple
7	Green
9	Yellow
11	Brown
13–21	Resolves

2. Clinical manifestations of neonatal withdrawal are similar regardless of the drug abused, and include:

   - tremor, jitteriness, irritability, convulsions
   - hypertonicity, hyper-reflexia
   - persistent and high-pitched cry
   - excessive sleepiness or wakefulness
   - hyperventilation, irregular respirations, apnoeas
   - nasal stuffiness, repeated sneezing
   - excessive yawning, hiccups, mouthing movements, fist sucking
   - diarrhoea, repeated vomiting, poor feeding.

3. Treatment involves the administration of methadone to the infant. This is titrated according to a standardised scoring system based on the presence or absence of the above symptoms and signs. High scores on consecutive recordings result in an increase in the dosage (in a controlled fashion) until a plateau is reached. Once stable, the methadone is gradually reduced over a period of several weeks or months (necessitating prolonged in-hospital stay). If the logistics of giving a controlled drug to such infants is problematic, the infant can be treated with chlorpromazine, again in increasing dosage until the symptoms of withdrawal abate.

4. Although these complications are almost certainly related to methadone withdrawal, sepsis including neonatal meningitis and metabolic derangements, in particular hypoglycaemia and hypocalcaemia, must be considered. Serum glucose, calcium and electrolytes are mandatory, and a septic screen performed if there is sufficient clinical suspicion.

5. Close collaboration with social services is required before discharge. You must ensure that the housing and social environment is adequate, and all support services that may be required are in place. Close liaison with the illicit drug rehabilitation unit is also necessary. Clear follow-up and supervision arrangements must be defined beforehand.

6. Given the sudden change in 'attitude' and recurrence of bruises on the mother, it is likely that the boyfriend has reappeared. The mother is probably being subjected to physical abuse. The implications of this situation on her own drug problem and the repercussions on the welfare of the child are now brought into serious doubt.

7. The mother needs to be confronted with your fears and social services alerted immediately. If necessary, it may be appropriate to involve the police at this stage. At any rate, the child is no longer in a place of safety and alternative accommodation must be found as a matter of urgency. In view of the child's weight loss and general state, admission to hospital for a short period is required. Following this, the child may be transferred, preferably together with mother, to a safe place of refuge while the case is investigated (and any charges brought forward) by the social services and police. Regular medical follow-up must continue to monitor the child's growth and neurodevelopmental progress.

Short notes answer

Truancy is the absenteeism or running away from school without a valid reason (e.g. ill health). It is not an extension of normal developmental behaviour and generally signifies an underlying problem. The child may be running away from a distressing situation at school or is attempting to draw attention to a similarly distressing situation at home. Hence, truancy follows problems in certain areas of the child's life.

Problems at school

- anxiety about fear of teacher, fear of peers, teasing and bullying
- failure to cope with humiliation, learning difficulties, inability to match peers.

Problems at home

- anxiety about separation from parents or siblings, parental discord, family strife, disagreement with parents
- social problems resulting from family disorganisation, unstable family environment, criminal, illicit activities at home
- child abuse including physical, sexual, emotional abuse or neglect.

Problems with the child

- personality problems
- inadequacy
- psychoemotional problems.

The management involves an in-depth investigation into the above possibilities during a series of sympathetic interviews with the child, teachers and family. The underlying cause should be addressed and eliminated. Child psychologists and social services should be involved where appropriate and supportive behavioural therapy instigated, depending on the cause.

Index

Preauricular sinuses, 23
Precordium, examination, 66
Prematurity, 34
    see also Preterm infants
Prenatal diagnosis, 22–23
Preterm infants, 22, 34–35
    feeding, 7
    morbidity and mortality, 22
    nutritional requirements, 6, 7
    temperature control, 37Q/40A
Protein energy malnutrition (PEM), 12
Protein requirements, 6
Proteinuria, 125–126
Prune-belly syndrome, 221
Pseudohypoparathyroidism, 150
Psittacosis, 189
Psychiatric disorders, 242–243
Pubarche, premature, 145
Puberty, 9, 143–144, 154Q/156A
    delayed, 142, 144, 154Q/156A
    precocious, 142–143, 144–145
    staging, 140
Pulmonary atresia, 73–74, 76
Pulmonary incompetence, 71
Pulmonary stenosis, 70–71
Pulmonary venous drainage, total
        anomalous, 72–73, 76
Pulse(s)
    assessment, 65–66
    congenital heart disease, 80Q/83A
    respiratory disease, 46
Pulsus paradoxus, 46
Pyloric stenosis, 222, 234Q/236A
Pyridoxine deficiency, 15

R
Rash, with fever, 191Q/193A
Red blood cells
    decreased production, 196–199
    destruction, 199–201
Reflexes
    assessment, 104–105
    newborn, 24
Reflux
    gastro-oesophageal, 89–90
    vesicoureteric, 123
Regurgitation, 88–90
Rehydration, 92
    burns, 244
Renal abscess, 125
Renal agenesis, 122
Renal dialysis, 129–130, 136Q/134A, 244
Renal dysfunction, 130–131
Renal dysplasia, 122
Renal failure, 128–131
    acute, 129–130, 132Q/134A
    chronic, 130, 132Q/134A, 133Q/136A
    end-stage, 130
Renal hypoplasia, 122
Renal transplantation, 130, 132Q/134A
Renal tubular acidosis, 130
Renal vein thrombosis, 128
Repetitive mannerisms, 240
Reproductive organs, abnormalities,
        224–225
Respiration, 44
    work of, 46
Respiratory disorders
    cystic fibrosis, 54, 57Q/60A
    examination/assessment, 45–47,
        57Q/59–60A
    infections, 45–51, 55, 56Q/58A
    newborn, 28–29, 36–37Q/39A
    signs and symptoms, 45
    see also names of specific disorders
Respiratory distress syndrome (RDS) *see*
        Surfactant deficiency disease
Respiratory rate, 46
    newborn, 23

Respiratory system, 44
Restriction analysis, 160–161
Resuscitation
    burns, 244
    neonatal, 26–27
Retinol, 14
Reye syndrome, 96–97
Rhabdomyosarcoma, 208
Rheumatic fever, 183, 190Q/192A
Rheumatoid disease, 229, 234Q/236A
Riboflavin deficiency, 14
Rickets, 13–14, 149–150, 154Q/157A
    renal, 130
Rifampicin, 190Q/192A
Rigidity, 104
RNA, messenger, 160
Rotor syndrome, 167
Rubella, 186–187
    maternal, 31, 186–187
Russell–Silver syndrome, 140

S
Sacrococcygeal teratoma, 23
Salaam attacks, 110
Salicylate overdose, 244–245
Sarcoma, osteogenic, 208
Scalds, 243
Scarlet fever, 191Q/194A
Schizophrenia, 242
Scoliosis, 227–228, 233Q/235A
Scurvy, 15
Seizure-like disorders, 111
Seizures
    epileptic, 110–111
    following asphyxia, 28
    neonatal, 33
    non-epileptic, 111
Sensory examination, 105
Septic shock, 179, 180
Severe combined immunodeficiency
        (SCID), 168
Sexual abuse, 247
Sexual differentiation, disorders of,
        138–139, 154Q/156A, 155Q/157A
Sexual maturation, 9, 10, 143–144
    see also Puberty
Shaking injury, 247
Shock, septic, 179, 180
Short bowel syndrome, 99Q/102A
Shunts
    Blalock–Taussig, 73, 74, 75
    ventriculoperitoneal, 234Q/236–237A
Shunts, cardiovascular
    left-to-right, 80Q/83A
    right-to-left, 65
Sickle cell disorders, 89, 200
Skeletal dysplasias and malformations,
        227–228
Skin
    neonatal assessment, 23
    neurocutaneous syndromes, 106–107,
        115Q/117A
    pustules, newborn, 30
    vesicular lesions, 191Q/193A
Sleep disorders, 241
Slide examination, 3
Small bowel atresia, 217
Small for gestational age (SGA), 22, 34
Smoke inhalation, 244
Social paediatrics, 240, 243
Social services, 243
Soft tissue injuries, 230–231
Somogyi effect, 151
Sorbitol, excessive ingestion, 89
Sotos syndrome, 143
Southern blotting, 160–161
Soy-based feeds, 7
Spasms, infantile, 110
Spasticity, 104, 107

Speech, motor disorders, 105
Spherocytosis, hereditary, 199
Spina bifida, 23, 105
Spinal abnormalities, 23
Spinal cord compression, 112
Spinal muscular atrophy (SMA),
        112–113
Sprengel's shoulder, 228
Staphylococcal infections, 182–183,
        190Q/192A
Stature
    disorders of, 139–143
    short, 140–142, 154Q/156A,
        155Q/157A:158A
    tall, 142–143, 155Q/157A
Status epilepticus, 111, 116Q/118A
Stillbirth, 22
Still's disease, 229
Stones, urinary tract, 224, 234Q/236A
Stools
    bloody, 99Q/101A
    normal, 88
    watery, 92, 99Q/101A
Streptococcal infections, 182–183
    group B, newborn, 31
Stridor, 45
Subarachnoid bleed, 112
Substance abuse, 243, 248Q/250A:251A
Suicide, 243
Supraventricular tachycardia (SVT) 76–77,
        81Q/84A
Surfactant deficiency disease, newborn,
        29, 37Q/39A
Surgery
    acquired abnormalities, 222–224
    congenital abnormalities, 216–222
Sweat test, cystic fibrosis, 54
Syndactyly, 170Q/172A
Syndrome of inappropriate ADH
        secretion (SIADH), 153
Syphilis, congenital, 31
Systemic inflammatory response
        syndrome (SIRS), 179, 180
Systemic lupus erythematosus,
        glomerulonephritis and, 127

T
Tachyarrhythmias, 77–77
Tachypnoea, newborn, 28
Talipes calcaneo valgus, 226–227
Talipes equino varus, 24, 226–227
Tantrums, 240
Tay–Sachs disease, 167
Temperature, sensation of, testing, 105
Temperature, body
    fever and, 178
    preterm infants, 37Q/40A
Teratogenesis, 162
Teratogenic drugs, 170Q/172A
Term infant, 22
Tetralogy of Fallot (TOF), 74–75, 76,
        80Q/83A
Thalassaemias, 200–201
Thelarche, premature, 145, 155Q/157A
Thermogenesis, non-shivering, 178
Thiamine deficiency, 14
Thrombocytopenia, 201–202, 209Q/211A
Thumb sucking, 240
Thymic hypoplasia *see* DiGeorge
        syndrome
Thyroid gland disorders, 145–146
Thyrotoxicosis, 143, 154Q/156A
Tonsillopharyngitis, 47
    exudative, 191Q/193A
Total anomalous pulmonary venous
        drainage (TAPVD), 72–73, 76
Total parenteral nutrition, 8
Touch, assessment, 105
Toxic neuropathies, 113

257